WHEN YOUR BODY TALKS,

Listen!

Healing Yourself
& Others

by

Allen Lawrence, M.A., M.D., Ph.D.

Lisa R. Lawrence, M.S., Ph.D.

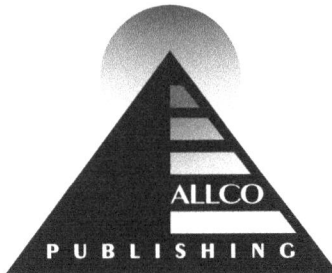

ALLCO
PUBLISHING

When Your Body Talks, Listen! Healing Yourself and Others
By Allen Lawrence, M.D. & Lisa Robyn Lawrence, M.S., Ph.D.

Library of Congress 2012.
Published by ALLCO Publishing
ISBN: 978-0615833392

This book is a reference work based on research by the authors.
The directions stated in this book are in no way to be considered as a substitute for consultation or appropriate treatment by a duly licensed physician.
Printed in the United States of America

How to Order:
Single copies or quantity discounts are available. If you wish to purchase multiple copies for distribution or resale or be eligible for our multiple copy discount program send a letter on your company letterhead and tell us your intended use of our books and the number of books you wish to purchase and we will contact you for mutual benefit:

ALLCO Publishing
18653 Ventura Blvd.
Suite #384
Tarzana CA 91356

If you have questions or require specific information you can reach us at
Questions@AllcoPublishing.com

For information regarding Drs. Allen and/or Lisa Robyn Lawrence,
go to: http://www.AllenLawrenceMD.com

Book design , layout, & production by abcDesignsLLC.com

Table of Contents

*Give your stress wings
and
let it
fly away.*

~Terri Guillemets

Acknowledgement

We would like to thank the many people who have helped us with writing this book. Those patients, several thousands of them, who sat and talked with us about their individual lives and their life experiences, how the stresses of their life affected them, how it made them sick, and how in many cases they healed themselves. I appreciate them and their extremely valuable contributions to this book.

I would like to thank my wife and partner Lisa Robyn Lawrence for her many contributions of time and effort in reading, rereading, editing and discussing the content with me. Lisa is an amazingly bright woman with many insights and a gift for saying things the way they need to be said.

Accolades to Kip Allen who shared editing with Lisa and Arlette Capel who executed the book production, including the book design, layout, and multiple edits and revisions. They both did an excellent job of helping us produce a work that provides easy to read information.

I would also like to thank our many patients over the years. Especially those who allowed us to use their stories. Our patients have been our greatest teachers and without them we would still be in the dark regarding the role of stress in creating illnesses.

*Stress is an
ignorant state.
It believes
that everything
is an emergency.*

~Natalie Goldberg, Wild Mind

Dedication

This book is dedicated to all of us who were born without an owner's manual for our mind or body. In writing this book, it has been our intention to help people better understand how our bodies, minds, and spirits work and how we can cause illness in ourselves and others. In addition this book shows us how we can be more responsible for creating our own good health and supporting the good health of our loved ones, our family, friends, and colleagues.

The process we use is simple. We recognize that we live in an Intelligent Universe controlled by an Infinite Intelligence, and that this intelligence has given us an infinitely Intelligent body. By becoming aware of this Intelligence and understanding how our Intelligent body works and communicates with us, we can easily take control of not only our health and well-being, but of who and what we are.

This Intelligence tells us when we are operating perfectly in tune with our nature. It also tells us when we are in conflict, out of balance, not optimally taking care of our bodies, and when we are being destructive to it.

When these communications are positive, in harmony and balance with ourselves, and our lives, everything comes together and we create what we generally think of as good health. Good health not only means that our bodies work correctly but also that we experience a sense of well-being, feelings of joy, prosperity, and internal serenity.

Illness, on the other hand, communicates that an imbalance or breakdown of some kind has occurred. The body cannot speak in words; it can only speak in physical signs and symptoms. These physical signs and symptoms are messages from your body providing information about the state of your body, life, lifestyle, activities, diet, stresses, positive and negative behaviors, mental and emotional attitudes, and beliefs. Through physical, mental, emotional, and spiritual signs and symptoms, which we commonly think of as illness, we can determine what is right and wrong, working and not working and what needs changing, fixing, or repair. In learning how to identify these communications, we learn how to protect ourselves. The more we learn, the faster and earlier we can begin healing ourselves and those around us.

It is our hope to change the way we, as individuals and as a society, look at illness. It is our greatest wish to make a difference in the lives and health of each of our readers. The message we wish to impart is the title of this book, *When Your Body Talks, Listen!*

*The greatest weapon
against stress
is our ability to choose
one thought over another.*

~William James

Introduction

Each of us wants to be healthy and live a full life. Unfortunately, from time to time, we may find ourselves suffering from illnesses. Once sick, we count on medical doctors to heal us, although they are not always able to do so. This causes distress and even anger for many people. While some people hardly think about illness, others are concerned and want to know how they can protect themselves, insure longevity paired with good health.

There is a large group of illnesses that the medical profession cannot cure. Medical doctors generally do not recognize these illnesses until late in the diseases' course. Because of this, many people suffer needlessly. Many of these illnesses are preventable. Unfortunately, a majority of the people suffering from these illnesses, and often the medical doctors themselves, are unaware that these illnesses are not only preventable, but also fully reversible especially if found and treated early.

This book is primarily about a group of illnesses caused by stress–those conditions we will refer to as Stress-Related Disorders (SRDs). Most people suffer from one or more Stress-Related Disorder. In fact, it is likely that you, my dear reader, may suffer from one or more of these illnesses yourself. You will also find that if you suffer from an illness where treatment has not been successful, your illness might likely fall into this category.

When we discuss Healing of illnesses, we are specifically talking about Stress-Related Disorders. However, the concept of Healing itself is not limited only to these conditions. In referring to Healing, we generally mean the innate capacity that we all possess to heal any condition of the mind, body, or spirit in which there is an imbalance or an illness.

If the terms "illness" and "healing" are unclear or confusing at this point, please, don't worry, we will define and explain them in much greater detail within the course of this book. Healing of the body, as you will soon recognize, also requires healing of the mind and spirit.

Fortunately, this process does not necessarily involve psychiatry, psychology, religion, or the occult. Instead, it simply involves acts of love, self-love, and caring. Healing is not performed by a medical doctor, medications, or even surgery. Healing always involves your efforts to create your own physical, emotional, mental, and spiritual repairs–and return to wellness.

As we begin delving deeper into the healing process, it is important that we have a clear idea of what is needed to create healing and an understanding of the problem or problems that have originally caused the illness process. It is also important to recognize that illness, no matter the type or cause, is an intelligent communication from the body, mind, and spirit that a conflict exists and requires a solution.

It also helps to have a plan and the willingness to carry out this plan. In this sense, healing becomes a process of resolution and completion. Conscious and subconscious conflicts need resolution so that the body, mind, and spirit can return to normality. Implicit in this intelligent process is that healing can help us grow, evolve and ultimately find our highest, healthiest, and best Self.

True healing is about learning, repairing, growing, and evolving. Healing goes on all the time. It is a natural part of who and what we are. The repair process has to do with returning injured areas to normal, harmony and balance with the whole person, nature, and life itself. It makes no difference whether what is to be healed is a body part, an emotion, a business, a relationship, or our connection to the Universe in which we live.

Learning has to do with understanding the factors that caused our problems in the beginning. Growing represents not only our basic physical, mental, and emotional growth, but also the opportunities that arise in everyday life. In the end, personal growth is necessary, and intelligent healing requires that we master this process and reach for and find our highest, healthiest, and best Self. This includes learning from our mistakes and using what we learn to support our future growth.

Most important of all is allowing—and vigorously encouraging—the healing process and healing. Healing will not occur if we resist it. To become healed, we must accept our capacity to heal ourselves. To do this, we must learn to have faith in our innate ability to heal ourselves. Those who have already experienced this process know that it does indeed happen. However, it is not always possible to explain how or why it happens. We ultimately need to know that we have the ability to heal whatever must be healed, and that we must be willing to do the work to make this healing possible.

Foreword

BY ALLEN LAWRENCE, M.D.

What we present in this work is entirely our own personal viewpoint. We present little or no scientific references in this work, as we do not intend it to be a strictly scientific treatise. Instead, it comes from our years of personal observations and from what we learned from the many patients who have been our teachers.

When I decided to become a physician, I made a pledge that my life would be dedicated to helping people get well. In the early years of my practice, I relied on what I was taught in medical school to help me heal people. During those years, I helped many people, and my patients seemed pleased. I treated many and even appeared to cure a few people. However, I cured far fewer people than I believed were curable. I ultimately found that medicine was not about curing people, but about treating them with medications, surgery, and other medical procedures. I eventually became disillusioned, and I developed illnesses that forced me to give up the day-to-day-practice of medicine.

As with many others through the years, "We ultimately find that our own illnesses are our greatest teachers." These works, as well as the other books Lisa and I have written are about a few of the many success stories. It is also about a willingness to look beyond the medical textbooks and see what is actually happening. It is about those patients and their families who were willing to go beyond their previous limitations and view their lives in a different and more productive way. Ultimately, it is about the exploration and the journeys these patients took to find their own wellness and healing. I believe that this approach will one day, be considered the standard for a new medicine–a medicine of healing rather than simply treating.

Currently, the medical profession concentrates on technological systems to solve its inability to cure patients. I believe this is the wrong place to look. It's not that technology isn't valuable, but rather that the answers are within each of us in an area where it is unlikely that any technological breakthrough will ever be of great value.

The answers exist within the interrelationship of our minds, bodies, and spirits. Certainly, the role of our brains, anatomies, physiologies, and biochemistries are all important factors. However, the part we are about to discuss is about being human, and how we actually work beyond our physical parts.

The principles we will discuss within this book are the basis of many healing systems, many of which are thousands of years old. One such system that we believe is extremely valuable is *Huna* (meaning "secret"), an ancient Polynesian and Hawaiian healing system that has been actively used for somewhere between 2,000 and 14,000 years. It is not only much older than Western medicine; it is much wiser and more sophisticated in many ways.

In this book, we will introduce you to some new ways of thinking about old problems. We will present a framework upon which the interaction of our minds, bodies, and spirits are described. No such structure presently exists in modern day medicine. This is a major problem for those of us who want to heal and those of you who want to be healed.

Because the information I am presenting here is so different from what you may already be used to, I decided that I must give you one extremely important instruction before we start: *believe nothing I say, unless you first know it to be true.* If, after you have completed reading our book, you are still unsure of what I have offered, do two things: First, live with it for a while without trying to prove it to be either right or wrong. Second, watch the world around you. Look at those people who become ill, and see if what I have said helps you to understand why some people heal spontaneously and why others do not and may subsequently remain ill or develop one or more chronic or even fatal illnesses.

I believe that if you do this, you will soon find out for yourself that what I say herein is basically correct. If you recognize this for yourself, then you will also recognize that you are the creator of your own life. Once you become aware that only you can cause your own illnesses, then you can learn how to heal yourself. Only you can heal your illnesses and change your life for the better. Only you can reach for and find your highest, healthiest, and best Self.

Allen L. Lawrence, M.A., M.D., Ph.D.

Foreword

BY LISA LAWRENCE, M.S., PH.D.

When I, Lisa, was very young I knew that I possessed the ability to heal myself and others. I knew and trusted that bodies could heal and get well. I did not need to understand the process at the time, I just trusted it. As I grew older, much of that system was taught out of me. Teachers, parents and doctors told me that healing was scientific, doctor stuff. "You have to go to special schools and learn to be a doctor in order to heal people." I was told it was a lot of hard work and that only doctors could cure you if you were sick.

I learned as a young adult that people who were sick with serious illnesses like cancer, heart disease, tumors, arthritis, infections or other types of illnesses usually went to see their medical doctors for help in feeling better or healing. My biggest question was who helps us prevent these illnesses and teaches us not to get sick?

It seemed that I first had to get sick before a medical doctor would help me get well again. No one gave me information about what I could do to help myself prevent and even cure illness. It was not until I was an adult and had a problem that my medical doctor could not cure that I took my life and healing into my own hands. This was when I started learning how to heal myself and how to prevent myself and others from becoming ill.

My husband, Allen, and I have worked together for more than three decades in presenting the tools necessary for healing to our patient/clients. We then gave them the information about how to apply these tools in their lives to help prevent illness and to improve their ability to heal.

Now we feel it is time to share what we have learned from this experience with a much broader group.

Listening to the wise communications from our body to identify and heal the underlying blocks, conflicts and misconceptions is the basis of this book. We hope that soon you too will have a better appreciation of how to listen to what your body is trying to communicate to you. Thus the title of this book, When Your Body Talks, LISTEN!

Lisa Robyn Lawrence, M.S., Ph.D.

*Stress is
the trash of modern life
— we all generate it —
but if you don't dispose
of it properly,
it will pile up &
overtake your life.*

~Terri Guillemets

Disclaimer

The ultimate goal for most healing professions is to identify illness and heal it. In order for this to take place the practitioner, and hopefully the patients, should have a clear idea and understanding of what illness is, how it is caused, the process of moving from its most minimal stage to its most maximum end result. With this information solidly in mind, one can then recognize even the simplest illness while it is still in its earliest stages. Early recognition then allows planning and development of a meaningful healing program which can resolve the causes and stop the progression of the illness, and finally, reverse the signs and symptoms that have already occurred. It is also important to recognize that even the highest level of well-being requires constant vigilance, regular maintenance, 24/7-365 protection of the individual's overall health and wellness. It is to these goals that our book is dedicated. Also, while we recognize that not all medical problems and health issues are caused by or made worse by stress and Stress-Related Disorders, some 70-80% of all medical conditions are either created by or worsened by stress which is more often than not 100% resolvable.

If you are ill or are in the process of becoming ill, see your medical doctor for evaluation and treatment if needed. We cannot stress this enough. Also, always ask yourself if your illness could be caused by stress and whether it is or is not a Stress-Related Disorder. If the answer is yes, then understanding the information we present in this book will allow you to better direct your overall health care and treatment program.

While we are proponents of alternative medicine and healing, we recognize first that some problems are better dealt with by medical doctors. Secondly, some problems can only be dealt with by medical doctors. Thirdly, at least —whether or not you chose to work with a medical doctor—healing requires a diagnosis, so that you actually know what you are dealing with and hence what you are treating. Finally, it is extremely valuable to know and understand your options.

Our book is an attempt on our part to present information about an area that is poorly dealt with on the part of the Western medical profession, many alternative medical practitioners as well as the general public itself. It is a sad fact that stress is poorly dealt with and treated by almost all aspects of the healing professions. This book is meant to convey information regarding stress and the Stress-Related Disorders which are poorly understood. It is our goal to help readers obtain more sophisticated health care solutions as well as attain healing as rapidly as possible.

There is no intention on our part to offer any specific diagnosis or treatment program for any specific medical condition or health problem. Our goal is to provide our readers with a basic understanding from which they can identify any role which stress may play in causing or worsening their illness, or in blocking results from their current treatment program.

While treating illness is generally the role of your medical doctor, chiropractor, homeopath or other licensed standard or alternative health care practitioner, the knowledge contained in our book will help you understand what is happening to you, why treatments are working or not working, and what you can do to help and support your practitioner and yourself in eliminating and curing your illness.

After a solid diagnosis has been made by a health practitioner, we offer information which can now offer additional help and support to your standard or alternative practitioner regarding how they can create a meaningful and appropriate treatment programs for reversing your illness and helping to heal you. Working with your health care professional, you can help identify the causes of your illness and find new creative solutions to heal yourself. The information we present is not offered to take the place of standard medical practices, instead it is meant to be used as an adjunct to a well designed standard medical treatment program offered by your health care professional.

Professional Disclaimer

The information contained within this book is intended to be wholly for educational purposes and is not meant or intended nor is it implied to be a substitute for professional medical advice, diagnosis or treatment. Always seek the advice of your physician or other qualified health provider prior to starting any new treatment or with any questions you may have regarding a medical condition. Nothing contained in this book is intended to provide a medical diagnosis or offer specific treatment without a competent evaluation by a medical professional.

The information in this book is offered by the authors Allen Lawrence, M.D., Lisa Lawrence, Ph.D., and Allco Publishing and is based solely their opinions and beliefs, observations and research and not that of the medical community as a whole.

The information presented herein is mainly based on proven scientific information, which is generally well known and well understood. While the greatest majority of what we present is based on the current state of the art for defining stress, illness and illnesses caused by or worsened by stress, we do believe that we also offer a new theoretical model for how stress can and does cause illness.

Within this book we discuss what we refer to as the Survival Center. This concept is not found in most scientific literature as the "Survival Center," rather most often what we call the Survival Center exists not as a specific place nor anatomical/physiologic structure but rather as a combination of processes, anatomical and biologic functions, which are generally assigned to various parts of the brain and the hormonal-neurological systems.

There is another area where we offer a new way of thinking about stress and the creation of illness is: the Wellness-Illness and Illness Wellness Continuum. This construct is based on our many years of observation of how stress ultimately ends up causing various illnesses. It is not a construct taken from any medical text book. A third area is where we take observational liberties in our breakdown and definitions of the various sub-stages of the Wellness to Illness process: distress, dis-stress, dys-stress, disease, dys-ease and some portion of the definition of disease.

These areas require scientific research and recognition so that the process by which stress leads to or causes illness is clarified and better understood. This is essential so that this information can be used again and again to help prevent and treat those suffering from SRDs.

The basis of the Wellness-Illness Continuum, the definitions and descriptions of distress, dis-stress, dys-stress, dis-ease, dys-ease and some portion of the definitions for disease are based on our observations over the past 40 plus years in medical practice as well as our day to day experience working with and helping those ill with Stress-Related Disorders (SRDs) and illnesses. We present this information as a series of observations that make sense to us and which we believe present a new theoretic basis for how SRDs are formed, how they can be recognized, diagnosed and ultimately treated. These portions of our work, the Survival Center and the Wellness-Illness and the Illness-Wellness Continuum are theoretical constructs that must be approached in the very near future to prove or disprove.

The case histories we have presented herein are based on fact and specific individuals. Some parts of their stories have however been changed (names, dates, time and places) to protect those individuals whose stories we ultimately used. Some parts of their stories may have been left out while others parts have been featured in order to make specific points as examples. We have made these changes to make sure that no person was compromised in any way or form. Changes were made based on relevance to their past history, to their overall health and to the medical problems they exhibited in order to protect them from recognition. In all cases the basic information is correct and appropriate and deemed sufficiently important so that the specific case history was selected to provide valuable information which we feel is relevant to the specific area of discussion the case history was selected to exemplify. Some information was left out when it was deemed neither significant nor relevant to the specific example as it was used in order to minimize space and also, more importantly, to direct the reader's attention to those issues relevant to the concept we are discussing regarding the creation and effects of SRDs.

We call for the medical profession and science community in general to take a brand new look at the process by which stress causes illness so that we can begin to not only better understand this process but create a meaningful system of early recognition of SRDs. Recognition early enough to block their formation and hence create a new level of prevention, protection and treatments for those who if not identified early, educated and assisted, would one day simply be another sick person whom it might, when finally diagnosed, be too late to help, treat or cure.

*The time to relax
is when
you don't have time for it.*

*~Attributed to both Jim Goodwin
& Sydney J. Harris*

Chapter One

TRANSFORMING ILLNESS INTO WELLNESS

In the process of practicing medicine and working to facilitate people getting well, we recognized that there is a large group of illnesses that are often missed by both patients and physicians. Even when recognized, these illnesses are frequently mistreated or often not treated at all. In the course of this book, we will discuss these illnesses and educate our readers on how to recognize them, how they are created, how they can be prevented, and healed.

In recent years, articles in both the lay press and medical literature have suggested that between 70-80 percent of all illnesses seen within medical offices are either caused by stress, made worse by stress, or related to stress. This group of illnesses, which we refer to as Stress-Related Disorders or SRDs, robs tens of millions of people of their well-being, health, and vitality each year. They cost society billions of dollars in medical expenses and lost productivity each year. Stress-Related Disorders often generate suffering and pain in those affected by them. Much to my dismay, the public and the medical profession know little about SRDs, why they occur, and how to eliminate them. In the following pages, we examine how Stress-Related Disorders occur, their effect on us, and how you can heal and ultimately eliminate them.

ONE PHYSICIAN'S STORY

After graduating from medical school, I (Allen) planned to set up my medical practice. I wanted to save the world. I believed that if I were just given the opportunity to work with sick people, I could cure them and heal their illnesses. I believed that their new found health and well-being would enhance their lives, and that they and their families would live happily ever after. How quickly my illusion was shattered.

Within a short while, I realized that the practice of medicine was not about curing people. Instead, it was about reducing their symptoms to a comfortable level. The problem was that although the patient's symptoms were treated and maybe even controlled, they remained sick. Conditions such as diabetes were often fully reversible through diet, exercise, and use of appropriate vitamin and mineral supplements. Year after year, I saw that many men, women, and even children who had diabetes were treated with medication but never really cured. At best, they were only brought under "good control." A large percentage still ultimately developed complications and many most likely even died of the complications associated with their diabetes. This was also true of most Stress-Related Illnesses. While the symptoms were being treated, the true cause of the medical condition was not resolved. This often led to chronic disease and death, even when this was totally avoidable.

The same is true of many other illnesses, even illnesses that are easier to reverse and eliminate. Through the course of this book, I will not only describe how illness is created, but also how it is too often allowed to progress from simple intelligent communications from the body that something is wrong, through more complex, dangerous stages into illness, disease and even chronic disease and death.

It became apparent to me that not every sick person wanted to get well. They often believed too strongly in their illnesses. Their doctors, family, and society's belief in illness too often held great negative power over them. Frequently, their illnesses became an integral part of them. Many felt powerless to affect their illness. In fact, many people could not even imagine themselves being completely well or entirely healthy. These people suffer from what I think of as an "illness mentality." They believed in illness and accepted its power over them to the point that they surrendered their ability to return to wellness.

It also became clear that for many people, there are significant secondary gains from being ill. Children who are ill don't have to go to school and sick adults don't have to go to work. Sick people surrender many responsibilities to others because of their illnesses. They often receive desperately needed attention from others. For some individuals, illness is a justification for their inability to succeed, to take risks, or to even try to succeed. For others, illness legitimizes their failure to function normally in life. Illness often provides a reason or excuse for why they have not turned out the way others wanted them to be or what they expected of themselves. Illness may also relieve them of obligations for social contact, friendship, and commitment.

After many years of practicing medicine, I recognized four different types of patients: Those who believed in illness and are frequently sick, those who are only occasionally sick, those who were at sometime in their life very sick and at some point later had become completely cured and finally, those who are never sick.

THOSE WHO BELIEVE IN ILLNESS - ILLNESS MENTALITY

The first group consists of many of the same types of people I just described. They believe in illness. They generally suffer from a wide variety of illnesses from recurrent colds and influenza to conditions such as headaches, neck and back pain, high blood pressure, ulcers, bladder infections, urethral irritations, abdominal pain, vaginal infections, and constipation all the way to heart disease and even cancer.

Often in the beginning of their illness process before the full pattern of their ultimate illness becomes defined, only vague and general symptoms are recognized. Some examples of these vague types of symptoms are fatigue, nervousness, anxiety, depression, constipation, diarrhea, difficulty sleeping, and so on.

These symptoms often seem to come from nowhere. They can vary greatly in degree, coming and going in irregular patterns, often seemingly random and unrelated to each other. In some people, they cause pain, suffering, and inconvenience. In others, they are simply a nuisance. Through the years, we have all experienced parents, relatives, neighbors, and friends being sick. We gradually learned to accept sickness as a normal part of life. Sickness has become expected. "Everyone gets sick from time to time," a patient once told me. "It is normal to get sick." I have heard these types of statements thousands of times over my years in practice.

Each of us has our own personal experience with illness. It generally starts early in life as we suffer the illnesses of childhood. These give us proof to believe that all illness is real. The problem is that we too readily accept this as proof that all adult illnesses occur for the exactly the same reasons, and that bacteria and viruses, "bugs" or genetics are responsible for illness.

As we age, there is a clear change in the pattern of illnesses that most adults experience. The causes become less apparent, and the circumstances are often ill-defined. Illnesses are no longer occurring because the individual and their immune system have been exposed to "childhood diseases" to which we have no existing immunity. As we reach late childhood and early adolescents, illnesses are more commonly associated with nutritional factors, lifestyle, and exposure to the elements, injury, accidents, and stress.

These illnesses differ in many ways from childhood illnesses. One way is that when medical attention is sought and after an examination, laboratory testing and other diagnostic tests are performed. Test results are often normal for the individual's age and sex. The physician's diagnosis is therefore often vague and imprecise, and related to his or her best guess based on acute or chronic symptoms more than a specific disease pattern. In fact, in the earliest stages, most diagnoses are simply statements of the patient's symptoms. The majority of times, when a diagnosis is ultimately assigned, it often reflects the physician's need to please his patient, the patient's family, or the patient's insurance company. Too often, the diagnosis and treatment assigned are based on the patient's and/or physician's need to justify the office visit rather than determining the real cause or problem at hand. Whatever diagnosis the physician ultimately chooses, it is likely that it will have little if anything to offer regarding the real cause of the patient's problem nor what factors underlie his illness.

The assignment of a diagnosis often validates the reality of the illness for both the patient and the physician. This frequently misdirects the physician, taking him away from the real problems that underlie the illness and leaving their patients feeling as if the symptoms they are experiencing are really bona fide illnesses.

Whether necessary or not, the sick person is usually given medication. Patients often demand medications to "fix" their "illnesses." It makes little difference to most people whether the medications they receive are appropriate or potentially dangerous. They may request and even demand antibiotics to treat conditions where antibiotics have little or no value. I have had this experience in the past, where patients demanded medications such as penicillin for minor, viral, upper respiratory illnesses. Even when I have explained that these problems are caused by viruses which will not respond to any antibiotics and that my prescribing antibiotics would unnecessarily place them at risk for potentially lethal side effects, they still want, even demand, being treated with an antibiotic.

The fact is many physicians eventually end up prescribing unnecessary even dangerous medications not just to relieve their patient's symptoms and anxiety, but also because they really don't know what else to do. In addition, the work and negative energy expenditure associated with arguing with the patient or his family about this is rarely worth it since they will merely go to another doctor to get what they are demanding. All too often, medications are prescribed because the doctors tire from arguing with patients' requests for unnecessary medications.

Just as with assigning a diagnosis, the ultimate effect of prescribing medication confirms and reinforces the patient's fears and ultimately their beliefs that "illness" really exists.

THOSE WHO ARE ONLY OCCASIONALLY SICK

The second group is composed of those who are only occasionally sick. These individuals may become ill on occasion. Their lives do not revolve around illness. They may disregard the signs, symptoms, and illnesses that they do get. They may or may not have an "illness mentality." If they do, it is considerably less developed than in the first group. Often, their illnesses relate to stress, exposure to the elements, nutrition, lifestyle, injuries, emotional or spiritual causes. I spend a great deal of time in this book talking about this group.

THOSE WHO WERE SICK AND BECAME COMPLETELY CURED

In the past, these people have had a serious, possibly life-threatening illness or series of illnesses. At some point, they recognized that they were not their illness and they no longer needed to be ill. Whether they take credit for healing themselves or give credit to the medical profession, to a healer, or just good fortune, they somehow in some way learned something from their illness and now using what they have learned they stay healthy. These individuals may or may not have had an "illness mentality" at or before the time they last became sick. However, if it did exist, it was no longer an issue once they were healed. It no longer affected them or moved them toward illness. In fact, once recovered, they often change to develop a "wellness mentality – health and well-being are my natural states of being." We will address this in greater detail later on in this book.

THOSE WHO ARE NEVER SICK

There is a small group of people who rarely get sick, even during childhood. They have consistently had and maintained a "wellness mentality." They simply do not believe in illness. Once again, I will also discuss this group in greater detail in later a later section.

ABOUT THE ILLNESS PROCESS

There are two general types of illness: acute and chronic. Acute illnesses generally have sudden onset. That is they seem to arise out of nowhere. They then often either resolve themselves and go away or progress over time to become a chronic illness. Chronic illnesses can be any illness whether it has an acute onset or starts gradually and builds up slowly over months and years.

Acute illnesses are generally short lived; one of several outcomes are likely to occur. The illness occurs and either heals spontaneously, or it transforms over time into a chronic illness, or the recipient dies from it or from complications associated with this illness.

When an acute illness strikes, it often causes signs, symptoms, discomfort, pain, inconvenience, loss of capacity, and more. In our society, one of the first things we do with acute illness is to wait and see whether or not it will go away on its own. If that doesn't occur, then we consult with our primary care doctor or go to an urgent care or emergency room. During the following doctor's visit, a series of events takes place, including the doctor or his assistant taking a medical history, the doctor then performs a physical examination, laboratory and other diagnostic testing will be done and finally the doctor will end the visit by offering a diagnosis and then some type of treatment and treatment plan.

The diagnosis may be clear or unclear to the physician. However, having a diagnosis is essential on many levels. The diagnosis helps the physician decide if treatment is needed and the type of treatment required. A diagnosis is necessary so that a reason for the illness can be given to the patient, or his family and friends. It is essential to rule out communicable diseases so that others are not exposed, or if already exposed, are treated as early as is possible. A diagnosis is necessary for medical record keeping, for if a physician does not generate a diagnosis, he could be liable for legal action by the patient or the state medical board for poor record keeping or even incompetence. Finally, if the patient wants his insurance to be billed, one or more diagnoses are essential since the insurance companies will not pay without at least one. The more diagnoses given, the more complex the visit, and the more the physician can bill and hence ultimately collect.

TREATING THE PATIENT

Once one or more diagnoses are made, the physician must do something about the illness, the symptoms, the patient's discomfort, pain, or risk to their life. Doing nothing could leave the patient or their family and friends doubting the physician's skill, judgment, and medical competency.

The physician must also deal with his own personal need to feel of value and feel as if he were "doing something to help the patient." Generally, he may utilize one of several alternatives. First, is the illness dangerous? Will it lead to an immediate death? If it is not life-threatening will it resolve on its own or with treatment or will it progress and ultimately transform into a chronic disease condition? If so, will it eventually lead to or cause a significant disability, a meaningful loss of function, a significant reduction in individuals' overall quality of life? Will it ultimately result in a painful or humiliating death, months or years down the road? Second, the physician must decide whether the process will heal itself spontaneously without any medical treatments and medications. (This probably happens more often than most people realize.) Third, the physician should be considering as to whether this condition or conditions are part of a larger process. Third, is medication necessary? Which medication? Does the physician have a medication or series of other treatments that can cure or, more commonly, relieve the immediate risks and dangers of the condition?

Unfortunately, one of the most common situations occurs when a series of illnesses, related or not, appear to come and go, changing their characteristics from time to time, presenting different patterns sometimes looking like recurrences of one or more minor or serious conditions, or sometimes appearing totally unrelated. As these complex signs and symptoms appear, one "condition" may appear in the moment to be "cured" when at a later time a "new condition" possibly appearing to be unrelated just seems to spring up. This is especially true of Stress-Related Disorders.

In the majority of such situations, the underlying causes of the patient's acute or recurring symptoms are never really explored. Physicians' often feel that since the symptoms do not suggest a life-threatening or dangerous situation, or that there is a specific "disease" pattern, or when the symptoms resolve easily with medication or even spontaneously, and because they are short lived, the physician may opt to simply treat the symptoms and never investigating their underlying cause or causes. The physician is generally looking for life-threatening illnesses, not for Stress-Related Disorders. By missing the causal events or conflicts that triggered these illnesses, the physician often misses SRDs that may later end up becoming a life-threatening illness.

**Physicians generally look
for Life-Threatening Illnesses –
not for Stress-Related Disorders.**

The patient often thinks of their symptoms as their illness. As time passes, these symptoms may begin taking form and eventually advance into specific, well-defined patterns. When this occurs, a defined diagnosis is eventually made. Since the real underlying problem is neither looked for, found, or resolved, a real illness or disease may eventually be the result. (We use the term illness to refer to conditions that are not harmful. Disease refers to a more defined condition that can cause or lead to harm.)

In my early years of practicing medicine, I, too, believed in the reality of illness. My classmates and I were taught all about illnesses and diseases in their acute and chronic forms. We were taught about their causes, pathologies, and medical and surgical treatments.

I learned that disease was not only "real," but that it was clearly "part of the human condition." What I was taught was tangible and believable. How could I, as a neophyte, dispute any of it? The problem was that I was not taught or presented with any detailed information regarding the roles of stress, nutrition, lifestyle, or exposures to toxic chemicals played in creating illness and disease. In most medial training programs it is rare that anyone ever presents or discusses any viable model for recognizing or preventing Stress-Related Disorders. It is even more rare that anyone would even talk about or deal with recognizing or identifying the stages (Stress, Distress, Dystress, Dys-Stress, Dis-Ease, Dys-Ease) which often lead up to and present information about most Stress-Related Disorder. It is even rare for anyone to talk about illness being created by or caused by stress. Hence, stress is rarely considered to be a consideration or cause of any illness before the illness reaches the Disease stage. In fact, stress was hardly ever mentioned at all.

With experience and the passage of time, it became apparent that the majority of patients who suffered from even the most common illnesses seen in everyday practice rarely behave the way the textbooks tell us they should.

There are significant and divergent individual and human factors that make the textbooks potentially meaningless for precisely diagnosing an exact illness in one person. Sometimes, people with life-threatening or incurable illnesses get better with no treatment at all. At the same time, other people who suffer from what initially appears to be a minor illness may suddenly die of unexpected complications even after rigorous treatment.

I noticed that there is a relatively large group of people who rarely become sick. Often, these people seek medical attention only for well-person examinations, such as a routine annual exam, a driver's physical, a pre-employment physical, or an annual Pap smear. This healthy group may actually make up a large percentage of the people in our country. Not only are they seldom sick, they have another interesting characteristic: they generally have little or no belief in illness or disease. They see no value in getting sick. In addition, they do not see themselves as "sick" people.

> **People who are seldom sick generally**
> **have little or no belief in Illness or Disease.**
> **They have a Wellness Mentality.**

The third group, those who, at one time or another were seriously ill and were completely cured, are more difficult to describe. This is a small, rapidly growing group. It is made up of individuals who transformed illness into wellness. These people either had a serious or a recurrent illness, or learned the secret of wellness. Whether they overcame cancer, diabetes, high cholesterol, recurrent bronchitis, problems with gambling, panic attacks, alcoholism, or drug addition, the people of this group healed themselves with or without the help of others. I am proud to declare that my wife Lisa and I belong to this group.

Those readers who have also healed themselves will recognize what I am going to tell you in this book. These readers will likely have already recognized, what the other two groups have not, that wellness is a state of mind, and that it is available to everyone. People who healed themselves often credit their healing to prayer, religion, or a strong belief in a higher authority. While there is truth in this type of belief, it is more likely that it was the changes they made in their lifestyle, their rejection of an "illness mentality," their desire for wellness, their adoption of a "wellness mentality," their problem solving skills and a host of new, healthy and problem-solving decisions on their part that ultimately made the difference.

This is clearly illustrated in the phrase, "God helps those who help themselves[1]."

Wellness is a State of Mind.

Ultimately, a cure takes place because of our own faith in ourselves and our willingness to heal. It depends on our ability to solve problems and willingness and then commitment to do whatever is needed to insure or regain health. While a strong religious or spiritual belief helps, it is our belief in ourselves, in our ability to heal (with or without the help of others or even God), and the problem solving we practice that cures us. Prayer is most helpful, especially when it helps solve problems, change a negative lifestyle and when it helps us feel that we deserve to be healed.

It is common to see that when people with one or another serious health condition do spontaneously heal that the medical profession calls this healing a "miracle." While there may be miracles of divine origin, it is more likely that when a physician tells a patient that their being healed was due to a miracle, it is an indication that the physician, and even the medical profession, really does not understand how the illness really occurred nor what these individuals did to heal themselves. If the medical doctors or the medical profession understood this process better, they would be creating and facilitating "miracles" all the time.

In the following chapters, we look at the basis of illness and wellness. You will then learn for yourself what many well people have learned as they transformed their illness into wellness.

AN INTELLIGENT UNIVERSE

The human body is Intelligent and we are part of an Intelligent Universe. I use this concept of an Intelligent Universe to refer to the highest order of Intelligence and Knowing, or "Universal Wisdom," which is the source of the Laws of the Universe. Some might call this Intelligence "God" while others understand it as physics, chemistry, Newton's Laws of Thermodynamics, Evolution, and that which makes science meaningful.

---

1   *Often attributed to the Bible, but not actually found anywhere in the Bible.*

It should not be difficult to recognize the fact that our universe is Intelligent and that we are Intelligent. The opposite, more common view is, that the Universe is random, dumb, uncaring, scary, and even cruel. This view results from people choosing not to see the Intelligence of the Universe operating. When the events of life don't turn out the way they think they should, this is used as evidence and proof that the universe is a hostile, random, unfeeling and uncaring place or situation.

> **The human body is intelligent
> and is part of an intelligent Universe.**

The Universe we live in, including our body, mind, and spirit, is Intelligent; we only need to look around us to see this Intelligence in action. Our Universe knows how to be a Universe. Our solar system knows how to be a solar system. Our planet knows how to be a planet. No one has to tell the Earth how to spin, or how to rotate around the Sun every 365 days (give or take a day or so). A rose knows how to be a rose; a mountain knows how to be a mountain. No one has to tell your digestive system how to digest, or a heart how to beat, or the endocrine system how to create and maintain a proper hormonal balance.

> **A rose knows how to be a rose, and
> a mountain knows how to be a mountain.**

All of these activities are proof that the Universe we live in, our bodies, minds and spirits, and ourselves, are all part of an extremely Intelligent process we call Life. As we progress through this book, the existence of this Intelligence and its depth becomes increasingly clear. Even if you are not yet convinced, keep your mind open to the possibility that what I say is true.

Many people see this Intelligence operating all around them, but instead of acknowledging it, they become caught up in the events and circumstances of their own lives. The order and intelligence they do recognize often appear to them as a fluke or an island of calm in a sea of chaos. However, once a person recognizes this Intelligence operating within and around them, the next step is to become more aware that they and their body, and everything that goes on within it, are also Intelligent. Once you acknowledge this, all doubt leaves and life takes on a new and higher meaning. The purpose of the journey we are about to take is to recognize that illness itself has a meaning beyond anything our past beliefs have led us to accept.

THE 'GERM' THEORY

Since the time of Louis Pasteur, the medical profession has operated from a set of beliefs generally referred to as the Germ Theory. That is, germs–bacteria, viruses, and other microscopic and macroscopic parasites–cause infectious diseases. This theory is interpreted in two entirely different ways. On one hand, it suggests that infectious diseases are "caused" by organisms that enter the body from outside, attack, and infect it. On the other hand, it suggests another possibility, one that implies that the body may actually "catch" these organisms and allow them to create disease.

In the first situation, it appears as if these aggressive organisms first look for, find, and consciously invade our body. This would apparently be done without the body's (or the person's) consent or involvement. In the latter situation, the body would appear to play a more active role in the selection and entrance of these "germs" as well as the creation of the resulting infection itself.

At first thought, we may react to this latter proposal with disbelief. However, if we look more closely at what actually happens, we find that the majority of microorganisms known to "cause" infection are generally simple and non-aggressive organisms. Most of them already live in or on our bodies symbiotically for months or even years before suddenly becoming aggressive, "causing" an infection. Most of the other organisms (those not already living in or on the body) enter the body only when they are looking for a warm meal, a comfortable place to live, and the opportunity to grow and multiply. The myth that paints them as "demons" waiting to attack us and take over our bodies is an exaggeration. Most organisms found in infections normally coexist with us in the same world. We usually have some level of resistance, antibodies, or other defensive system, which protects us from them and mediates their ability to "invade" us.

Germs generally live in harmony with us.

These "germs" generally live in harmony and balance with us. For the most part, they are like us–just trying to survive. Only once in awhile does one organism that is foreign to us and to which we have no immunity, enter us and cause illness.

When this happens, most of the time some type of injury or physical, mental, emotional, or spiritual trauma has been involved and precipitated their "attack."

There is nothing personal about this. However, even in these situations we still have many ways of protecting ourselves from their entrance and attack. To these organisms we are simply a host–any host–one that just happened to come along or be there at the right time. Since they have often lived in peace, harmony and balance with us for very long times, it looks to them as if we have opened our door and invited them in as our defense systems go down and are rendered useless against them. It is just as we might come upon a restaurant or a motel while driving along the highway looking for a place to eat or sleep and find the door open, no one in charge and lots of inviting food and restful rooms available for the taking.

PROTECTING OURSELF FROM ILLNESS

Our body has many built-in levels of defensive and offensive protection systems. These systems protect us against stray organisms setting up housekeeping. These defensive systems belong to an extraordinarily complex system that operates everywhere in our bodies, organs, and tissues. They operate 24/7 throughout our lives. They take no vacations. Being extremely Intelligent, these defensive systems do not require our conscious awareness to act when we have been invaded. They sense any invasion whether we are aware of it or not. With few exceptions, it makes little difference what organism invades. Our defensive systems respond to most organisms and substances, even when they are far smaller than we can see, feel, or consciously recognize.

Once these systems recognize that invasion has occurred, they operate swiftly and decisively. Any foreign organisms or substances are isolated and destroyed, as they try to enter our body or set up housekeeping. Although this system does not require conscious help, it can be seriously hindered by negative mental attitudes, beliefs, thoughts, and feelings. Similarly, positive mental attitudes, beliefs, thoughts, and feelings enhance and facilitate it.

Since the discovery of microorganisms, society has thoroughly integrated the Germ Theory concept into our day-to-day beliefs about illness and disease. It is quite common to see people rush to their doctor at the first sign of illness and demand antibiotics to kill the "bugs" they believe are causing their illness. The integration of the Germ Theory into our society is so complete that advertisements on television or radio warning us that the "bugs" are out there once again, are commonplace. Every winter, radio and TV commercials, and newspaper and magazine advertisements warn us that "cold and flu season" is just around the corner or already is here. These advertisements ultimately give people permission to get sick, to "catch" the flu, a cold or a "bug" of some kind.

DO WE GET SICK OR DOES SICKNESS GET US?

To understand the transformation from illness to wellness, we should ask ourselves several important questions. Do we get sick or does sickness get us? Since the bacteria, viruses, and other disease-causing organisms generally coexist in our living space, why are we not sick all of the time? Why does everyone not become sick when a so-called epidemic of influenza or the cold season occurs?

Many of these organisms enter into us on an almost continuous basis. However, our immune system with its multi-layered defenses is generally capable of protecting us, and controlling or even destroying these intruders. Most experts tell us that we have the ability to protect ourselves from most of these organisms. If we look closely, many people around us are never sick. This leads us to the core question regarding illness and wellness, "How and why, is it that individuals both do and do not get sick?"

When we say that we "catch" a cold or other illness, what we are actually saying? Is it that our immune system has failed to work or protect us? In this sense, the organism (and hence the illness) has caught us off guard. If we look at this situation closer, we may find that this failure is often a selective failure.

Our immune system actually seems to not only allow these organisms into our body, but it also appears to let them set up housekeeping with little or no resistance. It is as if we specifically let them into our body and then allow them to establish illness within us. With careful observation, we may see that the body allows these organisms to generate illness for a purpose. If our body is Intelligent, then it must have reasons for doing this. As we proceed, these reasons will become evident.

To illustrate the role of the immune system in protecting us against infections, considers "the boy in the bubble." A number of years ago, a young boy in Florida was born with no functioning immune system. Because of this, he had to live most of his life in a large, sterile room. He had no protective systems against infection except his sterile surroundings. This was necessary because virtually all organisms were dangerous to him. Fortunately, we do have defensive systems protecting us. When most of us become ill, there are only a small number of organisms and illnesses involved. If we were to have a complete immune system failure, then almost any organism could be fatal to us. In Chapter 3, we will discuss the role of the Immune System in protecting and creating disease, in much greater detail.

As I suggested earlier, there are groups of people who are rarely or never sick. Physicians, for example, are constantly exposed to sick people. Yet, most physicians rarely get sick. This suggests that germs–bacteria, viruses, and other parasites–are not the sole cause of illness. Failure or inefficiency of the immune system is the real culprit. Critics might suggest that day-to-day exposure to bacteria and viruses strengthens our immune systems. This may likely be true. However, I suggest that the reason most physicians do not get sick is that while their patients bring in their illnesses; these illnesses do not belong to the physician. The physician does not believe that he is going to get sick. Because the patient's illness is not his illness, he doesn't become ill.

I am rarely sick. I have been sick on only a few occasions in the past 30 years, and I know exactly why I became sick each of these times. On one of these occasions, I had just completed a brief vacation. During the entire time I was away, I worried about being gone from my practice. I felt guilty for having such a good time. Later when I recognized that I was getting sick, I realized that I had created a kind of self-punishment for enjoying my vacation and being away from my medical practice and the people who needed me.

My next illness came because I wasn't listening to my body when it was telling me that I was overworked and needed a rest. I now realize that I "Intelligently" got sick so that I would have to take time off. On another occasion, I became sick during a period when I was also overworked and depressed about my life. When a patient came in with a "terrible cold," I remember thinking to myself, "I am so run down, I just know that I am going to catch this cold," and I did.

The point is that not only is our body Intelligent and capable of protecting and healing us, it is also capable of using illness to communicate with us when we have an unresolved conflict, guilt, anger, frustration, or need help in solving certain problems that are causing us to get sick. When sickness occurs, it usually has a definite reason for occurring. Illness often is a direct communication to us from our Intelligent Body. It is a message about conflicts in our life that our body wants the conscious part of us to do something about.

> Illness is often a direct communication to us
> from our intelligent body, letting us know
> that we have one or more unresolved conflicts
> that need to be resolved.

In the next sections, I explain how this works so that you can better understand what your body is telling you when you get sick. I will introduce you to illness and healing by looking at the Intelligent systems your body maintains to protect you, your defensive and offensive protection systems, and the Fight-or-Flight Stress Mechanism. I then look at how disease is generally created and what you can do to prevent illness in the future.

Chapter Two

STRESS-RELATED DISORDERS

CREATING HEALING AND WELLNESS

Now that we have had a brief looked at the Germ Theory, let's move onto the focus of this book–Stress-Related Disorders or SRDs. We examined infectious diseases to see how they affect the way Western medicine looks at illness. In the following sections, we will investigate an entirely new way of looking at illness. This concept came to my attention because of the findings of a new medical field of study called psychoneuroimmunology[2]. This is simply the study of the interaction of mind and body with its own immune system. Its long name is necessitated by the fact that this discipline is made up of experts in many disciplines including, but not limited to, psychology, psychiatry, internal medicine, neurology, immunology, genetics, and biology.

What I am about to discuss relates to virtually every area of medicine and to all of humanity. This information can also be applied just as easily to legal and business problems, and family relationships. The Intelligence of the Universe is built into the very fabric of life, not just one or two aspects of it. I no longer feel that I specifically work within the field of medicine alone. I incorporated into my work an all-encompassing concept that I call "Healing." This includes the ability to bring all aspects of life into harmony and balance (See Diagram: 2-1, below). The goal of all healing work is creating well-being, prosperity, and good health in all human beings.

The facilitation of healing is not just the role of the physician, but of all other health care providers (physical therapists, nutritional consultants, radiologists, as well as alternative medical practitioners, etc.) Surprisingly, it can also be performed by our accountants, attorneys, bankers, and clergy, as well as politicians and storekeepers. In fact, it includes all of the functions of any person or group that helps others solve problems. In doing so, this also helps them to promote their own personal well-being.

---

2   *Also at times referred to as psychoneuroimmunobiology.*

Therefore, the role of the healer does not belong exclusively to members of the medical profession, but to anyone who helps others solve problems or conflicts. If we are to begin to solve problems and heal our community, the medical profession, and the public, must change their current viewpoint regarding what healing is and how it can be accomplished.

It is also important to believe that true healers (physician or otherwise) are constantly working toward facilitating wellness and health in all areas of their own lives. The Hippocratic Oath, which every physician takes, specifically states, "Physician Heal Thy Self[3]." The capacity for each of us to heal ourselves carries over into the lives and well-being of every person in our society. The physician/healer should always work toward healing. Their role should not be to just treat patients or clients through standard medical procedures, but to find out what life changes and problem solving they need in order to help them to be returned to complete wellness, and then to make sure their patients get it. This may require help with medical care issues, but this might also require financial counseling, relationship counseling, or even a good chiropractor or acupuncturist.

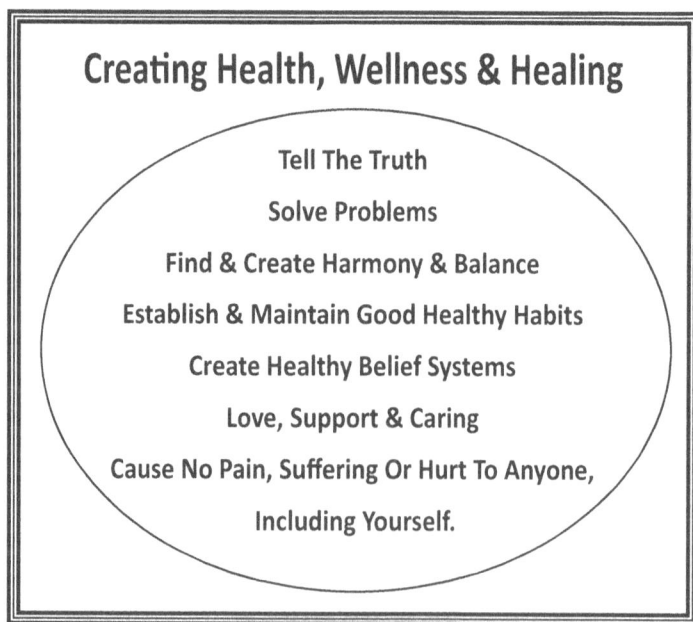

Creating Health, Wellness & Healing

Tell The Truth

Solve Problems

Find & Create Harmony & Balance

Establish & Maintain Good Healthy Habits

Create Healthy Belief Systems

Love, Support & Caring

Cause No Pain, Suffering Or Hurt To Anyone,

Including Yourself.

Diagram: 2-1

---

3   From the Bible. Luke 4:23. "And he said unto them, Ye will sure-
     ly say unto me this proverb, Physician, heal thyself: whatsoever we
     have heard done in Capernaum, do also here in thy country."

To create a totally healthy society, the medical profession must relinquish its claim that physicians are the only ones allowed to be healers. Ultimately, if the medical establishment and the individual physicians within it do not recognize and support other healers, including the healers within their own selves, they will be responsible for perpetuating a medical health system that is designed to keep people sick.

It is possible in the future physicians will be considered more valuable not just for their technical skills, but for their ability to solve problems and help their patients obtain complete and total wellness. One way that all healers, physicians especially, can best help the people they work with is in the area of stress and Stress-Related Disorders.

STRESS-RELATED DISORDERS

As suggested at the beginning of Chapter 1, somewhere between 70-80 percent of all people who visit medical doctors do so because they suffer from Stress-Related Disorders. These individuals are suffering from illnesses, "which are either caused by or related to stress." It is this group of illnesses and diseases which are the main topic of the remainder of this book. All too often individuals with Stress-Related Disorders–and their doctors–do not even know that their physical, emotional, mental, or spiritual problems are caused by stress. These problems are often fully reversible and even preventable in their earliest stages. Yet, their physician, to whom they turn for help, generally does not know this. Since most physicians are unaware of the role stress plays in creating illness, their patients may not end up getting the help they really need.

> **Healing is not the domain of the physician alone.**
> **Any person who works with or helps another**
> **to solve problems, promote well-being, prosperity,**
> **and increase their health & wellness,**
> **is a Healer.**

Stress-Related Disorders can reveal themselves from minor health issues all the way up to life-threatening illnesses. This list of conditions can include upper respiratory infections, colds, allergies, hay fever, and fatigue, but also more dramatic and serious conditions such as high blood pressure, heart attack, diabetes, injuries, ulcers, intestinal diseases, heart disease, pneumonia, bronchitis, cancer, autoimmune diseases, and acute life-threatening allergic episodes.

Included within the scope of Stress-Related Disorders are a large number of common and uncommon medical conditions. The common denominator among all these illnesses, and the people who suffer from them, is that the complex of symptoms or illnesses they are suffering from, are either caused by stress, related to stress or worsened by their unresolved stresses. This is explained in greater detail in Chapters 9 and 10.

It is impossible to cover more than a small number of the illnesses and conditions that belong in this group. What we will do now is to present you with an overview of Stress-Related Disorders, how they work, where they come from, why we have them, and how they generally need to be approached. You can then use this information to determine the specific relationship between the symptoms you might suffer and their relationship to the stresses of your life. Throughout this book, I refer to the many conditions that belong to this group simply as Stress-Related Disorders, or SRDs.

We suggest that there are three types of SRD illness processes: 1) those which are loosely related or connected to stress, 2) those in which stress is a significant or meaningful factor, but not the primary cause, and 3) those in which stress is the primary cause. Through this process we hope to clarify why 70-80 percent of all illnesses are stress-related. We will later define wellness. However, before going any further, we will give you a very basic definition of wellness. Wellness is not just the absence of illness, but is an active process of feeling good, solving problems, and creating mental and emotional clarity.

DEFINING ILLNESS

It must be made clear that not all illnesses are directly related to stress. Before beginning a detailed discussion of Stress-Related Disorders, it is important to compare the more prominent types and categories of conditions that are normally considered either "illnesses" or "diseases." While this discussion is brief, it provides an overview of the illness or disease process and allows you to contrast those illnesses caused by stress with those of other causes.

It is helpful to be aware that there are a number of categories of illnesses and diseases. The medical profession generally defines disease as, "those conditions that have a characteristic train of symptoms and causes which affect all or part of the body." There is usually a clear pattern of symptoms, causes, and effects within a specific disease process. The various diseases within a category and the various categories of diseases themselves are not always as well defined and often have overlapping symptoms, causes and effects.

In the following pages, I illustrate why definitions like this, which are commonly used by the medical profession, often create confusion and limit a clear understanding of the processes which lead to illness and disease.

THE MAIN CATEGORIES OF
NON STRESS-RELATED ILLNESS AND DISEASE

One can be born with certain types of illnesses and diseases. These are Genetic Diseases, which are transmitted from one or both parents to the individual through genetics. They include such conditions as Down syndrome, Tay-Sachs disease, color blindness and diabetes mellitus, to name only a few. These conditions represent a relatively small segment of the population.

Another important group of conditions, are those conditions caused by Congenital Diseases, Intrauterine Development Problems and Birth Injuries.

Congenital Diseases are illnesses transmitted from mother to infant during the period of pregnancy. These include conditions such as AIDS, Syphilis, rubella (German measles), nutritional deficiencies, fetal alcohol syndrome, and chemical dependency. These illnesses or conditions are either "caught" or "created" by the mother and then passed on to the fetus. They are not inherent within the genetics of the fetus or the mother as are the Genetic Diseases.

Intrauterine Injuries are those injuries that occur to the fetus while in the uterus. They can occur from a variety of causes including lack of oxygen, the umbilical cord being wrapped around the fetus' neck, or problems with the placenta leading to inappropriate development of the fetus while in the uterus.

Birth Injuries occur during the birthing process, labor, and/or delivery. Birth traumas can be the natural consequences of the birth process or can be caused by poor obstetrical management.

The single largest group of medical conditions is the Acquired Diseases or Illness group. These are not inherent in the individual, but are acquired through natural or man-made processes. The disorders that comprise this group represent the bulk of the conditions usually labeled as illnesses and diseases. In this category is the largest percentage of Stress-Related Disorders.

There are a number of subcategories in this group including injuries, infections, viral diseases, parasites, metabolic and endocrine (or hormonal) imbalances. Nutritional deficiencies are conditions caused by starvation, poor diet, excessive dieting, anorexia, bulimia, toxic chemicals in the food and water, or are caused by overeating and leading to obesity.

Another large group are the illnesses and injuries caused by the physician because of incorrect diagnosis, poor history taking, inadequate or wrong medical treatment, lack of providing proper medical care, the secondary effects of prescription drugs, inadequate or poor choice of medications or surgery. This group is called Iatrogenic Illnesses.

Acquired Illnesses occur for many reasons and have a variety of causes. They are often created imbalances due to excessive, diminished, or abnormal functioning of the body's chemistry, our immune system, the stress mechanism, or one or more of the other protective mechanisms of our body. Hence, they are often activated or made worse by life stresses.

Finally, we see that conditions belonging to this group may often signifi-cantly overlap with the other categories and subcategories. For example, diabe-tes is generally considered a genetic condition, but it is also a metabolic-endo-crine system disorder. It may be triggered by some form of life stress; obesity caused by a diet high in sugar, refined or processed foods, extreme dieting, or even a "normal diet" that does not contain sufficient essential nutrients. Diabe-tes can also be triggered by infection, certain medications, surgery, pregnancy, childbirth or even an accident or injury.

Injuries are often the cause of illness and disability. Falls, auto collisions, burns, electric shock, crushed body parts, or near drowning can cause loss of function, pain and suffering. Injuries can be created by other people, machinery or are self-induced, such as injuries caused while fighting, attempted suicide, intentional or accidental misuse of guns or knives, or chemicals.

Some injuries may occur when there is a need for a secondary gain. Stress is frequently involved and is commonly generated by the injury itself. When-ever there is an injury, we may even wonder why that person was in that particular place at that precise moment so that the "accident" could occur. Could there possibly be forces operating below the surface which take these injuries out of the realm of pure accident? Every injury creates some change in the injured person, his family or outside observers. It often presents an opportunity for the parties involved to change their lives in some way. So how can these injuries genuinely be considered accidents? This is a topic for a book of its own.

Bacterial infections, viral and parasitic illnesses are conditions caused by bacteria, virus, parasitic, helminthic, or fungal organisms. Many organisms live in and around us most of our lifetime. Most are generally harmless because we have some level of immunity or mechanism to live in harmony and peace with them. Only infrequently when a new, more potent organism comes around, when there is injury, or a breakdown in our protective powers or our immune system "fails," do we have to worry about invasion or infection.

The Stress Mechanism is a vital aspect of the immune system and the healing and repair systems of our body. The proper functioning of our immune system and other protective mechanisms of our body usually have a direct cor-relation with the degree and duration of stress in our life. When we allow stress to become excessive, chronic, or overwhelming, we may find our immune system breaking down. We may also disable the ability of our healing and repair systems to heal injuries that might be caused by these microorganisms or injury or even by natural causes. When our immune, repair, and healing systems are undermined by stress, the door is opened for illness.

> **Stress is responsible for many accidents.**

Metabolic Disorders are conditions affecting energy production within cells. Most metabolic disorders are genetic, although some are acquired because of poor diet, toxins, or infection. When genetically based, metabolic disorders are referred to as Inborn Errors of Metabolism. These genetically based metabolic disorders are usually caused by a genetic defect resulting in the absence of or improper manufacture of one or more enzymes that are important in the metabolic functions of certain groups of cells. The three largest classes of Metabolic Disorders are: 1) glycogen storage diseases, disorders affecting carbohydrate metabolism, 2) fatty oxidation disorders, disorders affecting the metabolism of fat and production of energy from fat, and 3) mitochondrial disorders, disorders affecting the mitochondria or central "powerhouses of the cells.

Endocrine Disorders include diabetes mellitus, a disease involving an endocrine gland, the pancreas. Other Endocrine Disorders include conditions involving the thyroid, pituitary, adrenal, thymus, testes or ovaries, and the parathyroid glands. All of these are endocrine glands. Any diseases involving the function of a specific endocrine gland would be considered a disease of that specific endocrine system. The endocrine-hormonal system is a complex arrangement of glands that produce numerous chemicals, each having specific and general effects on the body. When one of these endocrine systems breaks down, illness and disease often follow. The pituitary, thyroid, adrenal glands, ovaries and testes are the most significant endocrine glands. The endocrine system also includes lesser-known organs such as the pancreas, which manufactures and releases insulin and oversees sugar metabolism; and thymus gland, which produces and regulates certain white blood cells and a number of other cellular elements of the immune system. All of these organs and glands are involved in one way or another with the stress mechanism. All can be affected adversely by abnormal or chronic stress.

Digestive-Nutritional Disorders can affect us starting with the mouth and teeth, and then to the esophagus, stomach, the intestinal tract, the appendix, and the rectum. The liver, pancreas, and gall bladder are also part of this system. This entire system is involved with ingestion, digestion, extraction, absorption, and excretion of nutrients. The digestive system maintains the nutritional aspect of our body.

What we eat and what we do not or cannot eat is important. The human body requires fuel to produce the energy that runs it. Our body requires certain nutrients and micro nutrients, vitamins, minerals and enzymes to properly function. The foods we eat must contain all the essential nutrients and micro nutrients to insure that our body functions correctly. When our diet is inadequate or our digestive system is not correctly functioning, we can become ill. Nutritional deficiencies or excesses can relate to our choice of foods, whether we overeat, excessively diet, our environment, the time of year, or the stresses in our life. They can also be a function of our digestive system's ability to process the foods and nutrients we have eaten.

Together or individually, these disease processes (metabolic, endocrine and digestive-nutrition systems) involve the body's cells, organs, and organ systems that either directly or indirectly affect our ability to maintain normal bodily functions. These functions include the energy generation and release, body temperature maintenance, waste excretion, cardiovascular system regulation, as well as tissue growth and healing ability. They relate to the body's metabolism and ability to operate smoothly and appropriately. Generally, these functions are maintained through a joint cooperative effort in a coordinated manner with the endocrine or hormone-producing systems. When one system is thrown out of balance, the others may also malfunction.

CATEGORIES OF ILLNESSES AND DISEASE*

1. **Pre-Birth Illnesses**
   a) Genetic Diseases

2. **Birth-Related Illnesses**
   a) Congenital Diseases
   b) Intrauterine Developmental Problems
   c) Birth Injuries

3. **Iatrogenic Illness**
   a) Prescription Medication
   b) Surgery
   c) Counseling

5. **Mental-Emotional Illness**
   a) Neurosis
   b) Depression
   c) Bipolar Disorders
   d) Psychosis
   e) Chemical (as an Acquired Illness)

6. **Stress-Related Disorders**
   a) Illnesses caused by Stress
   b) Illnesses made worse by stress

7. **Organ, Tissue and System Diseases**
   See text for description.

8. **Spiritual Illness**
   a) Religious (Pseudo Spiritual)
   b) True Spiritual Illness

4. **Acquired Illnesses**
   a) Injury (Defined by location of occurence: Home, On-The-Job, Sports, Environmental, Transportation, War)
   b) Infectious Diseases (Defined by the type of organism: Bacterial, Viral and Survival particles, Parasitic, Fungus, Protozoa, Helminths (Worms)
      1) Communicable
      2) Non-Communicable
      3) Primary
      4) Secondary
   c) Metabolic-Endocrine Disease (Thyroid, Cardio-vascular and Diabetes to name only a few conditions in this very large group.)
   d) Digestive-Nutritional Diseases
      1) Vitamin-Mineral-Protein Deficiencies
      2) Starvation, Overeating, Excessive Dieting
      3) Dehydration
      4) Digestive Enzyme or Acid Deficiencies
   e) Drug Addiction
      1) Over-the-Counter
      2) Illicit Drugs: Heroine, Cocaine. PCP
      3) Prescription
   f) Environmental Illness
      1) Radiation
      2) Toxic Chemicals
      3) Pollution
   g) Mental-Emotional Disorders
      1) Suicide
      2 Depression

* THIS LIST IS NOT MEANT TO BE EXHAUSTIVE NOR ALL INCLUSIVE BUT RATHER ONLY AS A GENERAL GUIDE TO PROVIDE THE READER WITH AN OVERVIEW OF THIS SUBJECT.

TABLE: 2-1

Environmental Illnesses are another category. Within this group are illnesses caused by industrial and residential pollutants; contamination; improper disposal of human waste products; effects on the atmosphere from hydrocarbons, smog, climate change; and our ingestion of heavy metals.

We can also define illnesses in relation to diseases of organs, tissues, and systems. Examples are cardiovascular disease, gastrointestinal disease, neurological disease, kidney disease, bladder, prostate, blood disorders, and reproductive system disease. We can further categorize diseases by their degree of severity, such as marginal, minimal, mild, low grade, moderate, severe, acute, life-threatening and chronic. Tumors can be defined by whether they are pre-malignant, malignant, or benign. Finally, we can categorize illnesses by age, gender, emotional, mental, and spiritual criteria.

Iatrogenic Illnesses are conditions caused by medical or surgical intervention. While we usually consider medical treatment something desirable and necessary, it can be dangerous. Physicians can make mistakes. Even good physicians and appropriate medical treatment can create medication-related problems. These problems may be related to specific medications, combinations of medication, poor instructions leading to the inappropriate use or dosing of various medications, allergic reactions, side effects, and complications, as well as problems related by the natural consequences of medical, surgical or obstetrical management. Negligence can also cause Iatrogenic Illnesses. Unnecessary surgery, prescribing the wrong medications, using medications inappropriately or unnecessarily are examples. These problems can cause hardship and undermine the patient's health and well-being.

Even today, many medical doctors consider the adverse effects of the medications they prescribe simply as an unfortunate consequence inherent in their need to use these medications. Since physicians usually believe that the medications they prescribe are necessary, the side effects are generally considered a reasonable risk. However, millions of people are subjected to adverse side effects from medications they may not really have needed in the first place. Whether the medication is a tranquilizer given to calm an upset mother, an anti-hypertensive medication given to a stressed out father, or chemotherapy given to someone with cancer, every physician should consider alternative treatment methods. They should consider methods that encourage prevention and healing. No medication should ever be given without a well-justified need, as well as a clear understanding of their inherent risks and dangers.

Iatrogenic Injuries can be caused by accident. The right diagnosis is made, the right treatment is used, but side effects or complications occur that are reasonably unexpected. These side effects or complications may only rarely occur, or may be caused by various factor which were previously unknown to the physician or to his patient. For example, a surgery may be performed flawlessly and still infection may occur, adhesions may form, or an unexpected complication may occur.

STRESS-RELATED DISORDERS – OFTEN MISSED DIAGNOSES

Stress-Related Disorders as Iatrogenic Injuries are quite common. This is especially true if the medical doctor and the patient are looking at the illness as "real" and not recognizing the stress symptoms. This happens because most medical doctors and patients are not fully aware of Stress-Related Disorders, how to recognize or treat them. The typical physician is neither trained nor experienced in recognizing the characteristic patterns of Stress-Related Disorders. They may not recognize this process early enough to help their patients solve their underlying problems and stop, reverse or eliminate stress as a cause of illness.

> **Medical and surgical treatment**
> **can cause stress which can sometimes aggravate**
> **the situation and worsen an underlying illness.**

With the cause of the patient's stress unrelieved and conflict unresolved, the process persists, and the patient's symptoms progress and may advance to a harmful stage. This may take weeks, months, or years. Because the conflict is unresolved, the physician has not helped the patient reverse stress. The patient's condition gradually worsens. At some point, these patients will require extensive treatment with medications, potentially dangerous medical procedures, or surgery. All of this would have been unnecessary if a proper diagnosis had been made earlier.

Once again, the reason Stress-Related Disorders are not identified early is that most medical doctors were not taught about them. A significant contributing factor is that current medical practices are now commonly set up as business ventures. Time is just too scarce to allow doctors to properly evaluate their patients' problems. Another factor is that most physicians lack the interest to take the time to work with their patients to prevent illnesses. They are usually more inclined to treat early symptoms with medications rather than help their patients solve the problems causing these Stress-Related Disorders. Ultimately, this delay allows the stress process to create a full-blown disease.

The doctor is not the only culprit. Since the patient is unaware of the relationship between their symptoms and their unresolved stress, they are partially responsible for all of the problems that result from this lack of knowledge.

Every year, tens of thousands of people die or develop serious illnesses from the side effects or adverse reactions to medications which were given to them to treat misdiagnosed stress problems. This also occurs because most doctors have not been taught about the consequences of stress, or what SRDs are, or how to recognize or correctly treat them. This is a flaw in our current physician training system. For generations, the medical system has been drug and surgery oriented. They are so used to treating most illnesses with drugs and surgery without exploring the causative role stress plays in creating or worsening illness that they simply do not stop to consider the risk this presents to those patients with SRDs.

Most Iatrogenic Injuries can be prevented. This is especially true for those caused by SRDs where medications and surgery were not necessary to begin with. If doctors were aware of Stress-Related Disorder and were willing to be educated in the dynamics of SRDs, they could then teach their patients about prevention, wellness, stress management and self-healing techniques.

As we progress through the next sections, you will discover that because of this information, you know more about stress than most medical doctors, psychologists, and psychiatrists. In the past, SRDs were ignored by the medical profession. More recently, doctors who see a pattern of symptoms that do not fit a specific disease will tell patients, "Try to reduce your stress levels," "You're too stressed out," or "Your problems are all in your head." While these are often code words for stress-related problems, rarely do these physicians go further other than to suggest stress reduction exercises or a structured stress reduction program. Most doctors have only a rudimentary understanding of what stress is and how to deal with it. It's a good idea to choose a doctor who knows enough about Stress-Related Disorders that they can make an appropriate diagnosis and administer the most appropriate and specific treatment available for helping you eliminate your SRDs.

> The first step in learning about the incredible Intelligence inherent in your body is to envision your body as a resplendent symphony of life.

CREATING STRESS-RELATED DISORDERS

If you are going to listen to and trust your body, you need to understand it. You will need to learn how and why it does what it does, and how it communicates with you. You also need to appreciate how Intelligent your body really is. You need to recognize its Intelligence in action. Learning how and why you can trust your body is critical. To do this you must approach your body in a distinctly different way than ever before.

The first step in learning about the incredible Intelligence inherent in your body is envisioning your body as a resplendent symphony of life and no longer as simply cells, tissues, muscles and bones. You must see it for what it really is–a totally organized, integrated, and purposeful living being superbly designed not just to exist or survive, but also to be able to grow, learn and evolve. It is capable of protecting itself, finding food, reproducing, growing, learning, healing, and enlightening. Every cell and tissue has a purpose, every bone, and blood vessel a function. Most of these purposes overlap so that there are multiple failsafe systems making sure that we not only survive, but also thrive. We, as humans, are wondrous life forms. We are not only well adapted to our living environment, but we are also capable of changing and transforming our environment to suit our own purposes. Our body is a wondrous community with various specialists in each area of survival and thriving.

Life is a gift and our overall purpose is not just to survive but also to evolve and reach for, find, and become our highest, healthiest, and best Self. Our bodies, like our society and civilization, are directed not just to survive, but also to flourish. As evidence of this, just look at what human beings have accomplished!

The conscious, aware part of us has few answers about the meaning of life. Yet, our inner wisdom and Intelligence, combined with our spiritual and subconscious aspects, have all the answers to all the questions that our conscious Self may desire. Chapters 6, 7, and 8 discuss these three minds or Selves in detail.

As we proceed, we will look at some of the most important questions people have about illness and the answers that we have found. We will discuss whom and what human beings really are, how we get ill, and how we heal. We will define the roles of the personality or our conscious aware Self, that aspect of ourself which we usually think of as "me" or "I." We will also look at our subconscious mind or "body-mind." Throughout the remainder of this book, I will refer to this part of ourself as the body-mind[4], but please keep in mind the concept that it is the mind of our body, that is the subconscious mind. Finally, we will look at our super-conscious or Spiritual Mind, which we will also refer to as our Higher Self. As we proceed, we look at how these three minds, which we can also refer to as spirits, interact with each other, shaping us and helping us to be healthy and well, as well as helping us heal our illnesses. Using these tools, you will learn how to facilitate your own healing processes by listening to your body's communications and wisdom, and then taking appropriate action to resolve unresolved conflicts.

To help understand the full scope of the healing process, I will introduce you to an important law and two associated corollaries. They teach you what you will need to know in order to gain maximum benefit from this process.

---

4   *We prefer using the designation Body-Mind instead of the subconscious mind. This is because many people automatically substitute the term "unconscious mind" for subconscious mind. While the Body-Mind may be below the surface where it is not outwardly seen or recognized, it is never unconscious, except in rare circumstances of severe brain trauma. It is always active, aware, and alert, although the Conscious Mind is not always aware of it. This will be discussed in detail in a later section.*

This law and its corollaries are simply ideas. I would like you to think of them as belief systems, which can help you transform yourself from your everyday self to your highest, healthiest, and best Self. They provide you with a new way of looking at the processes of illness and healing. Once these corollaries are mastered, I will move on to describe what stress is. Then, we will look at the three levels of the Self: the subconscious (Body-Mind), the personality (Conscious Self), and the spiritual self (Higher Self). With this information, I then can demonstrate to you how illness and disease are created. Next, I will look at the many layers of the body's defensive and healing systems and at the genesis of Stress-Related Disorders. Finally, we will discuss a few simple steps of how you can heal yourself and maintain wellness.

Remember, everything that happens is part of the Intelligence of the Universe, the Intelligence of the body, and our own Intelligence.

THE LAW OF SURVIVAL

The Law of Survival is likely one of the most fundamental laws of the Universe. This law underlies our entire existence and every aspect of our life. Included within this law are the processes that create and heal illness and disease. This law's mandates are built into the very fabric of our being. Because of it, we are equipped with the necessary faculties to ensure survival in every facet of our life. The only exceptions to this would be extreme and unnatural circumstances. The Law of Survival is built into us. It exists as an inherent set of instructions within in our DNA, built into every cell, tissue and fiber of our body, mind and spirit, to protect and preserve our life and well-being. Included within this mandate are a number of subsidiary mandates: procreation, reproduction, and sexual drive. These constitute a deep-seated and potent set of drives to pick a mate, have sex, create pregnancy, and make children. These drives ensure that we carry on the species, that our family name continues, that family ties and lines of decent persist. All of this ensures that the species survives.

While all functions are important for the species to survive, they are only peripherally related to the Fight-or-Flight Mandate, or as we know it better, the Stress Mechanism which exists to make sure that we as individuals survive.

The following corollaries lay the groundwork for an understanding of the power of the Law of Survival and its interaction with the process of sickness and healing.

The Mind is all there is.

COROLLARY #1: THE MIND IS ALL THERE IS

This corollary represents a philosophical premise that has been debated for ages. For the sake of this work, consider "the mind is all there is[5]," as a statement of fact relating to all humans. As you will soon see, there are actually three minds operating within us at all times. The mind we are referring to when we say, "the mind is all there is," is primarily the conscious aware mind. The fact is that all three minds are always working together for our benefit.

What we know of the world is almost completely controlled by our sensory systems and our interpretations of our senses. We might like to believe that we think with our brain, but in fact, we think and interpret with our mind. While the physical brain performs many important biochemical-biological-neurological functions, it is our conscious mind operating within the laws of the Intelligent Universe that interprets everything our sensory systems hear, see, smell, taste, feel, and think. It is our conscious aware mind that registers and interprets what our sensory system experiences[6]. Our Body-Mind is responsible for integrating all of this information and integrating it with all of our memories of the past, recent experiences and our expectations of the future.

While many people believe that the mind and brain are the same, they are not. The brain is physical object, like the motherboard in a computer. It is more like a switching terminal for neurological events. The mind not only includes the physical brain and its functions, but the entire body and all of its functions. Since the majority of what we think of as the mind lies in the subconscious aspect of ourselves, we might more correctly think of it as the mind of our body or more simply our Body-Mind. Throughout the remainder of this work, I use this term, Body-Mind, to refer to the combination of our body and the subconscious part of ourselves.

It is the perceptions of our Body-Mind and its preliminary interpretation of its perceptions, which are mostly oriented to issues of threat and survival that are then sent up to our conscious mind where they are interpreted in relation to our immediate reality.

Our ability to grasp this is vital. If what we presume to exist is really only a projection of what our Body-Mind and Conscious Mind see and believe, then the way we see the world and our place in it is determined by how we interpret our sensory input and the belief systems we create about them.

---

5   *While we will only be talking about our human mind, consider that the Intelligence of the Universe implies an "Intelligent Mind" outside of ours, much greater than ours, one that we may not even be able to fathom. Call this mind "God" or "Intelligence Universe." It is everything and we are within it and part of it.*

6   *A superficial analogy that can be used here is a computer. Information typed into the keyboard or "seen" by its webcam is transformed from physical stimuli into electronic impulses, which are then stored on the hard drive and visualized on the computers monitor and interpreted by you based on what you see on the monitor.*

Our Body-Mind operates well below our levels of conscious thought. We are generally unaware of what it believes or how it sees the world. Therefore, we are at the Body-Mind's mercy, unless we learn to control it. The proof of this lies in the results we get in life.

If your life is giving you exactly what you desire and you are happy and fulfilled, you have programmed your Body-Mind perfectly for you. However, if your life is chaotic and out of your control, and you are feeling stressed or experiencing stress-related disorders, this is because of faulty belief systems, unresolved conflicts and inappropriate programs operating within your Body-Mind. To finally gain control and be the master of your life, you need to identify what your Body-Mind thinks, what it believes, and how it interrelates with your conscious mind to create who you are, what you believe, and how and why you make the decisions you make.

The corollary we have just described can only be recognized and confirmed indirectly. Take when a traffic accident occurs, as an example. A number of people in the vicinity may witness the accident. Each witness, when questioned by the police, may relate entirely different stories. Each of these witnesses is generally limited by a number of factors: such as where they stood at the time of the accident, their view of the accident, their past experiences, their prejudices, their expectations, and their capacity to fill in the blanks, understand, project and describe what they did and did not see. Each person will ultimately offer a picture of what he believed he actually saw. Most people will likely stand by what they believed did happen and consider it as an absolute fact, even when hearing or seeing that other witnesses may totally disagree with them.

In the end, what each witness thinks, sees, or believes is less a matter of what actually happened than what each perceived had happened as the events had unfolded. Therefore, our perceptions relate as much to how our sensory systems are designed, how we receive information, and how we experience sensory inputs, than what actually happened. As we suggested above, the interpretation of each witness is colored by what they believe they actually saw. They are often influenced by their past memories, emotional make up, and capacity to project what they believe happened during the accident. It is also important to understand that what people didn't see was automatically filled in from their expectations, personal and past experiences. In the end, their testimony is the result of these combined conscious and subconscious processes. To complicate the matter, what was perceived and remembered may have also been filtered, consciously or subconsciously, by how each person believed the accident would personally affect them. For example, what if they should have to testify in court?

The police can often reconstruct an approximation of the actual events from the similarities and discrepancies in the stories of the witnesses, the examination of physical evidence, and the application of the principles of science, physics, and mathematics. Using scientific methods to filter the stories of the witnesses, the police assemble a much more accurate approximation of what happened than was given by any one witness. Even then, the true story and most accurate picture of what really happened may never be determined. Each witness may fervently or tentatively believe that what they saw was what happened. The truth is what they saw was only part of the whole story. At best, we also only have a limited view of our own life. Our capacity to fill in the blanks of life often deceives us into believing that we are perfectly aware of the world around us.

We are what we BELIEVE we are.

COROLLARY #2: WE ARE WHAT WE BELIEVE WE ARE

If we can grant that corollary #1 is logical and correct, then we can open the door to identify Corollary #2. This corollary naturally follows the first: If there is nothing but mind and thought, then what we believe about ourselves and our lives ultimately governs who and what we are. This is true even when we accept other people's beliefs about the way the world is. In addition, you might notice that some of the things other people believe to be true are not necessarily true for you. It doesn't matter how true it is for them, or how loudly they declare it to be true. Ultimately, what is true for you is what you believe to be true. The world outside is a testing ground for our proposed realities. The world as we know it is not a basis for reality in itself. If it were, there would be no creativity or invention, no literature or drama. There would be only hard, cold facts.

It is important to recognize that what we think about the world and ourselves is derived from what we believe. These belief systems are produced from our perceptions, and our perceptions are based on how our nervous system works, past experiences, and what we choose to believe about our lives, the world, and ourselves. If you like apple pie, this is part of who you are and your personal belief systems. If you decide apple pie is your favorite pie, then you created this belief system. If you like the color red, then positive feelings about the color red become a part of your personal experience of life. Putting corollaries one and two together illustrates the fact that what we believe creates our own personal world and universe, as well as defining who and what we are.

Our intention here is making it clear that we not only create our own personal universe by what we think and believe, but that we can change this universe by changing what we think and believe. We can actually mold, create, and change who we are and how we relate to the world by choosing and directing what we believe. In a sense, we actually mold the physical universe by what we believe. No building was ever built by accident; no book was ever written without some forethought. Civilization is not a random occurrence and neither is our own personal development. Outwardly, all of this may appear to be random. We are always influenced either by our own personal belief systems or the belief systems of others around us. We either willingly or not adopt these systems to be our own, or we reject them and then created our own personal belief system defined by what we believe and how we read the world around us.

One impact of this construct is that when we believe in illness, we establish a process allowing it to enter into our minds, bodies, spirits, and lives. Our belief in illness can actually create that illness. In fact, our Body-Mind may even start looking for it or bring it to us. This is clearly spelled out in one of the most powerful biblical quotes, "Seek and you shall find, ask and you shall receive." In Eastern philosophy, it is stated as karma. We create our own fate or destiny as a result of our actions and our beliefs. We bring to us what we have by how we think and act. We get in life what we create for ourselves, both that which is positive (perfect health) and that which is negative (illness). It is important to be aware of what you are asking for and be mindful that what you are asking for is not negative. There is another old cliché that also fits, "Be careful of what you ask for because you are likely to get it."

WHAT DOES ALL THIS MEAN?

Who and what we are therefore depends upon what we believe, the decisions we make, and the beliefs we accept. Whether we are rich or poor, happy or sad, is dependent entirely upon what we believe about circumstances and ourselves. A poor person may be joyously happy while a rich person may be miserable.

While others in our society may give rigid credibility to false and contradictory beliefs, we must constantly carefully look and consider our own beliefs. We must examine them to see if what we are getting is what we really want out of our lives. Often, we may not know what we really want or believe. Because of this, we may not always get what we want. Instead, what we get may be what we think we want. As a result, we may end up feeling unhappy about how our life has turned out.

Sometimes, we lie to ourselves, as we will discuss in the next section. We create diversionary belief systems to keep us from seeing who we really are. We may do this for many reasons. It is important that we learn to sort out our real self and desires.

We must continually challenge the relationships of whom we think we are and who we really are, what we think we want and what we actually have. We must find our true direction in life. In my practice, I often tell patients, "It's not who you say you are that counts, it's what you do and the results you get out of your life that tells us who you really are." This is not a new concept. All the great teachers of the ages–the saints, gurus, sages, and other wise men and women–recognized this and tried to teach it.

Stress is something that we are not always conscious of; it can exist on a cellular level and hide, masked by our ingrained insensitivity.

~Garri Garripoli,
Qigong: Essence of the Healing Dance

Chapter Three

DISEASE IS A STATE OF MIND

A PHYSICIAN'S JOURNEY INTO HEALING

If the mind is all there is and we are what we believe, then health and disease are also seen as a state of mind. In my (Dr. Allen) early years of medical training, the last thing I was likely to believe was that the mind had anything to do with illness and disease. When I first graduated from medical school, the concept that our mind could play a role in creating, preventing, or even healing disease would have seemed absurd to me. Everyone knew that illness and disease are "real." The idea that our mind could have the power to prevent, control, create, or heal illness and disease was not often considered to be acceptable. This is commonly accepted even though our life experiences clearly demonstrate to us that everything we see, think and believe is actually products of our mind and not of our "reality." Since childhood we have had hundreds, if not thousands of opportunities to experience situations where, if we consciously thought back upon them, would clearly demonstrate to us that our mind plays an important role in the prevention, creation, control of our health and wellness. That we have again and again prevented or healed illnesses in the past, and that we actually do have the power and ability to heal our selves. Yet, we still often refuse to accept as fact the myth that we are not only incapable of being powerful, but that everything in life is happening to us and we have little or no power over what we are experiencing. What a loss to us and our ability to protect and heal ourselves.

Unfortunately, while people often profess their desire to get well, they do not always believe they will get well. They do not always have a positive mental attitude, and so do not get well. In addition, even when professing their desire to become healed, they do not always do what is needed to activate and maintain the healing process.

When we are sick, it is not just important that we follow instructions–that is, take our medications or do what we are told–but rather we must envision ourselves as well. When Thomas Edison was asked how he could have spent so many years working on inventing the light bulb, he replied that he could always see it working; all he had to do was to make it happen. Without a clear picture of wellness in our minds' eye, we are not giving clear instructions to our Body-Mind to help us do all that is necessary to stay well, to eliminate our illness, and to return ourselves to full and complete wellness. As you will see, without resolving the conflicts of our life and living a healthy lifestyle, we cannot hope to have complete wellness.

THE WILL TO LIVE

Many years ago when I was struggling with my own course in life, I watched a television series about a resident doctor and his personal and professional struggles. In one episode, the young doctor was coming out of a patient's room. He was perspiring and looked very haggard. A nurse walking alongside him complimented him on what a good job he had done in saving his patient's life. The young doctor responded that it was not he who had saved the patient's life, but rather the patient's "will to live."

This statement sealed my own direction in life. I often thought to myself that if I could understand and use this "will to live" concept, then I could really help people heal themselves. As the years passed, this concept remained elusive. Why did one person who said he wanted to get well do so, while another person who said the same thing did not get better? What people say they want is not necessarily what they truly want nor believe. I also noticed that people who really wanted to get well most often did. It was clear to me that these people often have a strong drive, and they usually do everything they can do to find and win their wellness. However, did those individuals who were not able to get well have less drive or maybe were they more confused about their goals? They talked about getting well, but did they always act on it or do exactly what they need needed to get well?

These are difficult questions to answer. Sometimes, they are just unanswerable. Through my observations, I learned that people often did lie to themselves, to their physicians, and to others about what they really want. I found that it was not at all unusual for patients to tell me what they wanted me hear, even though they may secretly have entirely different feelings and even very different long and short term agendas.

For many years, I searched for an answer to the haunting question, "What creates a will to get well, and to live?" When I could find no easy solution, I ended up losing my own will to live. For several years, my interest in medicine waned and I was less committed to the people I had once dedicated my life to heal. I lost interest in just about everything in my life. Even though I went through the motions and smiled at everyone, my heart was breaking because something was missing in my life.

For many years, I was aimless. Yet, I continued searching for the answers to why my life had no meaning. I asked myself thousands of times, "What is it that I want out of life? Is all this pain I feel worth it? Is life worth living?" I could find no answers. Yet, a passion burned in me to find the answers. Eventually the stresses in my life became so great that I inevitably ended up in a state of severe burnout. I experienced depression, anxiety, allergies, joint pains, fatigue, and irregular heart rate. Because of these symptoms, delivering babies and performing surgery were nearly impossible. If I kept providing these services, I felt I would be dishonest and possibly even dangerous. I decided it was best that I quit before someone's well-being was compromised. In order to survive, I began studying stress and the stress-burnout reaction. To find answers, I had to look outside of medicine to the people and literature of religion, philosophy, the ancient mysteries, alternative healing, shamanism, and even quantum physics. I learned a great deal, not only about my own symptoms and illnesses, but about the illnesses I was routinely seeing in my medical practice. I became clear that I was not the only one who suffered from stress-related health problems. During most of this journey, my wife Lisa was at my side and we learned together. This book is about what we learned.

During these years, I experienced a passion to find what I wanted from my life and to find what was making me so unhappy. What I ultimately realized was that my being miserable was the negative side of the will to live. The difference was that while our "will to live" comes from positive thinking, the negative side of this process ultimately comes from our burnout, our will to give up, to let go, to die and they all come from our negative thoughts, faulty belief systems and our fear. What I had been experiencing was not a real desire to die, but rather a lack of the will to live. I had become bogged down and even trapped by the negative end of the power to live and evolve. Eventually, I learned that once I could see this, my powers of positive belief and faith would enable me to transform the negative force, which I now think of as a "Death Wish," into its positive healing and evolving counterpart force, the "Will to Live," my "Life wish." I had discovered for myself the foundation of life and the primary secret for healing, think positively.

My journey has taken more than 30 years and is still in process.

When I started this journey, which I now refer to it as my Life Path, I had no one other than Lisa with whom I could talk or ask questions about what was happening. I found that few medical doctors, psychologists, or psychiatrists really understood the process of stress and illness as I was now able to see it. When I approached several colleagues to discuss my illness, they immediately wanted to start me on medications. My own natural instinct (my inner Intelligence) was against this, so I decided to trust my own instincts.

One day when I was particularly overwhelmed, I called a business acquaintance. He was not a close friend, but was someone I felt I could trust. I asked him to lunch and I told him my story. He was not a doctor, but an executive in a related field. At first, I felt ashamed that as a doctor I was still unable to solve my own problems. However, I needed help and he was a problem solver. I also had a sense that he too was on his life path. We talked for a while, and he suggested that I enroll in a consciousness-raising workshop. My first thought was, "A consciousness-raising workshop. How unscientific!" I knew that most of my colleagues would believe that this was a waste of time.

I walked back to my office thinking how embarrassing it would be to expose myself and my problems in public. How vulnerable I would be! I thought about what my patients might think, and how I might lose my practice. By the time I reached my office, I had just about talked myself out of doing the workshop. Yet, in the back of my mind, a small, weak voice said, "You asked a friend, someone you trust, to tell you what you need to do. You asked for help and he gave it. Now the part of you that is terrified wants to ignore that advice."

I picked up the phone and made a reservation. This was the beginning of my personal transformation.

During this time, I decided to give up my medical practice. Initially, I told myself this was because of the illnesses I had created. I later realized that it was the right thing to do because it was time to move onto a next phase of my life. I sold my medical practice. I started working on a temporary basis filling in for other doctors when they were sick or on vacation. I had no roots, and no responsibilities or attachment to the business part of medicine. For the first time, I was able to think about healing rather than treating. I was able to have time to put my thoughts onto paper and try to understand what illness and healing really were.

During this period, our lives changed significantly. Lisa and I had considerably less income and our life style became much simpler. We were much happier. I became more involved in understanding the people I was treating and then helping them see and resolve their faulty beliefs, fears, unresolved conflicts and the problems which were causing their illnesses.

FINDING OUR HIGHEST, HEALTHIEST, AND BEST SELF

A patient of mine once told me about himself, "I am trapped within the belly of the beast and I don't see any way out."

I saw this place from in my own journey. I told him, "In order to get well, you must do whatever is needed to create, find, and solve the problems that trap you and keep you from wellness."

You, dear readers, must also start somewhere, work toward, and become your highest, healthiest, and best Self. It is also advisable that you don't let your negative thoughts get in the way. They will eventually sabotage you. Learn what you need to learn, make mistakes, forgive yourself, correct the mistakes, and then practice telling the truth and making your life work. You must do this over and over again until you get it right. You must work hard until you are out of your confusion (the belly of the beast), until you know who you are, until you no longer have to lie to yourself (and others), and until you can find, accept and nourish your true Self.

This requires dedication to your life wishes, your will to live. This leads you to the next level on your journey to your highest, healthiest, and best Self. Each demon you face along the way is merely your own fear of moving forward. They repeatedly test your mettle and resolve to find and become your true Self. It is simply not enough that we are alive and have amassed material wealth. Rather, we must grow and better ourselves until we have reached our highest, healthiest, and best Self–our ultimate power and wellness.

For me, the battle was always about letting loose the healer that exists within me. This meant getting past my fears, feelings of inadequacy and of being different, as well as my anger at myself and other people. In the process of discovering my true nature as a healer and of thinking for myself, I also had to face my anger and frustration at other medical doctors, the medical profession, and all of the people who criticized me for not remaining part of the establishment. I was also angry and frustrated with my patients and the public for not wanting to become responsible and actively involved in their own healing process.

Eventually, as I let go of this anger, my focus turned to seeking a new understanding of those feelings. There exists a paucity of information in the medical field about the real causes of stress, illness, and disease. This is neither the fault of the present-day physicians nor the public, but of the history of mankind and medicine in general. I learned from this not to be so hard on myself and other people. I also acknowledged that life is a great teacher and that the anger and frustration, the fears, and inadequacies I experienced were all teaching me lessons I needed to learn. I had to master these precepts if I was to attain my highest, healthiest, and best Self.

I recognized that most people learn very early in life to suppress their feelings and beliefs. Often, conflict starts even in the uterus. Yet, it can also begin during the birth process, infancy, childhood, or any time thereafter. Emotional growth is often limited because of fear: fear related to solving or not solving problems and fear of facing the things you feared. I realized that what we say to ourselves and think about ourselves is crucial. What we think we believe is generally much less important than what we really believe. Finally, what we get out of our lives often relates more closely to what we really want and whether we believe that we are worthy of getting it.

Illness and disease–and especially Stress-Related Disorders–are the result of living in a society that forces people to hide and lie to themselves and to others. The same system educates children by bludgeoning them with information instead of bringing out what they know inside themselves. I could see that most people did not know how to reach their inner path to find enlightenment. I understood finally that healing is more a state of mind and living the "right" life than it is to simply taking the "right" medication.

Our "will to live" comes from being our own real and true self. It comes from being whom we really are under the facades used to protect ourselves from being hurt. Our "will to live" comes from our dedication, not only to what makes us truly happy, but also to what leads us to our total fulfillment as a human being. By our nature each of us will have different life goals. Each of us is unique, and yet we all belong to the mosaic that makes up all life and humanity. We have a free will and the ability to make decisions to grow and learn from our experiences, even the negative ones.

In my journey, I found the essence of the will to live. Through understanding this power, I was able to facilitate healing myself. Through teaching others to find this same power within themselves, I learned that I could help others heal themselves. All of us are healers. Even if we never use this capacity to heal our Self or another person, it is always available to us. While the essence of the power we hold is different for everyone, the power's source is always the same; it is our need to rise above our past and reach out to our highest, healthiest, and best Self.

Lisa and I believe that within our life journey our ultimate goal is to learn, grow, and evolve. To become our very best Self, our highest, healthiest and best Self. At the same time we strive to grown and heal our pain, suffering, and illnesses. The force behind this growth is an innate drive within us that is always pushing us toward reaching our highest, healthiest, and best Self. While we may deny its existence or work against it, this force ultimately empowers our desire to survive, live, grow, reproduce, and evolve. As each of us evolves, so does our society and so does humanity. We also help the Universe in which we live to evolve and grow toward its own highest, healthiest, and best Self. This is the heart of what survival (also survival of the fittest) and the Stress Mechanism really mean.

Chapter Four

THE BODY & ITS DEFENSE MECHANISMS

DISEASE IS BROUGHT ON BY
FAULTY INTERACTION WITH OUR BODY-MIND

The Law of Survival operates within us on a number of levels. The highest level of survival relates to the survival of the Intelligence of the Universe itself–the Godhead, God. Next set of laws relate to the Survival of the Laws that govern our Intelligent Universe and the physical and spiritual Universe. While these levels are way beyond the scope of this work, they can give us insight into the fact that the Law of Survival is not only important, but that it operates well beyond our needs in every aspect of life. The parts we are often most concerned with are those aspects that specifically include our body, mind and spirit as well as all beings and organisms that might threaten or attack us. The very first level we usually consider relating to us directly acts in a dual form. We commonly think of it as Survival of the Species and that it operates at every level of life from the single cell organism to adult grown human beings. The duality occurs in that it is divided into two essential divisions: the Fight-or-Flight or Stress Mechanism and Procreation, the Reproductive Drive. If we do survive as an individual but we do not procreate, our species dies out. If we do procreate, we further our own gene pool. Once we die, we can no longer create any more offspring, which then means that our personal genetic line will also die with us.

> **Survival is a primary Mandate,**
> **and Wellness is a primary goal of Survival.**

The Fight-or-Flight or Stress Mechanism is itself made up of a number of component parts. Many of these parts are not always easy to recognize. The main role of the Stress Mechanism is to protect us from attack, injury, and threats to our life or overall well-being. The Stress Mechanism acts to prepare and ready us to fight our potential enemies upon threat or attack so that we might survive and persist. We usually think of this as the Fight part of Fight-or-Flight. The other part of the Fight-or-Flight Mechanism is flight. This part of the survival mandate works to get us out of danger's way, as fast as possible. Some people believe that these are entirely opposite behaviors and contradictory. They believe you should either fight or flight, but why both? In reality, these are simply different strategies that animals and humans use to protect themselves. They both accomplish the same goal – survival. In some cases, the individuals might start fighting to protect themselves, but find that they are unable to win. At that point, their strategy changes from fight to flight and as they flee away from harm and possible destruction.

There is another rarely discussed aspect of fight-or-flight, and that is freeze. Freeze occurs when the individual is overwhelmed and can neither fight nor flee. The brain and body may become so overwhelmed that they can no longer function, so the individual simply freezes, much like a deer caught in the headlights of an advancing car. This process is most often a response to events of the moment, or it might also be a strategy in that freezing acts to prevent an enemy or adversary from seeing, hearing or recognizing you in that moment. It is often erroneously seen as indecision, depression, or immobilizing anxiety where an individual essentially shorts out because he or she is too overwhelmed to respond. However, when used as a strategy to protect our self, it can at times, be extremely valuable.

The part of the stress mechanism we are going to be concerned with is not the strategy responses to a specific threat, but what happens when the stress mechanism is triggered. This includes the response of multiple levels of our own bodily defensive, repair and healing mechanisms. We will also look at a number of very special processes involved with our physical, mental, emotional, and spiritual survival systems for completeness.

The totality of our human survival mechanisms includes our sensory system, internal defense systems, food acquisition and digestive mechanisms, excretory mechanisms, breathing respiratory systems, our muscular and nervous systems, our endocrine and reproductive systems, all of which are part of the overall survival and stress response protective systems. Finally, and most powerful of all of the survival systems is the mind/brain/body interaction itself.

You might think at this point that we have included just about every organ system in the body in describing the component parts of the Stress Mechanism and you would be absolutely right. This is exactly the point we are trying to make. Just about every part of our body, mind, brain, emotions, and spirit is involved and working for us to either ensure or support our survival. This gives proof that survival is a primary mandate, and that our safety, wellness and survival are its primary goals.

Since our minds decide everything we either are or will be almost all illnesses and diseases we experience must have a mental and/or emotional component, as well as a physical component. As stated earlier, the majority of illnesses, at least the 70-80 percent of all illnesses seen in medical practices, are caused by, related to or made worse because of stress, hence the Stress Mechanism, Fight-or-Flight, the Survival Mechanism and the mandates we have just discussed are all part of this process. While the Stress Mechanism is generally triggered by an acute or long term threat to our life or well-being, SRDs generally start as unresolved conflicts which are acting to undermine our immune and other defensive or protective systems. This causes our Body-Mind, which is trying to heal us, to communicate that there are unresolved conflicts that must be resolved in order to not only survive, but also thrive and hence optimize our wellness. When we do not respond, and do not solve these " unresolved conflicts," the resulting illness may then affect not only our physical body and organs, but also our Body-Mind. When we do listen to our body and hence resolve these conflicts, we may never even know that something had been wrong. When we simply deal with these issues and solve problems, these conflicts will not occur and we will usually, remain whole and healthy.

At our highest state of survival, we are perfectly healthy and nothing but extraordinary forces should penetrate our defensive systems. Within this state of survival, we have layer upon layer of defense mechanisms that are impervious to most kinds of enemies. Do not confuse this by believing that human beings are either superhuman or impervious to all hazards. We are part of an endless food chain. Fish eat plankton, sharks eat fish, and people eat fish and occasionally even sharks. On occasion, sharks eat people. There are enemies that can overpower us. This is where our mind, intelligence, and creativity come into play. They help us design, create, and implement external defensive systems, which have capabilities of working with our internal defensive systems to protect us far beyond what either can do alone. These external defensive systems include not only our ability to creatively solve problems but also all that living in a modern society can provide for us: police, the military forces, atomic bombs, burglar alarm systems, governments, building security, radar, bullet proof vests, and so on and on. What is even more important is that none of these are simply inherent in nature. Instead, over hundreds, even thousands of years, they were created and designed to protect and defend us. All are products of our mind and intelligence. All are created to protect us, keep us alive, and promote our optimal health and well-being. As you will soon see, all of this, everything outside of us, is uncannily based on reflections of our internal defensive systems.

Ultimately, each of us has the ability to prevent illness and to protect ourselves from these illnesses, which when our internal defensive systems are not optimally working, may have some form of dominion over us. You can now learn a way of thinking that can ultimately allow you to manage your life and attain the highest level of wellness you can desire. Using this new information, we can now tell you how capable you are of protecting yourself and at the same time, prevent and even undoing existing or potential illnesses. This is really what healing is all about and it is our life's goal to share this wisdom with you.

WHAT ARE OUR BODY'S DEFENSIVE SYSTEMS?

Within your body we have many layers of defensive and offensive systems protecting us. We categorize these protection mechanisms in a number of ways. One valuable way of looking at them is to recognize them as levels of protection. The first level, our Basic Defensive Systems, is divided into four separate layers: 1) Early Warning Systems, 2) Primary Defensive Systems, 3) Secondary Defensive Systems, and 4) Tertiary Defensive Systems. The Secondary Defensive Systems can further be broken down into the Strategic Defensive Systems and the Offensive-Defensive Systems. The Tertiary Defensive Systems may also be broken down further to the Clean-Up, Repair and Rebuilding Systems. As you read on you will learn even more about these four systems.

In Diagram: 4-1 below, we can visualize all of these systems as layer upon proactive layer, one on top of the other. Each defensive layer protects against invasion and attack. Much like a medieval fort with its many defensive barriers, each layer has a specific role, and when all are working appropriately only the most extreme or most violent of invasions can ever be successful.

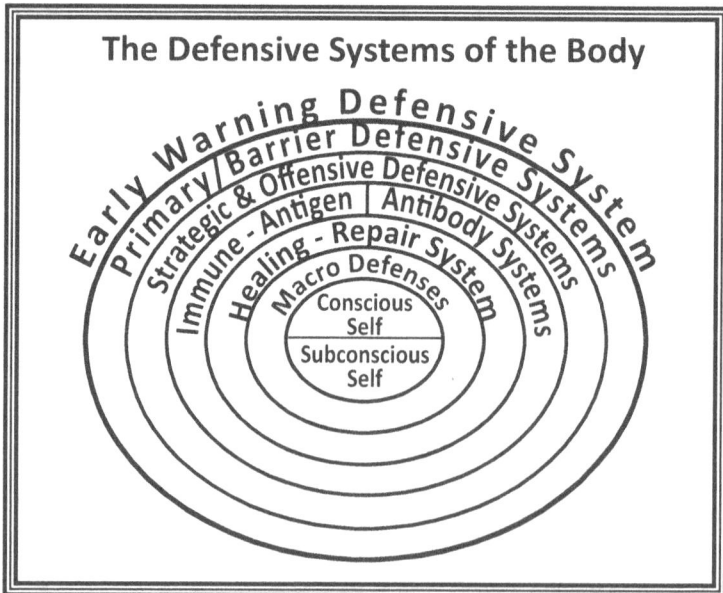

Diagram: 4-1

THE EARLY WARNING SYSTEMS

Our Early Warning Systems are made up of several layers of defensive systems, each of which warn us when external threats come too close, or potentially endanger us. The first layer is our Sensory System. Sight, hearing and instincts extend our sensory system far out from our core. Touch, vibration, and temperature can also tell us about the external environment and when danger might be approaching. These systems are important not only in protecting us from what we see and hear, but from more subtle dangers that we may only experience as feelings. They help to protect us from the natural and man-made dangers in our immediate environment. We are all familiar with situations where we sense danger is approaching. It is the combination of these defenses, the early-warning mechanisms along with our subconscious Body-Mind, which registers that "something," some potential danger, is approaching or is likely going to happen. Because of our sensory system, we usually brush off insects or other parasites before they have had time to invade us. We can turn toward enemies ready to fight, or we can turn and flee from danger long before they are near enough or capable of causing us injury.

The number one defense system in this group is our combined Body-Mind along with our brain. Earlier in Corollary #2, we explained that the Body-Mind is important because it integrates sensory input from events occurring outside of us with what is happening inside of us. This keeps us in contact and aware of what is going on around us and how that is affecting us.

Our Body-Mind can act without consultation, conscious thought, or deliberate decision making by the conscious aware self. This is the essence of the Fight-or-Flight Mechanism. Generally, it takes time for the conscious self to think through, interpret events, and make decisions. When it comes to protecting our life and well-being, there is often insufficient time to register sensory inputs, evaluate them, think them over, make a plan, then make a decision on what to do, and act in a safe and productive way. The Body-Mind, however, acts on its instincts, past experiences, reflexes, and training to preserve and protect us.

Our Body-Mind cannot however always use instinct to protect us. This is especially true when the choices are complex. In such situations, the Body-Mind often requires the help of our experiences and even our conscious mind. This situation may occur if information received by the Body-Mind is confusing, if sensory perceptions are questionable, or if inputs are too similar to draw meaningful conclusions or take meaningful actions. In situations like these, the Body-Mind usually calls on the conscious self to use its powers of deductive logic to sort through memories, and make enlightened decisions.

Our Body-Mind is in charge of protecting us. It makes almost all of the important decisions as to what may or may not be threatening us, based on its experiences and our present belief systems. In a sense, we choose who and what will be our enemy by the decisions we make, the thoughts we hold, and the belief systems we operate from. It also directs the sensory systems to what it believes might be the problem, controlling where we look and what we look for.

Our Body-Mind reacts to external stimuli. It integrates these inputs with the stored memories of past experiences, decisions, fears, intuitions, and even instincts. Our conscious mind then may be left to make the complex decisions the Body-Mind cannot make. The combined conscious and subconscious selves are always acting to defend us. They work together as our Early Warning Defensive Systems. When working together, they effectively extend our capacity beyond the range of our sensory system far out into both time and space.

Because of this, we are capable of sensing risks that do not exist in the present, but have occurred in the past or will occur in the future. What we have learned from our past experiences helps us anticipate what we might experience in the present and future. What we fear from our past or in the future often creates stress in the present. Because of this, we can bring forward false enemies, such as old fears based on memories of situations which may no longer even exist, or imaginary enemies that do not now or may never have existed except in our imagination or fears. Unfortunately, our conscious and subconscious selves are often willing to believe that these old or potential future threats, real or imagined, exist here in the now-moment, even though they actually do not. Because of this dynamic phenomenon, it is likely that you may have experienced feelings of apprehension because of old memories or expectations of some real or imagined danger which ultimately may never manifest.

THE PRIMARY DEFENSIVE SYSTEMS

The first physical defensive layer is our Primary Defensive or Barrier Systems. This is our skin and mucous membranes.

Skin and mucous membranes both act as primary barriers protecting us against bacterial and viral organisms, as well as from radiation, heat, cold, parasites, toxic substances, and foreign objects. The skin provides a physical barrier much like a castle wall or the brick and barbed wire barriers. In addition to keeping invaders out, the skin also keeps our bodily fluids and contents within our body. They define us from our environment. Below the skin are layers of fat, which insulate us and act as additional protective barriers to heat or cold and even physical injury. Skin and fat tissues cushion our bony parts and help us maintain comfort. Working together, these layers help regulate our internal temperature and protect us against dehydration and small traumas.

The way we look, our features, our size and shape act as a kind of barrier, a way of protecting us from smaller predators and from environmental risk factors. Our gender, degree of muscle mass, our overall posture and appearance, also act to protect us. Each of these aspects plays some role in our ability to defend ourselves, threaten potential enemies, and improve the likelihood of our survival. These factors determine who we are and how well we can survive.

Another important layer consists of our Mucous Membranes and the fluids they produce. This layer includes the wet, shiny tissues that cover or surround our eyes, ears, nose, mouth, throat, and sinuses, as well as the vagina, urethra and rectum. Mucous membranes act primarily as local defense barriers preventing the entrance of microorganisms and foreign bodies and secondarily improving functions such as ingestion of food, digestion, protection of the respiratory system, passage of digested waste, and sexual relations.

People are often more concerned about this route of entry for illness than any other. Today, these areas are especially important because of HIV/AIDS, sexually transmitted diseases, influenza, and certain bacteria that enter the body through the mucous membranes.

Our mucous membranes protect us from any number of illnesses that can enter our body including colds, the flu, tonsillitis, sinusitis, eye and bladder infections, vaginitis, urethritis, proctitis, and prostatitis. Maintaining a high level of protection in these areas is essential to our overall well-being.

The next layer of defense lies in our Lung Tissues. While this layer is part of the mucous membrane defense mechanism, it has other significantly broader capacities. The lungs act as a barrier protecting us from airborne materials that we are constantly inhaling, including foreign particles and organisms and toxic materials. It is actively involved in oxygen uptake. It also releases toxic products, such as carbon dioxide and excess nitrogen. This important part of our internal defense system also acts to purify our blood and discharges toxic waste products that could, if not removed, impair our ability to function, heal, and repair injured tissues.

Our Digestive System – mouth, throat, esophagus, stomach, small intestine, large intestine, and rectum–all act as barriers protecting us from organisms, foreign bodies, and toxic materials. They are all also essential in the processing of food and nutrients, which are necessary to run and feed all of our bodily functions, including our Defensive and Offensive Protective Systems.

THE SECONDARY DEFENSIVE SYSTEMS
- THE STRATEGIC AND OFFENSIVE SYSTEMS -

TISSUE DEFENSES

Our next major protection and defense level is our Secondary Defensive Systems. For this level to become meaningful our first level of protection has most likely already been breached, and we are under attack. This means that an organism or foreign invader has made it past our barrier defenses and entered into our body. At this point, our body responds with an immediate call to action by activating its Strategic and Offensive Defenses. These second line defensive systems are automatically activated and as a result they immediately become our most important line of defense.

The first part of this protective system, our Strategic Defensive System, is a group of local defensive mechanisms, enzymes, cells and cell walls that protect us against any invasion by organisms or foreign bodies that have gotten past the outer defense and barrier systems. The second protective layer involved with this group, the Offensive Defensive Systems, are aggressive attack systems that lay waiting within our tissues and the blood-circulatory systems to attack any unwelcome invader or threat.

Taken together, these structures are frequently referred to as our Tissue Defenses. They include many mechanisms that immediately respond when a foreign body, parasite, or potential infective organism enters their realm. This action is generally referred to as our Inflammation Process. These defensive and offensive systems operate by identifying that an invasion has occurred, localizing, and then destroying the invaders as soon as they are found. Elements of the tissue defense system encase anything that does not belong in the body within a thick coat of fibrous tissues. Like when you get a splinter in your finger that is not removed. The tissue around it becomes thickened in order to wall off and isolate foreign invaders. The tissue pressure can be significant enough to even eventually expel a foreign body, in this case the splinter, out from the body and away from causing further harm or infection.

BLOOD BORN DEFENSE SYSTEMS

Another part of our Secondary Defensive System, which works closely with Tissue Defenses, is the Blood-Borne Defensive Systems. This defensive system contains many different elements, such as white blood cells, macrophage, killer cells, eosinophils, and red blood cells. These mobile attack forces–the cavalry–attack and destroy anything that they deem to be an enemy. Much like city police, these cells are always on patrol and travel throughout the vascular highways and capillary side streets, policing and protecting. They can leave the blood system at will and travel deep into the body's tissues to join forces with our tissue, skin or mucous membrane defense mechanisms, adding an additional protection layer and at times finishing the job started by the others. This is much like a SWAT team, might do.

Another system essential for protecting us and healing wounds is our blood clotting/platelet mechanism. When a wound occurs, there is often immediate blood loss. This bleeding can be extensive and it must be stopped before excessive blood loss causes shock and possibly death. Even when bleeding is minimal, clotting is necessary to begin the process of wound healing.

As soon as our blood clots, the clot acts not only as a barrier to further invasions and bleeding, but it also acts as a matrix for the wound healing mechanism to lay down the protein substances bridging the wound, closing it and allowing it to heal.

ORGAN LEVEL DEFENSIVE SYSTEMS

The Organ Level Defensive Systems lie within and around the body's organs. All organs' have their own unique defensive systems. These systems are often integral to the organs individual make up and function. Many organs also belong to larger defense systems (the skin, lungs, mucous membrane and circulatory systems, etc.). These individual defensive systems often blend with those of other organ systems creating a network of defensive systems. Generally, each individual organ defensive systems are specialized for the specific needs of the organs involved. For example, the brain possesses a unique protective system called the Blood-Brain Barrier. The Blood-Brain Barrier consists of a physiological mechanism that alters the brain capillaries, preventing foreign organisms and substances, certain drugs, chemicals, even biologic hormones made by our body, from entering into the brain and its tissues. It does this to protect the brain while at the same time allowing or actively helping certain substances enter into the brain and its fluid tissues. The Blood-Brain Barrier protects the brain from substances that could impair its function. The same situation occurs with the fetus during pregnancy where the placenta creates a barrier protecting the fetus from harmful substances and organisms from the mother's system.

THE IMMUNE-ANTIBODY/ANTIGEN SYSTEM

If you think that all of what I have described so far is more than enough to defend us from danger, then you are in for a surprise. There's more. The next level of defense is the Antibody-Antigen System, more commonly called the Immune System. This is part of our Secondary Defensive Systems and protects us from invasion by foreign organisms and substances. It works throughout the body using the blood-circulatory system as its highway. Cells, which are constantly moving through our body, sense foreign substances or organisms by their chemical makeup. This level is even more sophisticated than the Blood-Borne Defense System, which is looking for whole organisms. This mechanism looks for even parts of organisms. It can find particles too small to be sensed by the other systems.

If an intruder or foreign body is identified, the body releases a series of proteins called Antibodies. These antibodies bind with the intruders' proteins or carbohydrates. The antibodies then either destroy the intruder or call in white blood cells or killer cells to attack and destroy the perceived enemy. This system is responsible for allergies, as well as the identification and destruction of microorganisms, parasites, and even cancer cells.

REPAIR AND REBUILDING – THE BODY'S HEALING SYSTEMS

This next group of protective systems is also extremely important. Without them, we would self-destruct. They are the Repair and Rebuilding Systems, which are responsible for our healing. Organisms invade and injure us through the process of daily living. Our tissues and defensive components are injured, break down, and are destroyed. Every cell in the body is willing to give its life for the body's overall protection. When organisms invade or injuries occur, the healing process is automatically initiated. The stress process is initiated by the release of a number of very specific chemicals and hormones. One of the most important of these is adrenalin. Once the emergency is over, then the healing must start. The repair process is triggered and guided by another stress hormone, cortisol, which is a steroid. Injured tissues and damaged organs must be repaired and returned to normal function. To accomplish this, the tissues themselves respond, they do so by enlisting several repair, rebuilding and healing systems which are now brought into action to help them. When we are injured, they repair the injury; when we bleed, they stop the bleeding and repair the area that was damaged. At the same time as the defensive systems are protecting the vulnerable and injured areas from further invasions, the repair process is aggressively working to restore the body's integrity as well as further strengthen its ability to protect us.

Without these healing and repair systems, we could not heal ourselves and return to our normal state. The entire process is orchestrated so that the defensive, repair, rebuilding and healing systems can continue to work effectively and at maximum activity all at the same time. Like army combat engineers, these systems work wonderfully under fire, under the worst of circumstances, and they diligently do their absolute best to get their jobs done right.

HOUSEKEEPING AND MAINTENANCE SYSTEMS
Several other systems have indirect roles in our defense and protection. Housekeeping and Maintenance Systems do the tasks necessary for the cleaning and maintaining balance and harmony within the body. Although they may not play a direct role in defending us against outside or internal invasion, none of the defensive systems could work effectively without them.

The Respiratory System, for example, is designed to exchange fresh oxygen for respiratory waste, hence cleaning and energizing the body.

The Cardiovascular System – the heart and circulatory system – pumps deoxygenated blood into the lungs and then pumps the freshly oxygenated blood out from the lungs to the body's tissues. The circulatory system with its miles upon miles of blood vessels, not only brings oxygen to the brain and other tissues, it also picks up waste by-products and toxic materials, and then brings them to the lungs, kidneys, intestinal tract, or skin for elimination. It also carries the Blood-Born Defensive System cells, hormones, as well as essential chemicals and nutrients to their destinations. It also maintains blood pressure and prevents shock when a major blood vessel has been injured and there is hemorrhaging.

The Digestive System is not only a barrier system, but also digests food and selects the nutrients necessary for good health and subsistence. It then excretes waste products, which can cause illness or injury.

The Endocrine System, as the main controller of the Fight-and-Flight Mechanism, controls and maintains the body's metabolism and energy requirements. It regulates the efficiency of all the body's organ systems. It communicates the body's needs to its organs, and the state of the organs to the body's hormonal glands. It does this through a process that maintains metabolic function by monitoring the release of the hormones of the pituitary gland (the Master Gland) as well as thyroid hormones, stress hormones, antidiuretic hormones, growth hormones, and others. The Endocrine System is ultimately responsible for regulating the flow of insulin from the pancreas, governing the body's ability to metabolize blood sugar and glycogen, the body's primary energy sources.

The Lymphatic System is part of both the Active Defense Systems and the Housekeeping Systems. It assists in the body's defense by producing blood cells and antibodies. The lymphatic system is important as a filtering and trapping system. Its lymphocytes entrap foreign bodies and remove debris from infected or damaged areas. The lymphatic channels act as a sewer system directing toxic products and remnants of destroyed tissues and cells out of the body.

The spleen regulates, stores, and manufactures blood cells and destroys old or damaged blood cells hence it maintains the Blood Born Defensive Systems and all other defensive systems.

The Skeletal System supports the body and allows for maximum strength and power based on leverage. Some of the larger bones also make blood cells and even stem cells.

The Muscular System not only moves the body and works with the skeletal system, but also helps move blood within the vascular system.

The Nervous System is one of two major communication systems of the body. The first sends, carries and moves electronic messages from one part of the body to another. The other major communication system, the hormonal system, sends hormonal and neurochemical messages throughout the body. This second system is also wholly integrated and works seamlessly with the nervous system.

MAXI OR MAXIMUM-DEFENSE SYSTEMS

The Macro Defensive Systems – our muscles, bones, and nervous system – are necessary to physically move us away from danger. They also enable us to use weapons, to fight, bend, turn, and lift to avoid danger. Without our muscles, bones and nervous system, we would be severely hampered in protecting ourselves from enemies. The macro-defensive system integrates several bodily defensive and offensive systems into one major system to perform the above-described tasks.

As if all these defensive, offensive, attack and repair systems were not enough, there is still one more helpful system. This system encompasses the entire defense, offense, attack and repair network. It coordinates and integrates all of them into what might be called our "Maximum-Defense System." It uses the sensory system, the mind/brain, the body, the endocrine system, and all of the other systems. This is the Fight-or-Flight Mechanism, also known as the Stress Response System or our Stress Mechanism. It is most important in Stress-

Related Disorders, since Stress-Related Disorders are born from real or imagined conflicts, as well as potential or imminent, threats to our immediate or long-term well-being. These unresolved conflicts can adversely affect this system and the systems that make it up as well as our body, mind, emotions, mental attitude, or spiritual aspect of us. The Stress Mechanism is a double-edged sword: one side may cut for the good of the individual, while the other side may cause injury or lead to Stress-Related Disorders.

DEFENSIVE-REPAIR SYSTEM OF THE BODY

I. **Early Warning System**
  1. Sensory Warning Systems
     a) Sight
     b) Hearing
     c) Vibratory Sensation
     d) Temperature
     e) Touch
  2. Body-Mind
     a) Integration of sensory system to create holo graphic picture of the world around us.
     b) Past Experiences
     c) The Survival Center
     d) The Stress Mechanism
     e) Instinctive Behavior

II. **Primary Defensive/Barrier Systems**
  1. Skin
  2. Mucous Membrane
  3. Lungs
  4. Digestive System

III. **Secondary Defensive Systems**
  1. Tissue Defenses
     a) Offensive Defensive Systems
     b) Strategic Defensive Systems
  2. Blood Brain Defensive Systems
  3. Organ Level Defensive Systems
  4. Immune-Antibody/Antigen Systems
  5. Blood-Lymphatic Systems
  6. Blood Clotting Mechanism
  7. Blood Born Defensive Mechansm
  8. Endocrine (Hormonal) System

IV. **Housekeeping Systems**
  1. Cardiovascular System
  2. Digestive System
  3. Endocrine System
  4. Lymphatic System
  5. Homeostasis Mechanism
  6. Clean-Up System

V. **Repair-Rebuilding**
  1. Protein Synthesis System
  2. Wound Healing System
  3. Blood-Lymphatic System
  4. Endocrine (Hormonal) System

VI. **Macro Defensive Systems**
  1. Muscular System
  2. Skeletal System
  3. Nervous System, Memory, Reflexes
  4. Reproductive System
     (Duplication of the species)

VII. **Maxi Defensive Systems**
  1. Integration of all of the above.

Table: 4-1

```
┌─────────────────────────────────────────────┐
│  ┌───────────────────────────────────────┐  │
│  │    Our Defensive System works best for us   │  │
│  │       when we solve problems &              │  │
│  │      leave no unresolved conflicts.         │  │
│  └───────────────────────────────────────┘  │
└─────────────────────────────────────────────┘
```

SUMMARY

All of the systems we have presented above (see Table: 4-1, above) working together account for a major portion of our defensive and protective systems whose job is to protect us from invasion, injury and disease. Many of these systems can be broken down into deeper levels of defensive systems. The sum total of all of these systems is at work for us on a 24/7-365 basis. If you think we are defenseless or that we just become ill, we hope that you now see that this is just not true. We hope at this point that you now have a deeper appreciation of just how difficult it is to become ill and how much your body is working for you.

If one or more of these systems should break down, this network can become disrupted. In the healthy individual, all these various defense, maintenance, housekeeping, macro and maxi systems, harmoniously work together providing a network that maintains life and facilitates health and wellness. They protect our body from injury, invasion, and external chaos.

If one or more of these systems temporarily break down in a healthy person, there is sufficient overlap for other systems to take over and maintain bodily security. However, in an unhealthy individual may become severely disrupted. Whether the network can be reestablished or not, often depends on the instructions it receives from the conscious and subconscious minds. If they tell the network that it can recover, it is much more likely that it will. If our instructions are negative, or they are conflicted by our negative feelings, faulty belief systems, feelings of helplessness, loss, depression, anxiety or fear, then a state of "overwhelm" may develop and the subconscious Body-Mind may be hindered in its ability to rapidly and effectively fix problems that may undermine it. If and when this happens, a lapse in protection may subsequently result. Our body, if given faulty instructions, may believe it is being instructed to fail and it may choose to listen to these instructions and give up.

It is at this point that we find it most important to disagree with the Western medical model, which suggests that bacteria or viruses have control over us. If we believe that they do have this degree of power over us, then we make it easier for them to penetrate our defensive network. This breakdown may then allow a threatened invasion by one or more organisms which can then ultimately lead to illness and even death.

We believe that it is through this mechanism that our immune and defensive systems are undermined. This leads to some or all of our immune and defensive systems becoming impaired. This not only allows infectious organisms to enter and invade our body, but it can also allow our body to turn and attack itself, which occurs with autoimmune diseases. While negative thoughts are at the root of many illness and health problems, unresolved stressors are a major cause of those illnesses we label as Stress-Related Disorders.

In the next chapter, we look at more of the many factors involved in causing people to become ill, how stress is involved and how undermining the stress mechanism can lead to illness. If we are to be fully capable of protecting ourselves from illness, then we must have a clear understanding of these mechanisms and how to protect ourselves from becoming ill.

Chapter Five

STRESS: THE FIGHT OR FLIGHT MECHANISM

STRESS AND THE STRESS MECHANISM

Stress is a total body defensive reaction to a physical or emotional threat. It makes no difference whether this threat is real or imagined. The stress mechanism, like the other defense mechanism, acts automatically without the need of thought or planning. This is very important, because in an actual life-threatening situation, thinking takes time and time may mean the difference between life and death.

The stress mechanism exists in nearly every living creature. Most people are familiar with the effects of a stress reaction, either having experienced it themselves or seen it in others. Some commonly recognized examples are the birds at the park that fly away when someone comes toward them, the kitten who is frightened by a loud noise, the dog that growls and crouches in an attack posture when approached. It might also be the person who becomes upset when things don't go their way. These are examples of actions that are mediated by the Fight-or-Flight - Stress Mechanism.

This mechanism has been with mankind since our first days on earth. In the jungle, the Fight-or-Flight mechanism protected us from danger. Consider your ancient ancestor who heard a noise in the trees behind him while walking through the jungle. Could it be a tiger ready to pounce or just a bird fluttering about? He probably didn't stick around to find out and potentially become a tiger's dinner. If that had happened, he would have been removed from the gene pool and would not have had descendants like you to read this book. Those who responded by either running away or fighting had a greater chance of survival.

This system still exists after thousands of generations. Yet, in today's jungle, the city, it is rare that we come across tigers waiting to pounce on us. Although we may rarely face any tigers, we still respond to threats. Today, the threats most people face are considerably different from the threats our ancestors faced. They are more likely to occur as threats to ego, livelihood, or well-being.

No matter the cause of the threat, however, today's threats are still mediated by our Subconscious Self, our Body-Mind. Today's threats may come in the form of too much debt; too many bills; losing one's job or not getting the job we want; not getting along with our husband, wife or children; too much pressure at work; or not getting something we desire or think we deserve.

The stress mechanism doesn't much care what the threat is; it reacts to anything and sometimes everything, we think, believe or feel might in some way be perceived as threatening to our present or future well-being. It is most accurate to say that stress can be created by any perceived threat, real or imagined, physical, emotional, mental, or spiritual.

DEFINING STRESS

Anything perceived as a threat, consciously or subconsciously, can have an impact on our overall well-being. This does not have to be a life-threatening event. It can be a situation that disturbs our ideal image of our self, the way we see our lives or the ideal way we want our lives to be. When a situation is perceived as a threat, it can trigger our stress mechanism. Today, long out of the jungle and far away from tigers or marauding bands of raiders, the things that cause or trigger stress today are very different from what our defensive systems were originally designed to protect us from.

> **Stress is the difference between the way
> we WANT our world to be
> & THE WAY IT ACTUALLY IS.**

In our new complex and civilized world, stress can best be thought of as the difference between the way we want our world to be and the way it actually is. This approach and definition is extremely important. In fact, this is the crux of the disease mechanism and Stress-Related Disorders. This concept is the focus of the remainder of this work.

If, for example, an individual believes that he should be rich and successful, but also believes that having bills means that he is not going to be successful, then having more bills than he expected can trigger the onset of stress. The more bills he has, the more stress he will likely experience. The more his situation differs from the way he wants his world to be (that is, the way he thinks or believes it should be), the more stress he will likely experience. It is important to recognize that the bills themselves are not the problem. The problem that triggers stress is the threat to his self-image and loss of what he wants in the present and in the future. These losses and treats are now represented by his bills. Stress is triggered when his ideal image belief system perceives these bills as a threat. Stress occurs not because of the bills, but because he fears that they interfere with the way he wants his life to be. He then fears losing his "ideal" or "desired" future. These thoughts, feelings, or beliefs create a threat to his overall well-being. His life, as he sees it or wants it to be, becomes threatened. Stress is created as a result of his belief that having bills somehow reduces his ability and vision of being to be successful. The issue becomes a "life-threatening" situation because if he does not get what he desires. At some level this will be just like dying. The part of him that holds his vision of success may well feel vulnerable, threatened, attacked, and even destroyed. This is not so far-fetched. Let us show you in greater depth, how this concept actually works.

CONSIDER THE FOLLOWING CASE HISTORY OF JOE N.

Joe N. had been working for a company that had just declared it would soon be closing down. As the days and then weeks after the Notice of Closure passed, Joe began feeling more and more nervous as he waited for his company to finalize negotiations with the workers over a closing date, severance packages, medical benefits, and pensions.

Not only had Joe's job and personal identification become threatened, but he also found himself fearing that he might lose his medical benefits and pension. When Joe first came to see us, he wanted medication to calm his nerves. Most of all Joe wanted to continue working for the company where he had worked for the past 20 years. He had planned to use his pension to buy a small piece of property in Oregon where he would retire. He told us that he couldn't picture himself looking for a job or going out on interviews "at his age." Joe repeatedly told us that he didn't want to have to start all over again. He was especially worried that even if he had to find a new job he would ultimately face a significant reduction in salary and possibly no meaningful benefits at all.

Joe had a very tight picture of the way he wanted his life to be. His conflict was that his life was no longer looking the way he had planned and believed it would turn out. At first, Joe couldn't believe that the plant would really close. He kept telling himself that it wouldn't happen "to him." He wanted to believe that the company would change its mind. However, as the days and weeks went by, his anxiety increased. Yet, he could do little about any of it.

Approximately three weeks before the closure, the company finally admitted it had no money for medical benefit or pensions. Joe's reaction first was devastation, but finally he admitted to himself that the end of this work situation was near and he would have to start over. At that point, he opened the job section of his local newspaper for the first time and started looking. He applied for a job in his field and was accepted for the position. He took a small salary decrease, but within six months was up to his previous salary level. The new job he was given was the last opening that the new company had. He later learned that a few of his former co-workers who procrastinated even longer than he did were left without jobs and had to go on unemployment.

It is important to emphasize at this point that the common belief that stress is caused by external events is only marginally true. Most physicians and therapists, as well as lay people, believe that stress is caused by what happens to us; this is wrong.

> Stress is **NOT** caused by the events of our life,
> but rather by our
> **PERCEPTIONS OF THESE EVENTS.**

Stress is caused by how we perceive what is happening to us, and this is always colored by the belief systems we hold or don't hold about what is happening. It was not the plant closure that triggered Joe's stress. It was how he believed the closure would affect him and the image he had created regarding how he wanted his life to look and turn out.

DISEASE IS A NATURAL STATE OF BEING, BASED ON THE INSTRUCTIONS WE GIVE OUR BODY-MIND

It is our belief that much of what we call Disease, and specifically Stress-Related Disorders, is really the result of a faulty interaction between our conscious and subconscious minds. At the base the cause or causes of these illnesses are often one or more unresolved conflicts. If an individual resolves these problems, the symptoms are likely to simply go away. What we see is a defined path from wellness to illness, and that this path is mediated by the Stress Mechanism. This path will be discussed in detail in Chapter 9.

Ultimately, these unresolved conflicts occur because of the difference between the way we want our life to be and the way our life actually turns out. Unresolved conflicts may also occur because of good or bad decisions we had previously made regarding events which take place during the course of our lives. These unresolved conflicts are often based on memories of real or imagined events. The origin of these memories and decisions may have occurred early on during childhood or even before our birth or possibly, as some people believe, during a past life. Usually these memories are faulty. This occurs because only part of what has actually happened is consciously remembered, or what is remembered or held onto is based on incomplete information. Also, our memories are often altered by us to be what we "remember," rather than what actually took place. We refer to these incomplete or inaccurate memories as lies. They are not the truth and holding on to them creates problems, even greater ones than simply triggering stress, hence they act as lies and they undermine us and ultimately act destructively against us.

The stress mechanism is an emergency system, which acts intensively over short periods. Built into this system is a process of resolution, the process by which the body ultimately returns to a state of normalcy, as each conflict is resolved. If this resolution phase is not allowed, the stress mechanism may be left turned on for extended periods of time.

Another possibility is that the stress episodes had become so frequent that resolution was ineffective. This ineffective resolution may now results in persistent or chronic biologic conflict, or "chronic stress." This chronic biologic conflict implies three results: In the first, the stress mechanism itself becomes uncoordinated or even chaotic and begins to malfunction. In the second possibility, the body and its organs become overstimulated, undermining their ability to function normally. In the third situation, both of these occur to some degree. When either of these happen, we generally refer to the result as "burn out," "disease," or "chronic disease."

These unresolved recurrent biologic conflicts can therefore ultimately lead to Chronic Stress, which is the foundation of Stress-Related Disorders. It is through this mechanism that our immune systems and other defensive systems begin malfunctioning. This is the reason foreign organisms are allowed to take hold within our body. When this happens, it is not the "invading" organism that is responsible, but us. We are the problem. We have not dealt with, resolved, undone, and eliminated these negative and destructive "unresolved" conflicts, before their existence acted against us by undermining our defensive and protective systems preventing them from operating effectively, hence allowing us to become ill.

When our healing and repair systems are so negatively affected they become unable to normally function. Healing becomes impaired. To make matters worse, if the unresolved stress reaction persists for an extended period, the resulting malfunctions can be learned by the body and subsequently then become the "norm." We all have seen examples of people learning bad habits, by becoming addicted to a substance or behavior, or are chronically ill. For example: smoking, alcoholism, and gambling addictions, but also chronic anger, anxiety, difficulty getting to sleep, heartburn, and stress headaches, are often learned behaviors created as we inappropriately deal with the stresses of our life.

While this may sound like a doomsday message, it is not. There is also good news. By understanding this process and how it works, we can find ways to eliminate stress; resolve previously unresolved conflicts; unlearn negative thinking; and reverse, eliminate, heal and even cure Stress-Related Diseases.

For the most part, it would seem that our individual life experiences, not to mention mankind's history, would prove that disease is real and exists within us and comes from outside. At first glance, it might even appear that disease is a natural part of mankind's experience of life. What is missing from this belief is the recognition of the untold millions of people who are rarely sick. Because illness is so poorly understood in our society, we often accept the belief that either people get sick for no reason at all, or because there are bugs and other things out there that are always ready to attack us and cause disease.

These beliefs also appear to support the view that life is dangerous, and that the Universe we live in is hostile. For people who believe these notions, there is always sufficient evidence to prove that illness is not only real, but also that it comes from outside of us to attack us. Not only do many people absolutely believe in illness, but also many of these people are also unwilling to believe that they have any role at all in its existence or occurrence. This is an illusion, which has been created by watching the circumstances of life and not fully understanding its essence. It is also dangerous because it leaves us powerless to either prevent or treat those illnesses, which we can and do really have power over.

My first experience with illness was during my childhood. I was told I was a "sickly" child. I had severe allergies, recurrent flu, colds, sore throats, ear infections, a constant runny nose, and other illnesses. Certainly, this should have proved to me that illness was real. However, I never really felt sick. As I grew up, I became aware of the thoughts, fears, and anxieties that were causing or creating my illnesses.

It was not until I was about 16 years of age that I really had a change in my circumstances. About that time, I remember tuning on a television program where a commentator was interviewing a member of the New York Polar Bear Club. The commentator was standing on the beach at Coney Island in the dead of winter. He was dressed in an overcoat, muffler, and hat. When he spoke, steam blew out of his mouth. Standing next to the commentator was a man who was wearing only a swim suit. This man didn't even look cold. He stood chest out and head high. Behind both men, the camera panned to the ocean where a number of bathers frolicked in the icy waters of the Atlantic Ocean. The beach was covered with snow. At one point, the commentator asked the man in the swim suit, "Aren't you afraid of getting sick exposing yourself to the elements like this?" The man smiled and answered, "No! No! Not at all! In fact we believe that this actually will make us healthier."

Up to this point in my life, I bundled up in sweaters, coats, hats, and scarves when it was cold. When it rained, I wore a raincoat and galoshes. I was told that it was essential to protect myself from the elements. Yet, this Polar Bear Club member now told me that I didn't have to do any of this. Many years later, I found that decisions I made at that moment would not only affect my life but also my patients' lives and well-being too. My decision to heal myself also included a decision to use what I learned to help my patients by neither accepting nor giving power to the illnesses they worried so much about.

During the years of my (Allen) medical practice, I had a rather unusual experience. Very few of my patients became seriously ill under my care. Those few who did develop illnesses often recovered quickly. Only two of my patients died during my years of active private practice. One committed suicide and the other was a 92-year-old woman who actually came to me to die. I only had to put one patient into intensive care when she came to see me with a severe, irregular heart rhythm. In the 14 years I practiced obstetrics and gynecology, I performed thousands of deliveries and never lost a single infant, either during delivery or after. I never lost a mother and I had only two serious postpartum problems. In both cases, the women involved recovered fully and rapidly.

Someone might say that this is the record of an exceptional physician, but I do not believe that this is the case. I think it is the result of my not believing in illness. I experienced other competent physicians who drew patients from the same geographical area, the same sources of referral, and the same age and socio-economic groups. Their patients suffered serious complications, extended illness, and some even died. What was the difference? It wasn't that these doctors were less competent, because in fact they were all highly competent. The only reason I could see was that these doctors believed in illness and I did not. I do not bring this up to flatter myself or criticize other physicians, but to make a point. While many of my patients believed in illness and came to me sick, they left feeling better or they left me to seek another physician, one who like them, believed in their illness. I refused to acknowledge that my patients had to be sick. I refused to believe that any problem they had was not entirely and immediately curable.

On the other hand, many individuals I saw needed their illnesses. They deeply believed in their illnesses, and made them the focal point of their lives. Many were unwilling or unable to solve the underlying conflicts that causing their illnesses. Often, their fear of dealing with their conflicts prevented me from even bringing up these ideas. Patients who worked with their conflicts often rapidly got better. Those who didn't either took longer or continued having recurring problems. Occasionally, patients would leave me to find someone who would either accept their sick self, or who would at least allow them to be sick. Conversely others "found" me and came to me as patients because they had heard that I generally got better results than their other doctors.

Today when we do wellness and healing work, we insist on working only with patients who truly are committed to getting well. We want to work with people who not only want to be well again, but also who are willing to do whatever is necessary to facilitate their healing. The process of becoming well and maintaining wellness requires the transformation from illness beliefs (the illness mentality) to wellness beliefs (the wellness mentality). This breaks the stress cycle and transforms the stress process into a healing process. Healing then automatically happens because once the stress process is halted, the resolution phase can proceed. Intrinsic to the resolution process is the activation of the body's natural healing and repair mechanisms. People can transform stress into challenge, negative stress into positive experience, and invoke resolution. With resolution comes release, relief and relaxation, and the healing mechanism's activation. They then get better and healthier.

On the other hand, those people who really, for whatever reason, don't want to do everything they need to do to get better, tend to procrastinate and refuse to take responsibility for creating their wellness. They may be critical of treatments that don't match their conception of standard medicine, which usually had not fully helped them to get well before they came to me either. It is as if they want to remain ill or that their conflict so undermines them that they just can't make the leap and get well. Most of us have seen this situation. Each of us has experienced similar resistance to getting well, accomplishing goals or solving problems as well. Not only does this kind of behavior keep many people stuck in their problems and illnesses, but it also demonstrates that their unresolved conflicts continue to have power over them.

> **Illness is an intelligent communication
> from our Body-Mind,
> telling us that we have one or more
> unresolved conflicts that MUST be resolved.**

Lisa and I believe that we always have power over our problems and illness. We believe that illness is an intelligent communication from our Body-Mind directed to us, telling us we have one or more unresolved conflicts that must be resolved. We have full control over them. We can heal ourselves by recognizing our unresolved conflicts and solving them. We can work on them, learn from them, grow and evolve from them while gaining valuable insights from our illness process.

We can go even further by stating that if you are willing to take full responsibility for your own problems, you can then attain full and complete power over your life and wellness. On the other hand, if you create conflicts by being dishonest with yourself and others, illness is one possible outcome.

As suggested earlier, it is our unresolved conflicts that trigger our stress mechanism. To prevent conflict, solutions must be found. If problem solving is avoided, then your problems will ultimately threaten your well-being and the stress-disease process may well be set into motion. If problem solving is embraced, then we can heal ourselves and prevent Stress-Related Disorders.

Chapter Six

THE BODY-MIND, CONSCIOUS AWARENESS AND SPIRIT

THE THREE LEVELS OF MAN — THE BODY-MIND, THE CONSCIOUS MIND AND THE HIGHER SELF

To understand the roles of the Body-Mind, the Conscious Mind (often referred to as the personality or ego) and the Higher Self (spiritual mind or spiritual self) in creating illness and healing, we must first understand each of these three consciousness components, and how they interrelate. If you try to understand these processes through our traditional approach with Western allopathic medicine, it cannot be done. "Modern" Western medicine evolved from its earliest days believing that everything meaningful had to be scientifically proven before it could be accepted or utilized. This process was designed to eliminate anything that could not be proven, including nearly everything that cannot be experienced beyond our physical senses or the current scientific instruments. In its early history, the fledgling field of medicine rebuked all that even remotely related to religion or spirituality. This was initially a reaction against the unseen and the unproven, the church and shamanistic healers.

Today, it is clear that without considering man's spiritual nature, true healing and wellness is difficult or impossible to obtain. The problem is that the present medical model is extremely rigid when it comes to anything that does not match its needs to maintain a strict scientific approach, such as the Germ Theory and the Faulty Body Construct; bodies are imperfect, everyone is different, illness is natural and becoming ill is an inevitability. Because of this, Western medicine is not able to allow a holistic understanding of the more subtle concepts of healing versus treating. The stress mechanism fits the challenges of the scientific approach. Understanding the rest and obtaining the highest level of results, prevention, healing and return to wellness after serious illness requires leaving the medical model and moving toward areas that are less rigorously determined and rarely recognized. This includes non-medical methods used for balancing body, mind, and spirit, and their accompanying energies. It also includes how unresolved conflicts can lead to illness, and how we can help others heal health problems, which are presently not capable of being cured using the current Western medical system approach to treating illness rather than healing.

Only by adding the unseen and the unprovable do all of the pieces of the puzzle fall into place facilitating healing. Only when we add these components to treating illness do we finally move beyond the confines of the old paradigm of "modern medicine" into the new, more integrated paradigm that is rapidly replacing it[7]. Only when Western medicine is finally able to integrate body, mind, spirit, intelligence and fundamental healing approaches, will the remainder of the puzzle of wellness and healing unfold. This unfolding will provide the answers we need to create healing and enable us to go beyond the current approach of simply treating symptoms, and not causes.

Through traditional Eastern philosophy, some Western medical practitioners have learned the concepts of mind, body, and spirit used in what is now being referred to as "alternative medicine." Even though the concepts of the mind, body, and spirit individually do seem clear enough, there is no simple way of integrating them into the present Western medical model. This leaves a great gap, which in turn creates a breakdown in the Western traditional medical practitioner's ability to understand illness and the healing processes. From the Eastern point of view, the body is seen as whole, and illness and healing are most frequently explained in relation to the flow and circuitry of energy within the body.

The Western model sees the body as a complex system of body parts, organs, and biochemical reactions within a series of physical and hormonal systems with each acting separately, yet affecting the whole at various times. The Western medical practitioner studies the body, mind, personality and rarely is anything presented about "the spirit." They study an assortment of body parts, organs, and tissues, each fending for itself and each relatively uncoordinated with any other body part, often as functioning against each other and the whole. The Western practitioner is not taught how all of these parts would work in a fully integrated organism. Instead of seeing the body parts working together in harmony with each other and the physical body, the Western practitioner is taught to emphasize genetics, body chemistry, function, and failure. Because of this, the Western medical doctor is taught that the human body and life in general, and the universe in specific, are random, hostile, cruel and destructive, rather than loving, caring and self-healing. For most Western physicians, the concept of the spirit relates to religion or manifestations of ghosts.

---

7   Capra, Fritjov, *The Tao of Physics, Shambhala Publications, Inc., Boston, MA, 1999*

The mind, body, and spirit are not recognized individually nor are they recognized as working together as an essential aspect of man's totality. Each aspect actually plays an integral role in the creation of illness and the facilitation of healing. This is still not well accepted by the Western medical profession or the standard Western medical model.

A NEW HEALING APPROACH

It is our hope that we show you a simpler way of understanding the roles of the Body-Mind, personality, and spirit and their relationship to the process of becoming ill and healing. We believe that this is simple, and it represents a direct approach to a new paradigm for understanding the creation of illness and our capacity to create healing. Our goal here, however, is not to prove the existence of spirit or our Body-Mind, but rather to explain to our readers how faulty belief systems and unresolved conflicts can and do lead to acute illness and chronic diseases.

To accomplish these goals, we must first learn that our Body-Mind, our personality, and our spiritual self are three aspects of the same entity – human consciousness, or what we think of as "life." Next, we must look at each of these three components separately, but without separating these components from the whole. In the following sections, we describe these components individually. Just be mindful that they are all part of one, integrated unit. We can think of this unit as the "being," the "Individual," the "I," the "me," or the "Self." It is also your "self," or you.

THREE LEVELS OF CONSCIOUSNESS OF MAN – AN OVERVIEW

Each of us, what we think of as our "self," is made up of three levels of mind. One level is the subconscious mind or subconscious self. The second level is the conscious mind, which is our conscious, alert, aware self. Then the third level is the higher self, sometimes referred to as the superconscious or spiritual self. All of these three selves inhabit one physical body. Together they comprise what we think of as our self.

These three consciousnesses or minds, what we like to think of as the "selves," work with three types of life-force energies, 1) our basic life-force energy, 2) our conscious or awake energy, often thought of as will-power, and 3) our spiritual energy. These three energies are the basis of who we really are. Combined, they are the "me" we often think of when we think about ourselves and who we are. Our physical body is not simply a machine, as commonly thought of in Western medicine. It is an intelligent and integral part of our being.

The body itself has no consciousness or awareness of its own. It needs all three of these "selves" and their energies to come to life and to function optimally. When one or more of the three selves or energies are out of balance, the body is in disharmony. This loss of harmony and balance is what Western medicine thinks of as illness and disease. The signs and symptoms of this loss of harmony and balance are generally the signs and symptoms of illness. Ultimately, we find that a substantial part of this illness process is mediated by the Stress Mechanism.

For the purpose of simplicity in our discussion, we would like to pick one set of terms for each of the three selves. For example, the subconscious self is often referred to by physicians and lay people as anything from the unconscious to the subconscious. We will call it the Subconscious Mind or the Subconscious Self. It is sometimes referred to as the Body-Mind or the Automatic Self. The subconscious mind is a combination of the autonomic nervous system (sympathetic and parasympathetic nervous systems) and the reptilian or primitive brain complex. It controls, oversees and runs all of the many functions of our body. It would not be accurate to think of it as "unconscious mind" just because it appears to not openly exist. The subconscious mind never sleeps or shuts down, except when it has been severely traumatized or injured. It operates quietly, without any fanfare, 24/7/365, always ready to activate our Stress, Fight or Flight, Mechanism. It is always alert and instantly responsive; ever alert, listening, remembering, and learning.

The conscious mind is also often referred to by different names including consciousness, personality, ego, self, and the aware self. We will refer to it as the Conscious Mind or Conscious Self. This is the conscious aware part of our mind and brain. It is only aware of what is going on as long as we are awake and as long as our Subconscious mind is functioning normally. It is, when we are awake and paying attention, consciously aware of our immediate circumstances and what is going on in the world around us. When we are aware of it, we often think of it as, "I," "me," or as "myself."

Finally, the spiritual mind is sometimes referred to as our spirit. In the deepest sense, this is incorrect, as all three of these selves are spirits and part of the "self." It has also been referred to as the spiritual self, super-consciousness, our guardian angel, supernatural spiritual self, our protector, the High Self, or the Higher Self. While all of these names can be used interchangeably, we prefer calling it the Higher Self. It is the highest level of consciousness of our being. It is always in contact with the Intelligence of the Universe or God. It is always in contact our spiritual guides and other guardian angels. Once again these are concepts which are rarely, if ever, recognized in Western medicine.

These three levels of consciousness at first may appear to be quite similar to the concepts of body, mind, and spirit. However, there are some significant differences. One of the main differences here is that each of these constructs is much broader than is simply implied when we refer to them as mind, body, or spirit. The exact differences are essential for refining our definition and recognition of these three concepts. This becomes evident when we look at and try to understand the many roles they play in creating or directing the causes and effects in getting ill and in understanding the process of how illness is healed and eliminated. It is also important that we understand how each of these three levels functions individually and how they join, creating the Self. I must reiterate once again that all three selves must work together. This is vital for our ability to function optimally on a day-to-day basis.

The Conscious Self has its center in the heart area. The Subconscious Self has its center in the solar plexus, which is located just above the navel just behind the abdominal cavity. Finally, the Higher Self has its center above and outside of the physical body, slightly above the head. The Higher Self is most commonly portrayed in religious art as the halo, ring, or bright light surrounding the head of Jesus, the saints, and other key religious figures.

The three selves are always part of an integrated whole and they can never be separated one from the other while we live.

Before starting the next section, it is best if you first review Table: 6-1. It is a thumbnail summary of each of the three selves, their functions, and qualities.

The Table is laid out so that you can see and compare, side by side, each individual function or capacity directly next to that of the other two selves. You can easily see both the similarities and differences of each. Once you have reviewed this Table you will almost instantly become an expert in understanding what each of the three selves do and how they all integrate to function as an integrated unit. To better understand the three selves, and their individual roles we will first start by discussing the self most familiar to us—our Conscious Aware Self.

SUMMARY OF THE THREE SELVES-1

THE BODY-MIND	THE CONSCIOUS SELF	THE HIGHER SELF
Automatic or Autonomic Self. The Body-Mind is also referred to as the Lower Self. All memories are stored within the Body-Mind. It operates 24 hours a day 7 days a week, 365 days/year, all of the time. It never sleeps unless seriously injured. Its center is in the Solar Plexus in the abdomen. Works automatically but it also takes orders from and can be commanded to action by the conscious self. Its purpose is three-fold: a) It manages all other than conscious bodily functions: It beats the heart, digests food and it maintains all memories. b) It supports survival. This includes managing the Fight or Flight, Stress Mechanism and the immune and defensive systems of the body. It manages the Healing and Repair Systems. c) It makes sure that the conscious self gets everything it wants and needs. All the conscious self has to do is ask for what it wants or even just create a thought of what it wants and the lower self will make it happen. Remembers everything, past and present. Maintains this information to help the conscious self to direct the future.	The conscious and awake self, the personality. The "me" or "I" we normally think of as who we are. It operates only while we are awake. Its center is in our heart area but it is not our heart. Involved with the business of the day. It conducts functions such as talking, thinking, planning and purposeful movement. Its purpose is two-fold: a) Maintain survival on all conscious levels. Finding food, shelter, ego pursuits such as hobbies, career and doing business. b) Creates civilization and civilizes the lower self. In doing so it makes judgments and has opinions. Since the conscious self is the personality its commands always inherently have within them its own particular viewpoint of the world, its likes and dislikes. To get what it wants, it makes suggestions and issues commands to the lower self and then expects that the lower self will give it exactly what it wants. It often confuses itself with the lower self. The conscious self operates only in the present moment. It has only short term memory and relies on the lower self for long term memory and recall.	The Superconscious or Spiritual Self. The highest level of human consciousness. Connection to the Universal Intelligence, "God". It is the connection to the Universal Intelligence (God). Operates all of the time. It exists outside the body above and to one side or the other of the head. Communicate with the lower self and with the Intelligence of the Universe. It makes our prayers or highest thoughts and requests come true. Its purpose is four-fold: a) Connection to the Godhead, the Intelligence of the Universe. b) Interconnection of the individual with Mankind and Mankind with all other conscious elements of the Universe. c) Makes the potential of "heaven" and the entire bounty of the Universe available to all through prayer or a specific construct of prayer called "Huna prayers." Can create "miracles" upon request.

SUMMARY OF THE THREE SELVES-2

THE BODY-MIND	THE CONSCIOUS SELF	THE HIGHER SELF
Related to the Western concepts of unconsciousness or subconsciousness, however, it is never really unconscious. Considered the nature or animal spirit of man. Ruled by natural and internal (genetics, biochemistry, physics) laws. Has an inherent wisdom. Constantly must learn from the conscious self. Can only think deductively. Holds all emotions and manifests them through bodily feelings, physical signs and sensations or symptoms. Serves the emotional aspects of the conscious self as well as the physical needs of the body. Manages sex and sexual attraction. Reactive to situations and stimuli. Has a very literal and linear mind. Always does what it is told, asks no questions nor resist reasonable instructions. Designed as a task-oriented achiever, to complete goals and tasks, as rapidly as possible. Essentially a child, a student, a servant, and even a robot. It is Programmed to perform tasks. Learns and grows from experience and rote. Its subtle body is an etheric body and its energy is life force.	The conscious self can be logical or illogical. Has likes and dislikes and possesses intellect, intuition, opinions and conscience. It is generally considered to be the human (civilized) spirit It is ruled by the heart and the head in its likes, dislikes, wants and desires. It is also ruled by external events and forces. It generally wants to be socially correct and craves love. Uses both inductive and deductive logic. Has some free will and free choice. Makes decisions about everything. Plays social roles, imitates, speaks in words, uses emotions positively or negatively, acts through emotions, feelings and physical actions. Reactive to situations and stimuli. Has a rational and intuitional mind; will think about and ponder questions. Designed as an achiever goal setter and problem solver, always looking for problems to solve. Most of the time the initiator, teacher, parent or master. Always feels it has to be in charge. Usually feels alone Its subtle body is the astral body and its energy is will power.	The Higher Self is beyond time or space. It has no equivalent of memory. It knows all and sees all and understands everything. The Higher Self is selfless and in the realm of what might be called Supra-conscious. Totally benevolent, totally trustworthy, parental spirit. Considered the "Spirit" or guardian angel. Operates under the rules of the Intelligence of the Universe or God, as well as Natural and Scientific Laws. Neither logical nor illogical. It is Truth and does not lie. It has no equivalence in earthly terms. It is just truth and does not lie. It has no equivalence in earthly terms. It is just truth and does not lie. Described as the "Totally Trustworthy, Totally Benevolent Parental Spirit or Self. Described as the "Totally Trustworthy, Totally Benevolent Parental Spirit or Self. Its subtle body is the auric body and its energy is the highest form of spiritual energy.

THE CONSCIOUS AWARE SELF

While the Conscious Self is the part of us that we most commonly associate with ourselves or our "I," it is by no means the most important part of us. The Conscious Self is the part of "me" that has written the majority of the text that your Conscious Self is presently reading. It is also that part of us that does business, talks, thinks, and interrelates with others and with the physical and mental realities of life. The Conscious Self is also the only part of us that relates to time and space in that it deals with yesterday, today, and tomorrow.

This is the part of us that makes most of our day-to-day decisions, although much of our decision making is influenced by feelings, emotions, and memories held within our Subconscious Self. Only the Conscious Aware Self cares about the past, present and future or how it relates to the other Selves. It thinks only in terms of experience, present events or short term and long term periods. On its own, the Conscious Self has only short-term memory.

Because of this, it relies almost entirely on the Body-Mind, the Subconscious Self, to provide recall of experiences and memories so that it can project and calculate the future[8].

The Conscious Self creates all of our likes and dislikes, desires, and obligations for us. It is the most illogical part of the three Selves, often operating from superficial appearances and faulty beliefs. Generally, it does what it believes is reasonable or desirable in that moment, but it can plan, even scheme, in order to get the exact results it desires. It uses anger, rage, fear, positive and negative feelings, guile and at time even logic and reason to accomplish its goals. It learns, though not always, successfully. It can rigidly hold on for years to what initially were just temporary emotions and beliefs, whether they were good or bad for it; or it can give them up in a second if that is what it feels is in its best interest. For the most part, it lives in the "now" moment and stores just about everything it does not need in the "now" moment within the Subconscious Self. Because of the enormous volume of sensory input and data entering into the Conscious Self every second, it tends to select out what it feels is relevant in the moment. It then sends everything it wants to keep onto the subconscious self. This would include what it either does not want to hold onto or any information, thought, beliefs or emotions it may not need in the now-moment but still wants to have available to it in the future.

---

8   *Using this model, Alzheimer's Disease (and possibly other dementias) could be thought of as a process of separation of the Subconscious and Conscious Selves, each essentially going its own way, no longer working together. Hence, It is a breakdown in their ability to work together. Possibly as death approaches, each prepares to go its own way. It could also be a break with reality as each sees it.*

The Conscious Self is our human consciousness. It possesses intellect, in-tuition, and the ability to reason. It thinks and feels. What it does best is make decisions and suggestions, or give commands to the Subconscious Self so that the Subconscious Self can manifest the personal reality the Conscious Self de-sires in the now-moment. In most cases the Conscious Self is only marginally, if at all, aware of the Subconscious Self.

While the job of the Subconscious Self is to survive in nature, the job of the Conscious Self is to support our survival in society. The role of the Higher Self is to relate and communicate with the Universal Intelligence (the God Spirit), to ensure our spiritual survival. While the Subconscious Self is primarily involved with physical survival, the Conscious Self considers survival an issue only when it is overtly threatened. Since it does not have to continually think of survival, the Conscious Self can play, have hobbies, create for the sake of creating, build, or simply enjoy life. While the Conscious Self plays the Subconscious Self is con-cerned with minute-to-minute survival and the Higher Self concerns itself with neither because to it, life is eternal. It exists outside of what we think of as time and space, and it is not at all involved with our earthly survival instincts and needs.

The interplay between the Conscious and Subconscious Selves is man's eternal struggle. Our Conscious Self is always looking to better itself and enjoy life. Our Subconscious Self is always working at maintaining necessary life pro-cesses, such as beating the heart, digesting food, excreting waste, and solving problems. At the same time, it is always working at fulfilling the needs, wishes, and directions of the Conscious Self. They are, in a sense, simply two aspects of the same Self, they are also very different. In the end, these similarities and dif-ferences feed the ongoing struggle that rages between these two selves – "Who is in charge?" "Who should 'I' listen to?" "What is happening to me?

In the context of our modern society, we see that the Conscious Self often lies to itself and to the Subconscious Self. These lies lead to deception and then act to create injury which can cause anger, shame and guilt which then acts to hurt us. When the Conscious Self lies to itself, it can easily lose its sense of reality. It may believe its own lies, then mislead itself and ultimately others as well. These lies promote negative and even destructive thinking and faulty belief systems which can lead us into make faulty decisions. When we create lies in our life, we ultimately cause harm to our self and to others. The lies we have created can now be thought of as "sins." Lies often lead to more lies and then more hurt. When we are aware that we are lying or living a life based on faulty belief systems we cause more hurt. We then know that lies and decep-tion exist and continue to accept and empower them we will ultimately create more and more intentional hurt to ourselves and others. This hurt undermines and negatively affects our Stress Mechanism. Also, it triggers the activation of our Stress Mechanism. The inciting conflict if not resolved, can and often does, lead to triggering the Stress-Illness-Disease Mechanism. This in turn leads to

Stress-Related Disorders, which if not resolved can and will eventually lead to illness, disease, and chronic disease. When we lie to ourselves or others, we set in motion a series of events which often lead to increased conflict, more guilt and more anger. If these conflicts are not resolved or corrected, over a period of time, they will eventually lead to more serious, even life-threatening illness, and eventually chronic disease and premature death.

The Conscious Self sees much of what it considers reality through the societal conditioning and programming in which it was raised[9]. Its ability to be obedient and honest, and to react to or consider the desires of others, and to live within the rules of society has all also been programmed into it. The Conscious Self is able to break or change these rules when conflicts occur between itself and its external programming or its Subconscious Self. From these conflicts, great poets, statesmen, artists, and scientists may arise. However, the liar, cheat, criminal, and antisocial behaviors may also arise out of these same conflicts.

These behaviors are to the societal self what illness and diseases are to the physical body-self, the result of unresolved conflicts. In essence, crime and the breakdown of our society are as difficult to deal with, as are physical illness and disease, as they often come from the same mechanism. To treat one is to treat the other. When we fully understand what the causes and reasons for illnesses are, we can prevent and undo them, then we may also be able to live in a crime-free world.

The Conscious self is constantly making decisions. When decisions are not consciously made, they may be unconsciously made by the Subconscious Self based on fragmented or incomplete memories from our past, non-productive habits, blocks and complexes that we have created while attempting to solve other problems or issues, and using inaccurate facts and understandings. These choices are often filtered through our social programming and the internal images or life pictures we have created because of our past decisions and current beliefs. Our self-image may be a clear representation of our true self, or it may be significantly distorted and bear little actual resemblance to who we are or what is actually happening around us in the now-moment. When self-image is true to the Self, there is little disparity between reality and the way the three Selves see the world. The result in such situations is harmony, balance, wellness, and well-being, which all lead to healing and wellness.

However, when our self-image is distorted, we then start out each day living a lie and there will likely be one or more unresolved conflict eating at us. This tells us, our Conscious Aware self, that these unresolved conflicts require solutions or else greater problems will result.

---

9   *Americans think and react differently than the French, Argentineans, West Africans, or Eskimos, each being brought up not only in different culture, but in many ways in different worlds. Each differs in many ways one from the other so that they each may see the world and other human beings in entirely different ways.*

Since we each have free will, each Conscious Self has the power to direct itself and its life path based on healthy, realistic belief regarding how it should live its life and solve problems. Through the decisions we make, we create either constructive or destructive results. We can overcome any negative social programming when we decide that it does not serve us.

We have the power and the ability to establish a more responsible and true self-image, or we continue acting from the lies that we ourselves or others (parents, friends, society, teachers or employers) have programmed into us. When we don't solve problems, this then further distorts both our reality of life and our self-image. If we choose to live with a distorted reality, we ultimately become confused, lost, unhappy, and unable to find our true joyful and healthy path. When this happens, we may consciously or subconsciously choose to protect ourselves. We may refuse to acknowledge that we created these lies and attribute them to others. We may project our negative thoughts and experiences to the world outside of ourselves. We may blame others for our problems. When we do not take responsibility for ourselves, our thoughts, and for the conflicts we have created and for the way our lives have turned out, we remain blocked from what we want in life.

Many people tend to hold on to their lies, mistruths, and negative projections, even when they recognize that these lies exist and even when they recognize their role in both creating or furthering these lies. Because of this, their lies remain unresolved and may persist for years. This lack of resolution often leads to illness as well as to also undermining their ability to survive and maintain their overall health and well-being.

Even when our Subconscious Self tries to communicate the existence of these conflicts through physical, mental, emotional, or spiritual signs and symptoms, which have now become messages and cries for help, some of us may still refuse to pay attention to them. In doing so, they are also refusing to solve their problems. This then leads to their conflict transforming into potentially solvable problems then into unresolved conflicts, which will then further undermine their ability to heal and return to full and complete wellness.

Since the Conscious Self is generally unaware of the existence of the Subconscious Self, it is unaware that the Subconscious Self usually takes its every thought and wish literally. Our Subconscious Self takes whatever we ask of it, right or wrong, as an order or mandate for it to create and manifest as asked. Hence, it often creates and manifests for us what we do not want; do not need; and what may in the end lead us into illness.

The Conscious Self, however, often misinterprets responses from the Body-Mind and interprets them as if they were coming to us from outside of us. In other words we create what others want from us, thinking it is what we want for us. When this happens, we miss out on creating what we really want and need and in doing so, we give away our right to free choice, free will, and having what we desire and need.

For example, an individual looking for a job may feel insecure. He may feel that he is unworthy of the job he seeks. At the time of the interview, his insecurity and lack of worthiness may be projected to the interviewer in many subtle ways. He may act or respond as if talking to an enemy, as he might when he defends himself to an unloving father. When he doesn't get the job, he may then conclude that the interviewer, "didn't like him," or that "she somehow knew," he wasn't worthy of the job.

When situations like this occur, the gap between our Conscious Self and Subconscious Self widens. The Conscious Self may soon believe that no one can be trusted, that it is all alone and separate from everyone and from the Universe. What is happening here is that the Conscious Self is walling itself off as a form of protection. After a while, the Conscious Self becomes isolated from the world. It sees itself as a failure. It begins seeing enemies all around. The Subconscious Self, believing what it is being told, initiates a withdrawal process. This is often seen as depression, internal withdrawal, or internal flight-or-freeze syndrome.

The Conscious Self creates another type of problem when it holds anger or is unhappy about its circumstances. These processes are registered as if the person or circumstance we are angry at is threatening our existence, and the existence of our Body-Mind. This threat triggers the stress mechanism. Anger eventually grows into rage and hostility. When we are unable to solve the problems that initiated this process, anger, rage, and hostility gradually turn to apathy, disinterest, and further withdrawal. All this time, the stress reaction builds while chemical and physical changes are occurring and the Body-Mind suffers.

As anger builds, negative energy is created; the more the anger and rage, the greater the internal pressure. At times, the person may look and feel like a time bomb, ready to explode. The Conscious Self may find one or more ways of releasing this internal negative pressure. One way is by periodically exploding. We often refer to these people as "hot heads." Another way might be taking risks and challenging our self and the world.

This can be done in a positive or negative manner. The negative way is through antisocial behavior, crime, hitting and hurting others, such as spousal or child abuse. Still others may let off negative energy in more subtle ways, such as creating a scapegoat, or following political, religious or spiritual leaders who are destructive for them. The positive aspect of this process is seen as problem solving, creativity, hobbies, or charity work. Here, the individual turns negative behavior into a positive and productive direction.

The negative actions transfer control from the individual to the anger. Hence, the power to control one's self is taken away from the Conscious Self and left to negative emotions that live within the Subconscious Self. This transfer of negative energy away from the Conscious Self often produces a temporary stress reduction. However, the Subconscious Self is also temporarily cut off from its normal ability to communicate that this anger now exists and is stored within it. At first, it does what it is told. However, it soon sees that the problem causing the anger has not been solved. When this happens, it starts its process of communicating that these conflicts and lies exist and that they are creating unnecessary internal conflicts that need immediate resolution. In time, it will send this message again and again, until the conflict is resolved. If it is not resolved, the Subconscious Self will increase its effort to communicate and eventually the Stress Mechanism is triggered. At this time, the conditions needed to create illness are ultimately activated and take over.

When we initiate problem solving, we change this direction in a positive way. Our anger and negative emotions are released. The Stress Mechanism is shut down and the Healing and Repair Systems are left to take over and heal any damage or injury that has been created.

If anger persists and seethes internally, the person may develop illnesses, such as high blood pressure, autoimmune diseases, or even cancer. These illnesses often "appear" to strike suddenly, "out of nowhere," even though this process has already been building for many years.

While we always have the choice of loving our Body-Mind and ourselves fully, we can fall victim to our unresolved conflicts and end up despising and hating ourselves and those we blame for our predicament. We may forget that our choices are always creating who we are and the world around us. Simply by changing our choices, we can change our entire being, as well as our direction in life and within the world around us.

Those who lack this level of self-knowledge often believe that they have little or no control over their own destinies. They may turn against themselves. Our inability or unwillingness to solve our problems and effect positive changes in our life or in our self-image may lead us to create great conflict between our conscious-aware self and our Body-Mind.

Remember, we always have the ability to change ourselves through using our free will and will power. By working through love, solving problems and conflicts, we can direct the Subconscious Self to create us to be healthy and well. It is this goal that we seek to accomplish through the information we are providing in this book. With a greater understanding of the power of our Conscious, Subconscious and Higher selves, working separately and together, each of us can transform illnesses into wellness, and transform our own unhappy lives into lives filled with joy and happiness for our loved ones and for ourselves.

OTHER IMPORTANT ASPECTS
OF THE CONSCIOUS SELF-BODY-MIND RELATIONSHIP

We each have the ability to use our conscious life-force energy (will power), to think, imagine, and create thought patterns that act as positive instructions to our Body-Mind. The Body-Mind acting on these instructions will then construct whatever we asked. An example of this is when we think of something we want to do and then we put sufficient energy, positive thoughts, planning and action into getting it, we usually end up bringing our desires to fruition.

For an illustration of how the Conscious and Subconscious Selves work together, consider the following: Suppose you desire a glass of water. You think to yourself, "I am thirsty. I would love a glass of water." Initially, this is only a thought, but it is also a communication and set of instructions to your Body-Mind. The Body-Mind, hearing the request for a glass of water, causes your body to get up out of its chair, go to the sink, reach for a glass, pour the water, return to your seat, and proceed to bring the glass to your lips so that you can drink the water. Once the water is consumed, the Body-Mind knows exactly what to do with it and does what is needed with no further help from the Conscious Self.

We ask and even demand what we want from our Body-Mind repeatedly, day in, and day out. It is the Body-Mind's job to give us everything we ask for.

To re-enforce this concept, let us look at another even more dramatic example. When you get into your car, you simply think where you want to go. You may or may not say it aloud. Your Body-Mind then takes over. It looks for the right key, places it into the ignition, turns the ignition on, backs the car out of the garage, and without the Conscious Self having to think or act, the Subconscious Self drives you to your destination. If you believe that you, your Conscious Self, is always in control, then answer this question: "How is it that you may start out traveling to a particular location and then once there not remembering the streets you took or the turns you made?" You may have been talking to someone, listening to the radio, or thinking the entire time you were driving. Yet, you arrived safely at your destination. You arrived as if the car was being piloted by an automatic pilot. In this case, the automatic pilot is your Subconscious Self, your Body-Mind.

While this is the mechanism of our successes in life, it is also the mechanism of our failures. Since our thoughts become the personal architects of our lives, we must truly be careful what we think about and what we wish for, because we will indeed get it.

Since the Conscious Self experiences reality through its conditioning, it is often programmed to accept the belief systems of others as law, allowing these foreign beliefs to have power over us[10]. The Conscious Self in turn programs the Body-Mind to create a self-image based on who it believes we are. This is often based on our past life experiences, past self-image, and prior life choices. If the choices created a view of life that is faulty, the Body-Mind will be programmed accordingly. Conflicts often arise when the Body-Mind recognizes that beliefs sent to it by the Conscious Self are faulty or differ from what it knows is true, and that a lie or conflict exists.

---

10   *Consider the motor vehicle laws set by your state legislature, how fast you can drive, where and when you can speed up or slow down, which lane you should drive in, what intersections you can make a U-Turn in and which you can't, or which side and when you can pass other vehicles. We drive by these rules following them relentlessly and soon they become so much of a part of us we do them automatically without even having to think.*

Once the Subconscious Mind recognizes that these views and beliefs are faulty or create conflict, it acts to secure your ultimate survival by letting you know you are operating from lies and potentially dangerous faulty belief systems. It believes and acts as if it is obligated to tell you when an unresolved conflict exists so that you can resolve them and in doing so increase your ability to survive.

Because the Conscious Self sees the world around it through various sets of filters (belief systems, previous decisions, memories, prejudices, biases, blocks and complexes and its own inflexibilities), it may at times misinterpret what it is experiencing – and because of this it makes mistakes. If it immediately corrects these mistakes, no conflict occurs. If it learns from its mistakes, it grows. If it does not correct these mistakes, the Body-Mind eventually signals that an error exists.

The Conscious Self only knows the truth it wants to know or is willing to hear. Without being willing to listen to the Body-Mind, we develop blind spots, hearing, feeling, or seeing only what we want to believe.

If we listen to the Body-Mind, we grow. If we don't, conflict may ultimately arise and our self-image may become damaged. When conflict occurs, the stress mechanism is triggered. If not resolved, illness and chronic disease can result.

Why are there such differences between these two parts of us? The answer is simple: the two Selves each have very different roles. Also, they are very different entities. The Conscious Self is awake, alert and alive in the now-moment. Its ultimate role is helping us survive in society. To do this, it requires us to be flexible and to be able to think on our feet. The Body-Mind, on the other hand, lives without time, and its role of protecting our individual survival allows it less freedom.

SUMMARY

The Conscious Self's role is looking for food, social contact, and shelter while the Body-Mind digests the food, uses shelter to protect itself, and social contact to feel accepted, loved, and protected. While the Conscious Self interacts socially, the Body-Mind stands ready to react if the combined Selves are threatened. The Conscious Self explores the world; the Body-Mind gives it the energy to do so. The two cannot exist without each other. In order to exist in the moment-to-moment reality, the Conscious Self requires an uncluttered awareness of its immediate circumstances. The Conscious Self counts on our Body-Mind to store within its memory banks, everything that it has ever heard, seen, thought, felt or experienced. To accomplish this, our Body-Mind filters all sensory inputs and then stores these sensory inputs along with all past memories in the Subconscious Self. It stores information so that it can remain clear minded and always ready to learn, grow, and protect itself. This information must be instantly available. Without this fund of knowledge, survival could be impaired.

When these two Selves are out of sync or in opposition to each other, a number of things happen. At the lowest level is anxiety or a sense of conflict, and the Conscious Self may not be sure what is causing it. Another result might be confusion. There may be memory blackouts, memory loss (long- and short-term memories). Because of this, memories may be partial and/or inaccurate and at the extreme is illness. This process will be discussed and illustrated in the remainder of this book.

Chapter Seven

THE BODY-MIND

WHAT IS THE BODY-MIND?

The Subconscious Mind is the "mind" of the body, or the Body-Mind, is always working. Subconscious Mind never sleeps. It is always working. It works 24-hours a day, seven days a week, 365-days a year. It works every day of every year of our life, from conception to death. It is always present and operating, and we have full access to it all the time, even when we sleep. It never sleeps. Only when the person dies, does their Body-Mind stop working.

Even with all of this, most people are unaware of its existence. In the previous chapters, we provided some general information regarding how we can know that it is always working for us. The illusion that our Conscious Self is much more dynamic or even more important than our Body-Mind is caused by the fact that during childhood the Conscious Mind learns how to tune out the Body-Mind and hence it will often stop paying attention to it. The fact is that there is so much going on in the Body-Mind if we were suddenly to become aware of all of this information and sensations operating within it at any given moment, we would likely lose control of our ability to function.

The Body-Mind checks through all sensory input on a microsecond-by-microsecond basis ensuring that there is nothing inside or outside of us threatening or negatively affecting our immediate survival. As stated earlier, the Body-Mind operates the automatic functions of the body – digestion, breathing; heartbeat; endocrine glands; body chemistry; maintenance; temperature regulation; and the body's defensive, offensive, healing, and repair systems. It easily and effortlessly runs all of our organ systems, endocrine glands, chemistry, nervous and defensive systems, and much more. If all of these functions were handled by Conscious Self, we would quickly become overwhelmed and bogged down simply from trying to cope with bodily functions even before we would be capable of starting to check sensory system inputs.

Another reason that we may be unaware of the Body-Mind's existence is that we don't know how to reach it in the now-moment. While we can command it to do what we want, we cannot talk to it and expect verbal responses to our questions. If you ask a simple question, such as "Tell me what you want from me?" Do not expect to get any meaningful answer in words. However, you may experience emotions, memories, dreams, or physical feelings such as fear, tension, and relaxation. The Body-Mind may give you hints, but they will be buried or hidden deep within sensory impressions and "feelings." This is the only way the Body-Mind can communicate or respond to your questions.

When we tell our body to run, jump, stand up or lie down and it does, the Conscious Self generally assumes that it had in fact made all of these happen. The Conscious Self, however, does not take these occurrences as proof positive that the Body-Minds actually exists. In our Western, science-based society, most people are unwilling to recognize the power and value of the Body-Mind simply because it functions behind the scenes, automatically, below their level of conscious awareness. What they can't see, they just won't believe.

The Body-Mind filters out everything it does not consider important. It takes the raw data presented by our sensory systems and it decides what is meaningful and then selects only what it believes is important in the now-moment. It sends only this information to the Conscious Self. It places only this information into our conscious awareness. All other information is stored for later recall, should it be needed. Generally very little information is either thrown away or lost.

The Body-Mind constantly takes in a large amount of information from the outside. Even prior to its next thought or sensory intake, it already has a vast body knowledge from past experience as well as from our genetic code. All this information and the instructions which run this process operate below the consciousness level. This leaves the Conscious Self to do the work it needs to do to maintain our life and intelligence. Our body's genetic coding provides detailed and specific instructions on how everything in our body will work. All of these processes are therefore mediated by the DNA of our genes to create and operate our body and our Body-Mind. This includes instinctive memories and species-specific memories, as well as what C.G. Jung called, "the collective unconsciousness." Unfortunately, our Body-Mind can and often does become conflicted, even with everything it knows. This is especially true when the Conscious Self gives it mixed or contradictory instructions. If the Conscious Self is confused or misdirected by its desires, likes and dislikes, it can eventually misdirect or confuse the Body-Mind. This causes conflict that it wants to resolve and undo.

While the Body-Mind is essential to the body's operation, it requires the Conscious Self to deal with making life decisions and social functioning. The Conscious Self must operate without worrying about automatic functions.

The Body-Mind's ability to do its job frees the Conscious Self to function freely and unrestricted within the conscious world.

It must be clear by now that the Body-Mind has many crucial attributes that are important to a healthy person's overall functioning. It makes no decisions. It simply reacts to instructions from genetics, built-in instincts, and memories specific to the species and most important, instructions from the Conscious Self. In a sense, it is a slave or robot in the way it reacts and deals with these instructions.

If the Conscious Self is strong and centered, the Body-Mind will better understand, evaluate, and work with its instructions. The Body-Mind can apply no new conditions or make changes in what has been asked of it. If it is told by you to create you to be totally healthy and well, it will do exactly that. If it interprets the instructions you give so that it believes that you believe that you should be sick or that you want to be sick, it will create conditions that ultimately lead to illness. It will do this just as faithfully as it would create perfect health for you.

The Body-Mind cannot make judgments regarding what is right or wrong, good or bad. This is why it is so extremely important to pay marked attention to what you say and think. If you allow illness to happen, especially Stress-Related Disorders, this will likely be almost entirely a result of poor or faulty instructions that you have or are giving to your Body-Mind.

The Body-Mind is extremely powerful. It can accomplish nearly anything we ask of it that is within the human range of possibility and even then, it can accomplish some things that are considered to be outside of what is considered normal. We have all heard of situations where an individual is spontaneously "cured" from cancer or when a 110-pound mother lift's a 3,000-pound car to rescue her child. These kinds of super-human accomplishments are facilitated by the power of the Body-Mind. It is this power which, if used poorly or improperly, can work against us.

The Body-Mind holds every memory that belongs to that individual. It stores these memories in deep storage until the Conscious Self asks it to recall them. Generally, memories are not sent up to the Conscious Self unless there is a specific request for information. However, it is usual for memories to rise up and even flood the Conscious Self during times of conflict, in dreams, or in the form of emotions when the Body-Mind is trying to communicate information about unresolved conflicts.

The process of recall is usually so fast that we often believe that the Conscious Self holds these memories. Hence, we may say, "I remember," when in fact we can only really recall memories stored by the Body-Mind. The Body-Mind can do nothing with these memories except compare them against current situations to see if we are being threatened. It simply holds them suspended in storage until the Conscious Self calls for this specific information.

The Body-Mind is also the seat of our emotions. Emotions are simply belief systems that are connected positively or negatively to physical or mental events. They are then transformed from potential electrical data into active information and emotions upon the release of specific neurochemicals that trigger their release. Upon release these emotions create either positive or negative effect on the Body-Mind, as well as upon other parts of our body. Emotions generally manifest themselves as feelings, such as love, hate, anger, rage, and desire. When emotions are experienced, they may encompass the entire body or only certain parts of our body. Healthy emotions are simply positive belief systems embedded in the form of complex physical-chemical patterns within the Subconscious Self and the physical body. For example, sexual love is a positive emotion associated with desires, physiological needs, and urges to mate along with hormonal discharges stimulating these urges and activating increased sensitivity within the genital organs.

On the other hand, anger, hate, and fear are negative emotions encoded within the physical body in the form of hormonal-chemical changes that increase muscular tension and produce generalized negative feelings. These neuro-hormonal-electrical changes prepare the body for Fight-or-Flight, for mating, for freezing, or for whatever will help us cope within the present moment. While negative emotions activate the Stress Mechanism, positive emotions often diminish and even eliminate stress. While positive emotions tend to lead to an increased state of well-being and joy, negative emotions tend to lead to anxiety, stress, tension, fear, withdrawal or Fight or Flight.

Understanding this process is crucial to understanding the creation of stress and illness. Positive and negative emotions have similar physical and chemical reactions associated with them. The difference appears only that positive emotions lead to positive internal changes, such as relaxation; negative emotions lead to negative internal changes, activation of the Stress Mechanism and tension. While the physical and chemical differences between them are only slightly different, their outcome and results are markedly different. Have you ever experienced loving someone one moment and then hating them in the next moment? If so, then you have some idea how this works. What happens from one moment to the next are two things:

1. We can, at a moment's notice, change our belief systems from ones that are positively oriented, to ones that may be negatively oriented.
   • Here is an example: Tim comes home to his wife after being away for a week on a business trip. Brenda, Tim's wife, sorely misses him and sexually desires him. However, as they come together Brenda notice's lipstick on Tim's collar. Her positive, loving desires quickly turn to suspicion, rage, anger, and jealousy.
2. Events can trigger memories of past positive or negative experiences.
   • Here is an example: Suzie is generally a happy person. However, every time someone brings up her ex-husband's name, her neck tightens and she becomes angry and upset.

In both cases, nothing changed in these people's life except that they suddenly changed what they were thinking or believing at a particular moment in time. Brenda was happy when she had positive thoughts about Tim. Her entire demeanor rapidly changed when she was suddenly confronted with the possibility that Tim might have been cheating on her. She had no real meaningful evidence, but she did have what we might normally think of as a "smoking gun," lipstick on his collar. The lipstick on Tim's collar instantly changed her belief about Tim's love and fidelity. While Tim may well have a perfectly rational explanation for this, Brenda's fears and jealousies grabbed her and she immediately changed her way of thinking, as well as her mood and emotions, in the moment.

Suzie is happy when her ex-husband is not in the picture. The mere mention of her ex-husband's name triggers a host of unresolved conflicts, fears, anger, rage and feeling of threat, as well as painful memories. In as little as one second all of the emotions and the physical discomforts that go along with them, may surface and take hold of Suzie's common sense and normal demeanor.

The Body-Mind is in charge of most if not all of the negative feelings or thoughts our Conscious Self has repressed into its memory. The Body-Mind is often filled with unexpressed and unresolved feelings, emotions, and thoughts from our embryonic stages of life and throughout our lifetime. These unexpressed emotions, feelings, and thoughts cry out for their fulfillment and completion, which if they still exist has been denied to them during the process of living life. Some are associated with fear and previous threats (real or imagined) and may generate negative feelings; others are associated with positive feelings.

These emotionally loaded thoughts and belief systems can control the individual. In times of conflict or stress, these negative memories may suddenly rise to the surface. We refer to those unexperienced memories formed during childhood as belonging to the child part of us, or the Child Within. These unexpressed forces can have an effect on every important decision we make as adults, as well as many of the belief systems we ultimately hold. We will discuss this concept, the Child Within, in Chapter 8.

When the Conscious Self is disappointed or when the self-image doesn't match our desires or needs, there may then begin a process of denigration, insults, and self-depreciation. When these negative thoughts are sent down to the Body-Mind, they are ultimately integrated into the Conscious Self and Body-Mind's image of the "self." If this happens often enough, a framework is created within which our Subconscious Self begins feeling unloved, unappreciated, inferior, and diminished.

This presents a problem for two reasons. First, the Body-Mind needs love and truth for stability. These are as important to our Body-Mind as food and air are to the body. Second, since our Body-Mind believes almost everything it is told, a conflict may be created between older, positive memories and the newer, negative information or vice-versa.

This may cause significant conflict that destabilizes the body-mind and undermines its ability to function positively.

For example, a young boy feels conflict when his father is unable to spend time with him. He may come to his father and say, "Daddy, why don't you play with me like Paul's father plays with him?" His Conscious Self is experiencing rejection because it holds memories of Paul's experience with his father and compares this to his own experience with his father. Since his own experience doesn't match Paul's, a conflict occurs. The child's Conscious Self may believe that something is wrong with him. This may lead him to feel unworthy or believe that his father doesn't love him, or that his father doesn't love him as much as Paul's father loves Paul. With time, his Conscious Self may look for other evidence to determine how much his father does or does not love him. He may create other comparisons. If he finds no clear evidence that his father loves him, he may conclude that his father really doesn't love him at all. He soon forgets about Paul and Paul' father and simply tells himself, "My father does not love me!"

If we accept the belief that there is only one real sin, "the intentional hurt or injury to ourselves or to others," then this young man's new way of thinking may cause him pain and hurt. He may feel that he has done something wrong, that in some way he has "sinned." Yet, the only sins he may have committed were the lies (misinterpretation of information – faulty comparisons) that he now believes about himself and his father.

As we are exposed to more of the real world, our Body-Mind begins finding it increasingly difficult to believe and also hold on to some or all of these negative thoughts, belief systems, and lies. At this point, wisdom begins setting in. The Body-Mind begins uncovering and knowing the truth about life. Eventually, it may refuse to believe some or all of the lies and faulty belief systems it previously accepted without question. However, since it cannot specifically do anything about it, a state of conflict arises between the Body-Mind and the Conscious Self. To remedy this, the Body-Mind begins questioning its negative self-image. If the Conscious Self remains afraid or mired in its own negativity, conflict occurs between what the Conscious Self is telling the Body-Mind and what it knows to be true. Soon, the Body-Mind tries bringing the conflict up to the Conscious Self. While this can occur at any age, it often is associated with certain passages in life. Often, these passages are associated with marital or job problems, or other periods of stress.

At first, the Body-Mind might send this information to the Conscious Self in the form of dreams. These dreams may create strange emotions or fluctuations of emotions while asleep and later while wake. In the dream state, our Body-Mind may try communicating what it wants for us to know. These dreams may present clues. Unfortunately, they may be in a language or code that while known to the Body-Mind, is difficult for the Conscious Self to interpret. If the dreams are understood and the conflict is resolved, the process ceases and the individual grows and evolves.

If the dreams are ignored or we are unable to understand them, the Body-Mind begins invading the Conscious Self in its waking state. Sudden remembrances, overwhelming feelings, daydreams, and flashbacks may occur, as the previously suppressed material forces its way to the surface. Emotions, such as anger, depression, and memories of past traumatic experiences, may surface causing anxiety and even panic. This often occurs when least expected and most undesired. At first, the individual may resist these events. He may even begin thinking that there is something wrong with him. Because he does not understand this process and what it means, he may attribute it to "nerves," or to "going crazy," or he may externalize it and blame others.

This process has been given many different names. Some have called it anxiety, while others may call it "panic reactions," or "nervous breakdown." This is often what is happening when we see a teen going through a teenage rebellion or acting-out, or an adult is going through a midlife crisis. It may also be the basis of criminal behavior by those who are unaware of what and why it is happening, and then act out in antisocial ways such as breaking windows, shop lifting, bullying, drinking binges, even homicidal rages.

If still ignored, war may eventually break out between the Body-Mind and the Conscious Self. As we will see later, in its earliest stages, this war manifests itself as a series of vague physical signs and symptoms that are often the first consciously recognized concrete indications of conflict from within. The individual may not be capable of deciding whether physical, mental, emotional, or spiritual processes are involved. While the conflict's substance lies deep within the Body-Mind, the physical symptoms, and emotions that surface, tell us that the Body-Mind is trying to communicate with us.

Medical doctors are often unaware of the meaning of these symptoms and signs. They generally do not consider it their role to become involved in this type of process. Commonly, the medical profession ignores these vague symptoms and signs, or chooses to use drugs to reduce or control them rather than treating the problem's root cause. When the root causes are not found nor treated, these medical doctors' are actually working against their patients.

By prescribing medication, usually anti-anxiety or anti-depression meds, their treatment acts to cover up the Body-Mind's messages that there are unresolved conflicts, hence leaving the problems and associated conflicts unresolved. This process then progresses through its natural course and illness is often the end result unless resolved. The symptoms which are now being manifested may be perceived by the individual and others, as signs of physical, mental, emotional, or spiritual instability rather than as information about unresolved conflicts which desperately need resolution.

The overlay of various combinations of physical, emotional, spiritual, and mental symptoms and signs are often confusing to both the patient and physician.

It is hard for the individual to know whether his problems require a medical doctor, a psychologist, a psychiatrist, clergy, or good counseling by an accountant, lawyer, or other professional.

When this person first sees a medical doctor, if this doctor is not knowledgeable about what is happening or what to do, the doctor may end up hurting the patient rather than helping him. While the physician's motives may be good, the result is that the Conscious and Subconscious Selves are first impressed that they are going to be seen by a doctor but then recognize that once again they are being ignored or abandoned and simply they are left all alone to do battle with each other. Ultimately, depending upon who wins – the Body-Mind by re-establishing harmony and balance or the Conscious Self by suppressing the truth – the result is either increased health and well-being, or increased illness and eventually chronic debilitating disease or even death.

If external forces, such as parents, teachers, siblings, friends, spouses, or employers, denigrate the individual or support his illness, the process may quicken. To what extent this affects the process depends upon how well the normal, healthy parts or our self are able to restore or maintain balance in the face of adversity.

GUILT, HATE, ANGER AND HOSTILITY IN CREATING ILLNESS

A frequently asked question is about the role guilt, hate, anger, and hostility play in creating illness. In an otherwise emotionally healthy person, guilt may occur from within the Body-Mind or within the Conscious Aware Self whenever that person intentionally or unintentionally causes hurt to himself or to another. This hurt does not have to either actually happen or be real; guilt can occur when the individual fantasizes about causing a hurt, or when they think they have caused a hurt even when no hurt ever actually occurred. Guilt can also rise out of not making proper amends for a real or imagined hurt. When guilt is not dealt with appropriately, it may lead to shame. Shame occurs when we do not meet our own "Personal" criteria or life ethics. This may occur even when our personal criteria and ethics may be created by us for us or if they may have been adopted from others and taken as our own. When we create an intentional hurt, we may feel dishonored or ashamed of our behavior and of our self. That is, one or both the Body-Mind or the Conscious Aware Self may feel dishonored or ashamed.

From shame and frustration arises anger. Anger is most often generated from either unexpressed hurt about an event or action of another or ourselves, whether real or imagined. Anger can occur when we do not get what we think is due to us or what belongs to us. It can occur either as anger directed inwardly, self-anger, and arising from our own actions, real or imagined, as well as from faulty beliefs we hold against ourselves or others. It can also be directed at someone or something outside of us, such as anger at a parent, child, boss, or stranger, or even an object or place we believe caused hurt or harm to us. When this happens, it is often because we believe that something this other person said or did or didn't say or do or their actions cause hurt to us or someone or something we love or care about. When this happens, we may become angry at them. For example, becoming angry with a parent for not giving us what we believed we needed or wanted, hence causing us or our life to turn out differently that we thought that it should have turned out.

THE STORY OF MARTIN R. IS AN EXCELLENT EXAMPLE OF THIS CONCEPT:

Martin R.'s parents were immigrants. They spoke with heavy European accents; their ways were very Old World. Martin was the older of two children. He was conceived before his parents arrived in America, and was born in New York shortly after they arrived in the United States.

From early in his life, Martin was ashamed of his parents. They were different from his friends' parents. His father was authoritarian. He would yell at Martin in his Old World tongue, wave his fists, and threaten to whip him whenever he believed that Martin was threatening his authority. His mother, like an Old Country peasant woman, was also different from the mothers of the other children Martin knew. She was subservient to his father, yet she was also outspoken, having opinions about everything.

Once Martin started school, he became a loner. Even when other children tried to be friendly, he would ignore them or tell them he was too busy to talk or get together. One day when his mother came to school, he ignored her and pretended that he didn't know her.

Throughout his formative years, Martin had been a dreamer. He would go to his special hiding place and think about how wonderful his life would be in the future. One morning, his father told him that the family was going to a family affair, but Martin was so ashamed of his family that he refused to go. He and his father argued and Martin was finally left at home. That night he had the first of many blinding headaches. During the next several months, his headaches became progressively more severe. He was taken to the family doctor, who told his parents that Martin was just a very high-strung child and wrote a prescription for pain medication.

By the time Martin was 20, he was taking two different medications for his "migraine headaches." While the medications reduced his pain, they didn't stop the headaches from occurring.

By age 30, he had undergone just about every test known to science to find out why he was having these headaches. One doctor told him that he had a brain tumor, another that his headaches were a form of epilepsy, another that they were stress headaches, still another that they were due to sinus problems requiring surgery. All tests done on him were normal. They showed no tumor, no sinus problems, or any other reasons for the headaches.

Once we started working with Martin, it soon became clear that his headaches were caused by his own guilt and the shame he felt over hating his parents. At first, this was hard for him to believe, as he could not see a relationship between these two things. We helped him look back to the first time he had a headache and remember what he was feeling at that time and immediately after. Soon, he was able to see the relationship between his negative feelings and the tension they created, and how the tension and guilt he experienced triggered his headaches. Once he was able to see these relationships, he was able to begin the process of forgiving himself and his parents. He was soon able to live without any further headaches or pain and without any need for medication.

Martin had been angry with his parents because they were not the way he had wanted them to be. He was angry with himself because he could not accept his family, and because deep down inside, he knew that they were good people who loved him. His inability to reconcile these issues created a significant internal conflict. Through our working with him, Martin soon realized that his loneliness during childhood was self-imposed because of his shame about his parents, his not wanting to have other children meet his parents, and his feelings of unworthiness for being ashamed. To protect himself from feeling guilty, he projected his self-hate to his parents, "It was all their fault!"

This was almost entirely a Conscious Self process. However, his Body-Mind recognized the conflict, his lies, and the many faulty belief systems from which he was operating and initiated a process communicating to him that a conflict existed that needed resolution. His unwillingness to deal with this issue, his displeasure, and negativity undermined his Mind-Body's intention to resolve these inappropriate actions and beliefs. The whole conflict is simply "a headache!"

The Conscious Self does not always want to deal with negative thoughts or belief systems, especially when these experiences or beliefs have strong emotional roots. In order to avoid dealing with unpleasant issues the Conscious Self may simply push the memories or thoughts about them into the Subconscious Self, out of its awareness. In this case this hurt him and his parents and this lie went on for years and decades, pushing up periodically from the Body-Mind as headaches when it wanted to encourage solution to his conflicts and create peace and harmony in the family.

When solutions are not created, the Body-Mind may force the issue, trying to get the attention of the Conscious Self so that it can solve the previously unresolved conflict or conflicts. It may do this in the form of strong emotions (anxiety, depression, anger, guilt, etc.), dreams as well as physical signs, symptoms and illness. It wants these issues resolved, and it will do whatever it needs to do to make this happen.

Unresolved suppressed anger often generates feelings of hostility. Eventually, this hostility may lead to anger and then eventually, rage. Rage wells up, pushes, and creates more conflict, which if not resolved, will once again lead to loss of power and control by the Subconscious and Conscious Selves. This does not necessarily happen at the same time. When the Body-Mind loses control, the person may experience episodes of anxiety or even panic attacks, helplessness, illness or all of these and more problems. When the Conscious Self loses control, it may have temper tantrums, confusion, obsession, exhibitions of anger, or acting out.

Hostility, unlike rage, is often expressed internally and against the "Self." The suppression of emotions limits the expression of true feelings. Because of this process, we lose control over a part of our self, who and what we are, and our place in the universe. This loss of control, anger, rage, hostility, anxiety, panic, or depression may each present a threat to our ultimate survival. Because of these threats, our Stress Mechanism is likely to be activated.

The continued suppression of feelings, thoughts, and emotions caused by unresolved negative emotions and conflicts can lead to further loss of control and may eventually become transformed into external outbursts of violence. If not positively directed, these outbursts may lead to more hostility against the Self or toward others or the community as a whole. When this happens, there may be suicidal thoughts or actions, or antisocial or even criminal behavior. In one sense this may be good , since, as the individual moves to his or her "dark side," their Body-Mind may become so overwhelmed with the many issues it is processing that it simply gives up. Should the individual become a sociopath neither his Body-Mind or Conscious Aware Self may be able to take care or muster action to try to control what this individual now thinks or does.

When our internal conflicts are not resolved, and they are of sufficient magnitude for the Body-Mind to want resolution, lack of resolution may trigger the Wellness-Stress-Disease Mechanism. While illness and disease are internal manifestations of faulty belief systems, lies, crime and lawlessness, antisocial, homicidal and suicidal behaviors are all external manifestations of these same processes.

Another possibility may occur when anger, shame, guilt, and rage are not handled appropriately and hence ultimately lead to a state of depression, hopelessness or apathy. When unresolved conflicts are left unresolved the Conscious Aware Self or Body-Mind may give up or begin to recognize and believe that they will never be resolved, maybe even that they can never really be loved nor fully do their jobs. Over time this is what leads to feelings of depression, hopelessness and eventually apathy. When depression or apathy are extreme, the person may be capable of suicidal acting out or trigger lethal processes, such as cancer or autoimmune disorders.

The Conscious Aware Self lives in a world of duality, us versus them, good versus bad, right versus wrong, and love versus hate. The Body-Mind lives in a world of singularity. The Body-Mind literally builds our personal world for us. It does this based mostly on what the Conscious Aware Self believes and occasionally what it feels or experiences. Since most of what we believe is based on social programming – our education, past experiences and the belief systems of others that we have adopted as our own – the Conscious Aware Self can easily find itself confused and conflicted.

The Body-Mind's knowledge of the outside world comes from two main sources. These are, first, what it learns from its sensory systems and the information they provide, and second, what the Conscious Aware Self tells it. What it receives from the sensory organs is direct information; what it receives from the Conscious Aware Self is indirect information. The Conscious Aware Self makes decisions and establishes belief systems almost entirely based on its life experiences and what it learns from others: history books, newspapers, media, etc. It may, however, pick and choose what it wants to focus on and eliminate whatever it considers either uninteresting or unimportant to its survival. In doing so, it creates a personal and a global or world view, most all of which is either belief or opinion. This filtered information is not necessarily always real or meaningful.

On a daily basis we are constantly bombarded with sensory input, much of which is not important to the Conscious Aware Self. For example, since our sensory system extends out many feet from our body, we often hear things that are neither important to our survival nor to the Conscious Aware Self. When we read books, magazines or newspapers, watch TV, listen to the radio, visit with friends, or walk through public places, the Body-Mind is constantly receiving information and sending what it believes is meaningful up to the Conscious Aware Self. The Conscious Aware Self then selects what interests it and ignores the rest.

The Conscious Aware Self may decide that some piece of information is superfluous, and eliminate it or simply store it for future use. If it needs this information at any time, it is likely available through recall. However, if not requested, the Conscious Aware Self may never even be aware of its existence. This process can lead to conflicts and dualities when others may believe that we are aware of certain information when our Conscious Aware Self does not openly remember.

The same is true of suppressed memories and thoughts. We may think thoughts or feel emotions that are either fearful or violate our moral code. Rather than dealing with these thoughts or feelings, we often simply suppress them – out of sight, out of mind. This immediately creates the potential for a conflict. If not resolved, it can create problems sometime in the future. This also creates another potential duality between the way the Conscious Aware Self sees the world and the way the Body-Mind sees the world. Since the Conscious Aware Self lives in the now-moment, it may feel the need for some sort of immediate action while the Body-Mind may disagree.

An example might occur where the Conscious Aware Self sees something it wants and decides that taking it is acceptable. However, the Body-Mind, reviewing its data banks, may find that this is stealing and conclude that stealing is wrong. Since the Body-Mind does not have the power to tell this directly to the Conscious Aware Self, it can only express itself in feelings, emotions, and thoughts. If the Conscious Aware Self then gives a command to the Body-Mind to create the actions necessary to steal the item, the Body-Mind must obey. While the Body-Mind does what it is told, it may still experience guilt, as the action it has just taken or has been instructed to take, will likely cause hurt to another. At this point, the Conscious Aware Self has two alternatives: one is to continue with the theft, the other is to heed the Body-Mind's voice and move away from the item. The Conscious Aware Self may then override the Body-Mind, "I want it. I have a right to it. I am going to take it. It is mine!" Or it can suddenly come to its senses, "Stealing is wrong. I know I will feel awful if I do this." "I know I could get into legal problems as a result of this and I don't want that stigma or expense."

Another problem created by these dualities is that the Conscious Aware Self sees the world the way it wants to see it rather than as it actually is. An example occurs when one person sees a certain action performed by another as person as cruel and/or dangerous, even while another person might well see this same action as loving and kind. For example: a parent allowing a child to do something that is dangerous, while the parent feels that the child needs to take risks in order to grow up strong and survive. Through the years, repeated experiences with such dualities can confuse us as to who or what is right, and who or what is wrong. Both the Conscious Aware Self and the Body-Mind can become confused about who they are and what they are doing. Hence, we as individuals may easily become confused about our purpose, goals, and experiences of life.

This is the construct of duality within which the Conscious and Subconscious Selves live and operate. Often, their confusion is more because they are unaware of each other than it is caused by external events that occur around them. The Conscious Aware Self's confusion and ambivalence may manifest as strong emotions, physical signs, and symptoms that may seem to surface from out of nowhere. The Body-Mind, in its attempt to maintain harmony and balance, may find itself frustrated, angry, outraged, or ill while also experiencing love and caring and a desire to live and be healthy. Understanding the existence of these two aspects of the two Selves is an essential key to re-establishing harmony and balance, and wellness for both.

Ultimately, our world view (our totality of belief systems about the world around us), is created from the input and values we accumulate during our life process. It is also significantly influenced by the beliefs and teachings of a few important authority figures in our lives as well as by school, literature, movies, TV, music, and the like. Certainly, our parents, teachers, and society in general each play an important role in determining who we are and who we will ultimately become. While the Body-Mind learns from all sides of issues it faces, the Conscious Aware Self may choose to give positive or negative power to one side or the other, or ignore both or any information it does not like or believe. Since the Conscious Aware Self wants to please others, it may change its view of the world instantly, usually in order to be accepted and loved. The Body-Mind is more consistent as to what it recognizes as right and wrong, or good and evil. This is another example of a duality that can ultimately lead to conflict.

While the Conscious Aware Self craves love and approval from other humans, the Body-Mind can only get love from the Conscious Aware Self and the Higher Self. The Higher Self always loves both. However, if the Body-Mind is contaminated by fear of loss of love from the Conscious Aware Self, it may well feel needy and even unloved. When this happens, it may totally disregard the "voice" of the Higher Self, feeling so needy for the Conscious Aware Self's love. This may lead to what we commonly think of as a "spiritual conflict." Many people's Body-Minds or Subconscious Selves live their entire lives starved for love and feeling unloved. When feeling unloved, the Body-Mind may not be entirely capable of acting in a loving way to itself, or even to the Conscious Aware Self, whose love it desperately desires. When the Conscious Aware Self desires or needs love, it may search for love everywhere and not find it. It may look for love where it can never find it. It may lose confidence in itself and it may give up become depressed, hopeless, and even apathetic.

Alternatively, when the Body-Mind is filled with warmth, caring, approval and love, its level of consciousness expands and it radiates love outward to include all the people in its world. This is often thought of as inner love or as self-love. The Body-Mind reflects the love it gets from the Conscious Aware Self back to the Conscious Aware Self and often to others. The Conscious Aware Self's appreciation of the Body-Mind is returned to it in the form of periodic surges of great energy and enthusiasm toward life, work, and the Conscious Aware Self's goals.

While a person who feels unloved may hide, contract, or pull away from others, the person who feels loved returns its bounty many times over to all around him, greatly benefiting his life and well-being.

Self-love is possibly the single most powerful tool we have for creating harmony, balance, and wellness. When we experience self-love, we are unwilling to tolerate lies or dishonesty in ourselves or in others. We are much less likely to allow negative thoughts, fears, or creation of any type of actions, beliefs, or thoughts that might cause hurt to ourselves or to others. When we experience self-love, we do not allow conflict, and we are much less likely to be afraid of anything. Love is an important tool for preventing and healing illness.

THE BODY-MIND, HEALTH AND WELLNESS

The interrelationship between health, wellness, and illness should be clear by now. The Body-Mind is the guardian of our physical well-being, health, and survival. It is the part of us that either keeps us healthy or causes us to become ill. It controls illness and wellness by its power over our immune and defensive systems, and its control over almost all of the bodily systems it governs. It controls the Stress Mechanism and how it affects us. It controls the autonomic nervous system and our critical bodily functions.

Through the instructions it is given, the Body-Mind decides how the physical body will fare in this life. Thus, it creates a strong will to live, or it sets us on a path toward illness and death. If we are unable to express our true feelings in the outer world, this will likely cause conflict within us, which then may be turned against us. If we lie to our self or others, this reflects back on us and how we think about ourselves. If we think angry thoughts, this can turn the world against us. If we are unloving, this can create our world to become an unloving place. If we are depressed, this can depress our nervous and our immune systems, and almost all other bodily functions. If we feel no energy, none will come to us. The Body-Mind directly reflects our will to live, and the realization of our potential.

While the Body-Mind has a good deal of creative power concerning how we experience the world, the Conscious Aware Self still has the final say. The Conscious Aware Self governs the Body-Mind, either directly or indirectly, even if it is unaware that the Body-Mind exists. If we recognize that the Body-Mind exists and we work to create healthy communications with it, it becomes healthy and keeps us healthy. If we ignore it, we may well find our self (the Conscious Aware Self) trapped in an unhealthy, confused, and helpless body, which is often the way people who suffer illness and disease describe themselves. The Body-Mind is our genie as it gives us what we desire, good or bad.

SUMMARY

The primary way the Conscious Aware Self helps the Body-Mind is through its communications with the Body-Mind and the factors to which it is exposed. The quality and character of the information and instructions sent to our Body-Mind is the key. While it is forming in uterus, during infancy, and childhood, we must give it love and truth. In our early formative years, this is the parents' role. If our parents themselves are emotionally and spiritually well, this is easy. If not, we suffer. This is the genesis of the so-called dysfunctional individual. Possibly, this is one of the more important meanings of the biblical saying, "The sins of the parents are visited on their children[11]." When we deal with parents who were themselves raised by confused, angry, or conflicted parents, it is common to find that their Conscious and Body-Mind Selves may be damaged and split, sometimes irreversibly so.

To prevent this breach, we must train our Conscious and Body-Mind Selves to work together. The Conscious Aware Self must operate from truth and love, and it must tell the Body-Mind exactly what it needs to know. It must not knowingly lie to or deceive the Body-Mind or itself.

---

11 *A prevalent idea of both Christians and Jews is in accord with the Ten Commandments, the 'sins of the parents were visited upon the children." While this may be recognized as religious law today; it by no means follows that all afflictions are the result of sin, at least as sin is described in the Bible.*

Whether we ask for what we want directly or indirectly is not the issue. What is important is creating a clear picture of what we want from our Body-Mind. Whatever our mental picture of our life looks like is what we will eventually get.

If this picture is vague, unclear, or confused, the Body-Mind gives us what it thinks we want – vagueness, loss of clarity, and confusion. If our picture is clear and realistic, it gives us clarity of purpose and real results. It is in this frame of reference that self-love is most important. If we love ourselves, then we are more likely to want the best and we will create a clearer picture. These pictures are welcomed by the Body-Mind and we will be more centered and comfortable with whom we are. When this happens, it gives love back to us. If we dislike or are unhappy with ourselves, the Body-Mind reflects our unhappiness with emptiness, or loss of self. Remember, you get what you ask for in life, so be careful of what you ask for.

Our Body-Mind needs the help of our Conscious Aware Self to live in the external world. We also need a caring and balanced Conscious Aware Self to maintain our inner world in harmony and balance. As suggested earlier, our Body-Mind does its job with or without our help. With the right help, it does it better. When we are injured, our Body-Mind heals us. It doesn't have to ask the Conscious Aware Self what to do or how to do it. It has built into it a clear picture of what we look like healed and well. It already has this blueprint and needs little outside instruction. It knows exactly what to do to return us to a complete, normal state of well-being.

However, this process may not work correctly if our Body-Mind is given confused and negative messages, or messages that are contrary to full and complete healing. Illness is a sign of discord and imbalance, of negative thoughts and lies, or of living an unhealthy lifestyle. When we live with negative messages, chaos, lies, and faulty belief systems, and negativity, we ask for imperfect results. Illness is not just the result of these conflicts, but is also part of the way the Body-Mind communicates with us that our lies, conflict, imbalances, and disharmonies exist and need resolution.

Health and wellness are signs of harmony and balance, positive belief systems and a positive lifestyle. Self-love and truth facilitate harmony and balance. Our Body-Mind wants us to survive and it will do everything it can to help us survive. All we need is to help it do its job well.

Chapter Eight

THE BODY-MIND AS THE CHILD WITHIN

THE CHILD WITHIN

In the previous chapter, we introduced the concept of the Child Within. We explained that since the Body-Mind possesses all our memories, it may at times respond from memories belonging to the child part of our self. The Child Within exists as a series of memories, real or imagined, resolved and unresolved. They may be good, loving, healthy memories or memories of conflicted events and experiences, even traumatic conflicts that are held within the Body-Mind.

One of the Body-Mind's primary roles is to help us resolve these persistent conflicts of childhood. We must do this to "clean our slate" so that we free ourselves from the obstructions and limitations that these negative, unresolved memories ultimately force upon us. This process is essential so that we maintain memories that protect our survival. It is important that we resolve all conflicts, memories, and experiences that could undermine our ultimate survival. It is an essential part of helping us to learn, grow, and evolve toward our highest, healthiest, and best Self. These old, negative, unresolved conflicts must be resolved so that we can safely and healthfully move forward into adulthood toward wisdom. They must also be resolved since they are our teachers. From them, we learn valuable lessons to help ensure our ultimate survival.

As described earlier, the Body-Mind will bring up to us these unresolved conflicts for our inspection and resolution when it feels this is necessary. When we resolve these conflicts, we free ourselves to move forward. When we cannot resolve these conflicts, they may act inappropriately and block healthy, sound decision-making. This of course can impair our ability to survive and thrive. This process triggers our Body-Mind to work as hard as is possible to notify the Conscious Aware Self that these conflicts exist and require resolution. We have tried to make it as clear as possible in subsequent sections why not dealing with these unresolved conflicts activates the Stress Mechanism and that this can lead to illness, increased risk of injury, chronic disease and even premature death.

The Body-Mind cannot always differentiate between the messages that come from the Conscious Aware Self and those that come from external sources. It is programmed to accept everything it hears, sees, feels, or experiences and register all as "fact[12]." It then organizes, files, and cross-files all of this information into an enormous and complex database of cross-references and relationships, which all must be remembered in order to ensure our survival. The Body-Mind associates each bit of information with every other piece of information already present in its database and classifies them accordingly in relation to time, place, situation and potential risk so that they are instantaneously retrievable at the first sign of danger. All this is done to provide instantaneous protection during times of emergency when our survival could be at stake.

Most of us are entirely unaware of the mass and bulk of all of our memories, thoughts, and feelings stored within the Body-Mind. A large number of these old memories exist since childhood when we were dependent, helpless, and had little understanding of the world around us. A time when we also had little, if any, experience solving problems. We know from scientific studies that humans start reacting to their environment, possibly even thinking, feeling, and remembering, almost from the instant of conception. We also know that this process continues until the last second of life. We think and remember when we are asleep, at rest, active, busy working, and even when we are under stress. Since, every thought, feeling, and experience is stored as a memory hence these memories can influence us long after we have experienced them.

Many of our memories are positive and come from love and the many nice things that happen to us, and what we learned from resolving day-to-day conflicts. Some memories, however, also originate from negative conflicts, painful, and often repressed experiences, as well as from traumas left unresolved or "incompletely experienced." When this happens, these memories often remain charged with negative emotion. They can later act as blocks that can prevent us from getting what we want in life. As previously stated, many of these memories come from our childhood when we were less understanding of the world and less capable of expressing and defending ourselves.

---

12   *As humans evolved, we did so living in very small groups, isolated from other groups. There were no newspapers, books, radio, or TV, only relatives, friends, and enemies. Generally, relatives were your allies and friends. You counted on them for your survival, and they counted on you for their survival. While there may have been castes, power struggles, or even backstabbing, when danger occurred, clan members worked together and could be trusted. Trust is in our genes and is essential for our survival. Hence, we frequently may trust what we hear, see, feel, think, and experience as truth, even when it is not.*

To Understand This Better, An Example May Be Helpful:

When we first saw Mattie L., she was 41 years old. She came to us with a list of illnesses that would take the next two pages to list. She had high blood pressure, heart problems, was obese, and had serious marital and emotional problems. She was unable to let go of her only son who was just graduating high school. Because of an extremely low self-image, she hadn't held a job for many years.

She suffered frequent anxiety and panic attacks. Mattie had been seen by many different doctors and was taking a shopping bag full of medications each day. She was under psychiatric care. In spite or all of this Mattie was also an extremely bright woman.

Mattie was one of those people neither of us could ever forget. When we first met her, she was wearing a tight pants suit. It was white and had two crossed six shooters embroidered over each shoulder. It was an outfit more like what a 6-year-old girl might wear when role playing at being a cowgirl.

Mattie was looking for another doctor, one who could finally "cure" her of all her problems. Her first words were, "I've seen many doctors and none of them have cured me. Do you think that you can cure me?"

Mattie was very unwilling to assume responsibility for her life and current health situation.

After working with her for a short while it soon became clear that Mattie was fixated within her 6-year-old self and that her 6-year-old self controlled her. It took several visits to understand why. When Mattie was six, her father walked out of her life and divorced her mother. Mattie felt abandoned. She could never let go of the fear, anger, hurt, and rage that her 6-year-old self experienced. Her Body-Mind decided to stay at 6 years of age and wait for him to come back to her and make everything right. She also blamed herself (actually her 6-year-old self), as she believed that she must have done something to make her father leave.

In one discussion, she openly confided that she was unwilling to accept her father's leaving and always believed that he would return. When we asked her whether he ever did "return," she quickly answered, "No! But I always knew he wanted to."

It was clear that her child within was so badly hurt that it was trying to control her life so she would never be hurt again. As her father's leaving had been out of her control, relinquishing control would leave her open for further hurt and pain. Her 6-year-old self remained the dominant force for the next 35 years of her life. However, her problems had recently intensified when her husband (who had been extremely standoffish to her for the past 15 years) got tired of her childlike behavior and told her that he would be leaving when their son went off to college.

Mattie could not change. Her 6-year-old self would not relinquish control, and soon she was off to another therapist and another doctor searching for someone who would solve her problems for her. Her husband left her soon after their son left for college, and then she lived all alone.

I, Allen, recognized one such dilemma within myself a number of years ago. However, until recently I had no way of "fixing" it that is, until I began understanding the relationship between my Conscious Aware Self, my Body-Mind, and the concept of the Child Within. Then, I was finally able to overcome my own conflicts and really begin solving my own unresolved childhood conflicts.

When I was seven, I was an awkward kid, not at all sports minded. I was one of those kids who was always among the last chosen to play baseball. On one occasion, after all of our baseball team players were picked, it was decided by the team captain, that I was to be the first-base umpire. For the first couple of innings all went well, but in the fourth inning, I had an experience that changed my life.

A runner came toward first base – and so did the ball. I saw the ball reach the first baseman just before the runner reached the base. I saw the first baseman tag the runner out, and so I called the runner out.

The runner's team surrounded me, yelling at me that I was wrong, that the runner was safe. I stood my ground, sure of what I had seen.

Suddenly the first baseman's team surrounded me also and, instead of arguing with the runner's team, they were yelling at me saying that I was wrong. I became extremely confused. Everything slowed down until everything seemed in slow motion. I knew what I had seen and I fully intended to stand by it, but at that point, I didn't know what to do. I was overwhelmed, confused, and disoriented. I remained insistent that the runner was out. I was the umpire; it was my job to make a decision and stick to it. The players then threw me out of the game and put the runner back on first.

This was a child's game, insignificant in the scheme of things. Yet, for years after, I was unable to confidently make decisions. I became paralyzed in decisions dealing with one or more people. I didn't want to fail again. I didn't want to feel threatened again.

This crippled me emotionally for many years. Then, as I began to understand the relationship between my Conscious Mind, my Body-Mind, and the Child Within, I finally realized that this was only one day, one moment, in my history. Initially, I believed that I had only two choices. Either agree with the players and admit I was wrong, or stand behind my decision and insist that I was right. Yet, I ultimately recognized a third way – one in which no one and everyone were right. There were no winners, no losers; no one would ever really know what was true.

I chose to make no one wrong but rather to recognize that I did my best. I called it as I saw it and that I was being my highest, healthiest, and best Self at that moment. I accepted their apologies (in absentia) for not being willing to recognize that I did my best. I forgave them for the differences we held, and then I forgave myself for all the negative feelings I felt about them. The incident was closed. I returned to the now-moment where decisions had to be made and I was ready to make them, whether my decisions were popular or not. I swore that I would always operate from my inner truth, highest, healthiest and best Self. The situation was resolved and other than for relating this story in this book, I have not thought about it in many years.

These two situations are demonstrations of how the Child Within operates. However, in most situations the effects of the Child Within may be more subtle. There may be no conscious memory. The individual's behavior may not be so severely affected. The only indication might be illness. For example, take the individual who is brought up believing that every winter he is going to catch a cold, and so he does. Think about the young girl whose parents told her that she was destined to be married and have children and that she should have no aspirations beyond this. Think about the child who is told repeatedly that she is stupid or that he is a failure. Alternatively, the child who could never make anything of himself in school and decides that he is worthless. Think about those who feel so unloved as children that they spend the rest of their lives trying to find love, in all the wrong places.

Everyone reading this section will likely have one or more stories of their own to tell. The Child Within is still affecting them, whether for their good or ill. It is part of growing up and reaching adulthood. It is important that we learn how to eliminate those negative forces that act against our well-being. Constantly re-balancing and re-harmonizing our lives are also part of the process of growing up. If people are unaware or unable to do this on their own, they should seek help.

Our Body-Mind has no concept of either time or space. Everything that affects it does so in the now-moment. The past is now, the present is now, and the future is now. When you think about something that happened years ago, you feel the same emotions as you felt then. This demonstrates the power and effect of the Child Within on you at any moment in time. This is why we may experience feelings of hurt and pain today because of something that happened many years ago. It is also why we can experience fear, frustration, anger, and hurt for something that has not actually happened, but might happen in the future. It is why the pain and emotional sensations feel so real when we are reliving long-repressed experiences or we anticipate events occurring in the future.

WORKING WITH THE BODY-MIND

The way to work with the Body-Mind is simply to ask for what you want and create a clear picture of the end result. This picture acts as a template that the Body-Mind uses to construct what you desire. This is the key to working with the Body-Mind, freeing it from negative influences.

Your Body-Mind loves you. It wants you to survive. It will do anything to help you. It will give you anything you ask for that is in its power to give. It will even tell you answers you need to free yourself. All you need to do is ask it to tell you what is upsetting it or making it unhappy and it will tell you.

There is however, one hitch in this. You must be willing and ready to hear its answers. Often, the Body-Mind may not have had as good an experience as it would have liked to have with you listening to it in the past. It is likely that many times in the past it has tried to help you or communicate with your Conscious Aware Self, only to be rebuffed or ignored. Most of us have lied and cheated our Body-Mind so many times that it may not believe that we really are interested in hearing or believing what it has to say.

It is possible that many times in the past when situations like this occurred, you may well have sworn to yourself that you would do something about it but in the end you took no action at all. You had lied to your Body-Mind. Each time you made a promise to yourself and didn't keep it, you lied again and again. Each time you acted in a way that was detrimental to your best interests, you cheated it. In fact, you may find that you have lied to it more often than you realize.

If you are a smoker, an overeater, a gambler, or a drinker, you are not only putting yourself at risk, you are also putting your Body-Mind at risk. If you keep saying you are going to quit but don't, you are lying to it. If you are a business-man with good intentions that you never fulfill, or a mother who forgets your promises to your children, a father who can't keep his word; in each case, you have been lying, cheating, and undermining your Body-Mind as well as the others involved in this process.

You dishonor your Body-Mind every time you accept a faulty belief system and every time you listen to or believe someone when you know they are wrong, or when you know what is right and do not do it. Every time you criticize yourself without learning from the experience, you cause it pain. Because of all of these lies, your Body-Mind may no longer take your requests very seriously. It may not take your desires to get well seriously. It may not even take you seriously.

To get answers to your questions, you must first show it that you are serious about wanting truthful answers. Fortunately, since it wants you to have the information and to get well and be well, it will not be very hard to get it back on your side. This may require you proving to your Body-Mind that you really mean what you are telling it.

We will now share with you some of our techniques for getting truthful answers from the Body-Mind and how to get it back working for you.

TECHNIQUE FOR GETTING ANSWERS

First, it is important that you ask the right questions. If you want to know why you have a recurrent fear, don't ask about something else. For example, ask, "Why do I feel fearful whenever I have to make a decision?" Don't just ask why you had a problem at some particular time when you want to know why you have it each time. Be as specific as possible.

The second and most important point is being ready to hear the answer. If you are not prepared to hear the correct answer, it will not come to you. If you ask the question but really don't want to hear the answer, then asking the question is just another lie. Therefore, work on yourself until you are ready to hear the answers. Remember the old proverb, "The truth will set you free![13]"

It has been my personal and professional experience that the Body-Mind will test you even when you are completely ready and willing to hear the answer. If you have not made it easy for the Body-Mind, it will not make it easy for you. While it won't lie to you, it may throw you curves. For example, when I, Allen, asked it whether my experience at age 7 was the cause of my discomfort in making decisions, the answer, "yes," didn't come to me initially. Rather, a series of possible reasons was presented in a sea of seemingly meaningless statements. "Well, maybe it was because your dad didn't love you the way you wanted to be loved," "Maybe it was because you didn't get all A's in school," "Maybe it was because you are too cocky and think that you know everything," and so on. While all seemed to have a bit of truth, none really answered the question.

I learned to listen to the answers and gradually, painfully, learned not to judge them. I learned that all the answers given to me had a piece of the truth. Finally, after months of listening, accepting, and not judging, an answer came that I immediately recognized as correct, "You wanted everyone to agree with you. When they didn't, you lost confidence in yourself."

It was truly just like the flash of light when a light bulb is turned on. I knew that this was what I needed to know.

When I asked my Body-Mind, "How can I get past this," once again it took months for the right answer to materialize.

Then one day it came to me, "Trust in yourself." I realized that not making decisions leaves us powerless. Even if you make the wrong decision, you at least tried. With each wrong decision, you have an opportunity to learn. Don't throw away this opportunity.

Taking risks is the only way you gain experience in making decisions. With experience, right and wrong, being accepted will mean less and being your best will mean everything."

---

13   This comes from John 8:31-2: "If you hold to my teaching, you are really my disciples. Then you will know the truth, and the truth will set you free."

In time, even that answer refined itself, as I learned that I had many more options to get what I wanted out of life then I had previously believed. I could ask for help. I could research whatever I needed or wanted to know. I could learn from other people's experiences. Perhaps what is more important, I learned that being an adult means taking risks and committing one's self.

The process for getting answers is as follows: Ask truthfully and be willing to listen honestly, and then use the information to better yourself. Under these circumstances, the Body-Mind answers any question you ask almost immediately. If it believes that you are not yet ready to hear the answers to some questions, it will take longer to answer. If you want answers, you must be willing to wait as long as it takes. Those answers that are part of your life's quest will unfold only when you are ready to move on to the next level of your life.

The Body-Mind becomes considerably more helpful if you are not judgmental of its answers. For example, don't say things like, "That's stupid," or "I don't believe that I am thinking this." Sometimes, it is difficult to not be judgmental. Sometimes virtually any response appears judgmental. One way of getting around this is to respond with, "Is that so? I will consider that," to each answer the Body-Mind gives you. This response is nonjudgmental and simply tells the Body-Mind that you will consider the response. Of course, you must mean it when you say or think it, as the Body-Mind always knows when you are lying and when you are telling the truth. You can't hide from it and you can't fool it, so don't try.

> **Ask truthfully &
> be willing to LISTEN honestly**

THE WISE PARENT - HEALING THE CHILD WITHIN

While the Body-Mind knows most of the answers to the important questions of our lives, it can still become stuck in a child aspect. This irritating dichotomy often confuses people. In one moment of their lives, they seem to be fully functioning, wholesome, intelligent adults who know all the answers of life. Then suddenly, it may seem as if they are an out of control child, upset, angry or having a tantrum. People are often unwilling or unable to admit to this Jekyll-and-Hyde transformation. They may even resist the idea; however, in order to overcome this duality, they must first accept both parts of themselves. It is hard for us to see our many parts, especially the ones that we don't like. It is often hard to admit to our self that we may at the same time be part wise man/woman, part child, part brilliant and part fool, yet this can and is sometimes the case.

Frequently, the wise part of us knows all the answers necessary to protect us, but the child part makes life fun. Together, they are a perfect combination of the whole. However, sometimes as discussed above, we can be stuck in a child part whose growth has been blocked or stunted. Then, we have a child in pain, a child who feels the need to control us, or one who is confused and stuck, similar to Mattie L.'s situation.

The question now becomes, "How do we handle this child part of us?"

If the child part is creating no problem, then nothing need be done. If it is healthy and playful, this is good, even ideal. However, if it is unnecessarily rebellious or destructive to the adult part of us, we may act to resist it. This then may create a battle and this can cause both sides to lose—or we can do the next best thing—we can parent it.

Every child needs love. This is true of the child within as well. The child part of us, which is out of control, generally needs more love. It is likely that it is out of control for one of two reasons. First, there was some traumatic experience during which it separated from us, and decided that it needed to take on a life of its own (hence take over and maintain control). It does this because it believes that it has to protect itself. In doing this, it may end up suppressing certain emotions, feelings, or thoughts that if left intact might well have allowed it to learn and grow from its current experience. The second reason is that it feels unloved and unheard. Because some parts are suppressed, it is no longer whole. This may create feelings of loneliness and being alone. Now, years later, it still wants and needs to be acknowledged, heard, and loved so it can feel whole.

In the first situation, almost any trauma can cause withdrawal. This means that almost any event or situation, anything that has happened to the person, anything that the child's Body-Mind believes is actually or potentially a threat affects it and potentially undermines its existence. Its fears along with the degree of trauma may be increased by its sense of loneliness, isolation, or abandonment by the Conscious Aware Self or its parents. In such situations, the Stress Mechanism has likely been invoked and, depending on the power of the experience or memories that drive it, there may be a wide range of responses from minimal distress to life-threatening fear.

Consider situations such as post-traumatic stress syndrome (PTSD) or the after effects of molestation, rape, abuse, growing up with alcoholic parents, or divorce. The separation of the Mind-Body, the Child Within, from itself or the Conscious Aware Self may occur because at the time of the trauma, the Conscious Aware Self moves into a state of altered consciousness. It may blank out, become numbed, withdraw, experience fear or even extreme terror. It may even be rendered unconscious or enter into a fugue state. The Conscious Aware Self separates from the Body-Mind, leaving the Body-Mind to fend for itself. The Body-Mind now does whatever it must to survive, even create a separate identity or personality. When there are recurrent traumas for a long period, multiple identities, one or more Child Within may be created.

At some point when a decision is needed and yet not made, one of these identities, often the strongest or most fearful one, may take over and do whatever it deems is necessary to assure your survival.

When lesser conflicts occur, such as a new child in the home, moving, changing schools, being bullied, or losing a pet, the separation may be partial or limited. The exact incident or time when these traumas occurred or when it was decided that they were no longer loved is important and will likely be remembered in detail whether we are conscious of it or not. The fact that it has happened is important. When this happens, the Child Within may become stuck, threatened, or significantly traumatized. Once again, this triggers the Stress Mechanism. Years later, these memories, even while consciously forgotten, may suddenly rise from deep within to affect the adult, conflicting our life and impairing our health. How, then, do we diminish this process, reduce conflict, and create harmony and balance?

The answer is simple—give the Child Within our love. This is best done when we come from the Wise Parent part of ourselves—our Higher Self. Since we live in an Intelligent Universe and our body and our mind are both highly Intelligent and we can draw virtually from any aspect of our Self that exists within the Universe, why not then draw from the Wise Parent part of us? Within us, this Wise Parent waits to be utilized and valued. Just as the Child Within is part of us, so is all of the wisdom and knowledge that we have already gathered from our life experiences.

Most of all, the child part of us wants love, stability, and a sense of security. The Wise Parent part of us can best confer these gifts. It knows what the child needs. Often the child part of us will not respond to the present adult part (our Conscious Aware Self), for it either has "lied" or "cheated" the Body-Mind, or is confused, angry and unhappy because its life is not going the way it wants. The Wise Parent often has the answers the Child Within needs. It is through the Wise Parent part of us that this child part fully feels protected, loved, and heard. It's like a grandparent coming to the aid of the injured grandchild.

While the Child Within may not trust the Wise Parent immediately, over time and with our own total support, it will eventually recognize that the Wise Parent can help it, survive, heal and become totally healthy once again. The Child Within may be hurt or damaged, but it is never a fool. It recognizes truth and it will eventually accept a genuine opportunity to heal itself.

THE VALUE OF THE WISE PARENT

To help those areas wounded within you, you may find gaining access to the Wise Parent part of yourself valuable. All you need to do is tell your Body-Mind what you need and want. You can only do this by creating a clear mental picture of what you desire and then asking for it. With this done, you must next open your consciousness up to hear what it needs to tell you.

The Body-Mind needs to know that you really want its help. Once you ask for its help, start working with the Child Within as if you are the Wise Parent.

Sometimes, it is helpful to think of having a wise old grandfather or grandmother within you and ask this wise part of you what to do and then listen to its answers.

It is important that you let the Wise Parent within you give the Child Within all the love and care it needs. When loved and cared for it eventually calms down and allows the adult part of you to re-assume control. Let the Wise Parent talk to the adult part of you, too. Let the Wise Parent teach you and give you love and respect. The adult part will also grow and become increasingly wiser and happier from this experience. The Child Within desires your attention, but it wants truth, caring, and love even more.

You will know the Wise Parent by its caring and love. You will know when it is telling you the truth, not only by the fact that what it says (what you are thinking) is correct, clear, loving, and supportive, but also because it will help you to solve problems and decrease conflict. Work with this part of you, and activate the Wise Parent and use it to help you solve your most daunting problems and undo your most painful and difficult life conflicts.

These techniques are valuable for returning your Body-Mind to harmony and balance. Every part of you can benefit from the Wise Parent's love and caring. It can also help you by completing certain important messages and instructions that the Body-Mind needs you to hear and understand. It can help you apologize for past mistakes and denigrations. It can help you take responsibility for creating a better future. The Wise Parent can fill a role that might not have been previously available to you. It can help the Child Within solve old problems that have been keeping the Conscious Aware Self stuck and out of control. It can give advice and answer questions that needed answering for a long time. By definition, the Wise Parent never lies. It always tells the truth, and of course, the truth will set you free.

These techniques are also valuable for people who are no longer able to communicate with their parents or whose parents have been negative forces in their life. If you never had the parent you wanted, or felt that one or both of your parents did not want you, then the Wise Parent part of yourself is ideal. It can ultimately become the parent you always wanted and needed, but never had.

With the help and love of the Wise Parent, the adult part of you will grow, become wiser, and learn how to tell the truth. Eventually, this now-wise adult part of you can join with your Wise Parent and they will become one. If the Child Within also grows and evolves, it can then also merge with the now healthy and wise adult part of you. Gradually, as all of your many parts merge, you can once again become a whole and fully healthy person.

*To be "on edge,"
you are literally
not centered
not being
in your
spiritual center.*

~Carrie Latet

Chapter Nine

THE HIGHER SELF

LOVE AND SELF-LOVE

The three Selves, as well as all of the various parts of the whole person, require love. Love is life's elixir. While our society has created many substitutes for love, such as money, power, friendship, possessions, sex, drugs, or evil-doing, love is still the supreme force, the glue that binds human beings. Without love, only fear and emptiness would prevail. Without love, lies endure. Love is important to healing, and the loss of love often leads to illness and disease. Love is the substance of why we really want to survive. Love adds color to our lives and gives us a reason, other than simply procreation, for wanting and fighting to survive.

Today, many healers write of love as the "best medicine" and that true love is the very best facilitator of healing.

Even after I (Allen) decided that I wanted to be a healer, my only concept of love was my love for my parents, wife, and family. It was difficult for me to understand the meaning of love, especially self-love, and what possible role it could play in healing my patients. Western medicine does not even include the word love in its vocabulary. In fact, the notion of love as a part of the healing process is purposefully avoided. The concept of love exists only as a psychological entity.

During my first few years as a physician, I believed, as most of my colleagues still do, that the idea of love as a currency of healing was only a romantic notion. When anyone, even another physician, even suggested that there could be a relationship between love and healing, they were laughed at. The belief that love is essential was sometimes dismissed as being either idealistic or just plain nonsense.

Understanding the true meaning of love and the importance of self-love in healing came to me through a crisis in my own life. One day, I realized that I didn't love myself. For many years, I tolerated myself and sometimes even liked myself. I occasionally accepted myself, but I never really loved myself.

When I loved others, it was always with the expectation that they would love me back. Because of this, I never truly felt loved. When any other person told me that they loved me, I usually wondered what their motivation was. I believe now that I never actually loved another person with the exception of my mother, father, wife, and children. Even though I loved them, I could not understand why they would love me.

I could see all of my shortcomings and lies. The things I feared or disliked in others were the things I either didn't like in myself or feared. I was afraid. I was stubborn. I was selfish and arrogant. I considered myself above everyone else; if I didn't then I would have to have believe that others were above or better than me. It wasn't until later in my life that I realized that all of these characteristics were really defense mechanisms protecting me because I felt unloved and unlovable.

I distinctly remember the night it all came to a head. Unlike most crises, there was no significant event tied to it. It affected no one else. It happened in silence, while I was alone.

For several months, I had been mulling over the concept of self-love. By that time, I was willing to accept that self-love was important in healing my patients, but I could neither explain it nor feel it myself.

I kept asking myself, "What would it take to feel love for myself? Is it simply a way of thinking? Is it the words you say to yourself? Is it something you believe about yourself? Does it just happen or do you have to do something to make it happen? Once you have it, can you see it, feel it, or taste it? How would I recognize it, if I did have it?"

I asked the questions and I waited for answers. Day after day and week after week, no answers came. Then one evening, I came home from work feeling very alone and very lonely. I wanted to go out, but also wanted to stay home. I wanted companionship, but I also wanted to be alone. I didn't want to be by myself and at the same time, I really didn't want to be with anyone else.

At this point in my life, I had been divorced from my first wife for several years. I opened my little black address book and started thumbing through it. I started at the beginning of the A's and went through to the end of the Z's. In this book was every person in the world I called a friend. Yet, I could find no one with whom I wanted to be. Nevertheless, the thought of being alone was painful.

I then asked myself, "Why was being alone with myself so distasteful and so upsetting?"

I realized that I was rarely alone and usually sought the company of others to keep from being alone.

At first, I thought that maybe I just didn't like my own company. Slowly, the picture clarified until finally I realized that I felt uncomfortable being alone. I asked myself, "Why?" And the answer surprised me – I didn't love and appreciate myself enough to enjoy my own company.

"Why not?" I asked.

The answer that made the most sense was that I was not willing to accept myself for whom and what I was. I wasn't even sure of what I liked and what I wanted to do. I was always looking for others to tell me that I was okay and to help guide me. I made others responsible for my feelings.

That night for the first time, I took responsibility for myself, for my entertainment, for what I chose to do, and for doing what pleased me. I recognized for the first time what self-love was. It was being myself and liking myself for who I was and not wanting or needing to be different. I did not need someone outside of me to tell me what to do or whether I was okay. I finally was just fine being me.

With this recognition, I found myself taking a series of steps that completed the process. The first step was finding out what I liked, what I enjoyed doing, what gave me pleasure, and what made me feel good about myself. I started living my life as a kind of exploration to find out who I was and what gave me joy.

The next step was the easiest – and the most difficult. It was easy because it felt right; it was difficult because I didn't entirely know how to do it. This step involved telling the truth at all times. If I didn't want to go somewhere, I would say, "No, sorry, I don't want to go," instead of lying or needing to offer an excuse such as, "I have to go to the hospital," or "I am too tired."

The hardest part initially was telling the truth without hurting anybody. Gradually, I learned that whether someone was hurt or not depended more upon them, than me. So I just decided to tell the truth all the time and let others decide how they wanted to accept it. What I found was that you never really hurt anyone if you tell the truth, except for those people who are looking for a reason to feel or be hurt.

The final step took longer. It started when I finally decided that I was going to dedicate myself entirely to helping people get well, rather than keeping them sick by practicing interventive medicine. I could finally be my own true self and do what I wanted to do with my life. Upon making this final decision, I could feel that my life and I truly had value.

As I learned that I had full power over my life, I felt like the circle of self-empowerment was closing. I could do what I wanted, and go where I wanted. I no longer had to lie to myself or to others. I didn't have to hurt anyone's feelings. I could reach for and attain my highest, healthiest, and best Self. I discovered that for me, self-love is being entirely true to myself, liking myself, and feeling valuable for what I do and for who I am. Self-esteem and self-direction all came from within me and from telling the truth. That's what it was and still is for me. I had finally connected with my Higher Self.

MEET THE HIGHER SELF

The Higher Self is frequently compared with the super or supraconscious. This interpretation has limited the Western medical establishment from understanding the full meaning and value of the Higher Self. The Higher Self is that part of us that connects us to the Intelligence of the Universe. Think of it as our "spiritual self." In addition, that part of us is aware of our connection to all other human beings, plants, and animals, and to the planet Earth itself. It is also that part of us that is in contact with the spiritual realm, with our spirit guides, angels and God(s). This last aspect however, is a concept that is quite threatening to Western medicine and is better understood from the perspective of religion, so we will not talk more about it here.

Healing easily occurs from this level, and often this healing may be spontaneous, when it happens at this level. The Higher Self cannot communicate directly with the Conscious Aware Self. It can only communicate with the Conscious Aware Self through the Body-Mind. The Conscious Aware Self is generally only aware of the Higher Self through the Body-Mind. Hence, the Higher Self is not a thinking experience; it is a feeling experience. When the Conscious Aware Self accepts that the Higher Self is present, it can communicate with it only through the Body-Mind. It does this most often though feelings, and when on occasion, we hear words in our head, the voice of the Higher Self (God). This is because we have transformed our feelings into words and given them a voice.

While we can only have an experience of the Higher Self, at the level of the Conscious Aware Self, though the physical and emotional experience of our Body-Mind, there are two ways the Conscious Aware Self can more directly experience or communicate with the Higher Self. One is through prayer and/or meditation, and the other through living life fully and honestly. Occasionally, it may also occur through revelation at a time of crisis or through a spontaneous awareness of our connection to the Intelligence of the Universe. It is through our connection with the Higher Self that we most easily create healing in our self and others.

We only connect with our Higher Self when we believe in it and trust it. Prayer is generally a combination of trust and faith. There is also an element of meditation. Prayer is asking the Body-Mind to accept and bless – even energize and create – what we want. When we pray, we are sending our prayer requests up to our Higher Self so that it can act upon it and help us obtain what we desire.

The Higher Self is "our totally benevolent and totally trustworthy parental spirit (or self)." We could think of our Higher Self as our spiritual protector or guardian angel. The Higher Self appears to live outside the limits of time and space. It is capable of bringing or manifesting almost anything we ask for. It can manifest whatever we ask for, but only as long as what we ask causes no harm to another. The Higher Self is more likely going to provide us what we want or ask for when it is for a good reason. Asking for something that benefits us or others and when it causes no hurt to us or to others, or when it facilitates good for all involved, at all levels.

The future has already been partially formed based on our previous decisions and actions. Thus when we ask our Higher Self to help us manifest what we are asking for we can change the fabric of time and space and bring to us everything we ask for.

In spite of our past decisions and actions, we can create a new direction for our future by what we now ask of our Higher Self.

The Body-Mind controls this process to a degree. If the Body-Mind is unwilling or unable to give energy to what we are requesting, then the prayer or request never reaches the Higher Self. However, if the Body-Mind is willing but blocked by the energy of negative feelings of unworthiness, guilt, shame, anger, faulty belief systems, or unresolved conflicts, then it may not be capable of doing all that is necessary to create what we desire. These blocks are the primary reason why we do not get what we want out of life.

When our Higher Self is not able to give us what we want, either because our requests are unclear, too complex, or outside of its range of power, our Higher Self may then call upon other Higher Selves. These other Higher Selves are referred to as our "totally benevolent, totally trustworthy family of parental spirits," (possibly something like "Archangels" or the "Heavenly Host"). We might think of these concepts as religious, the ancient masters viewed them in much the same way as we think of science today. They were provable by the deeds these Higher Spirits performed and the results they accomplished. When the ancient masters used this knowledge in the correct and appropriate manner, it worked.

The goal of all of these levels of spiritual helpers is to protect the Conscious and Body-Mind Selves, ensuring their survival, and helping them evolve so that they eventually move up from Subconscious Selves to Conscious Selves, and from the Conscious Aware Self to ultimately evolve to become a Higher Self. One might think of this process as a kind of Universal Survival or Evolutionary Mechanism. Working together, all these levels create a future that gives us everything for which we ask. It transforms man into a very special being, above animals and at the threshold of godhood.

This concept also differs from religion in that it involves no priesthood. The entire process is between you, your Body-Mind and Conscious Aware Self, and your Higher Self. Only you are responsible for how your life will turn out. We might also consider it an ultimate construct of free will.

We pray directly to God in most modern religions. When we get what we want, we believe that God heard us. When we don't get what we want, we believe that God wasn't listening. We may wonder what we did to prevent God from giving us what we have asked for. We may pray harder or just give up at this point. If we believe that our prayers are blocked, we might want to talk with a priest, other religious leader, to ask what we should do, think, believe or say in order to get our self back into God's good graces. What we believe is that there is no need to ask anyone but yourself, specifically your Body-Mind. No one else can know what is in our heart. No one else can fix our problems except us, unless they completely understand who and what we are together with the interrelationships between our body, our mind, our mental and emotional states as well as our spiritual state, and the existence and relationships between our three Selves.

We first must make a friend of our Body-Mind by giving it love, removing our blocks, undoing our past sins and transgressions as well as making amends for our past wrongs. This then shows our Higher Self that we are free of physical, mental, emotional and spiritual debt. Only then will we feel worthy of getting what we truly want and need. On the other hand, by its own nature, our Higher Self loves us just as we are. It is nonjudgmental. When we see others as bad, negative, evil, or disruptive, this is primarily because they are in conflict and manifesting their inner negative feelings to the world around them. In a sense, it is a cry for help, but the untrained sees it as negative behavior. It is not because of evil spirits, the devil, or anything outside of them. The truth is that everyone has the ability to change. The fact that people can change does not mean that they will change or want to change. It only means that if they did the work we have just described, they could change. We all possess the power and ability to change. All that is needed is the will, intention, and support to make changes.

It is important here to repeat that the Higher Self never judges us. It can grant us anything that we ask. It can only act if our prayers reach it with sufficient energy from the Body-Mind. Once it receives our prayers, everything we ask for is granted, as long as it causes no intentional hurt to us or to another. If we do not get what we want out of our life, it is because we have created blocks and limitations, which prevent it from happening.

Through this process, cleaning up our lives and making friends with our Body-Mind, we may heal ourselves, and also heal others, even when they are at great distances from us. While this may seem impossible, it is not. Indeed, it is a relatively common phenomenon. There are many medical studies that clearly back this up.

Lisa and I believe that it is through this method that we assisted others in healing since the early days of our practice. Our strong belief in the body's innate ability to heal itself, along with our lack of belief in illness, has actually healed and cured people. We believe this wholeheartedly. We believe that every patient we see is going to get completely well, and they generally do. As we look back now, we realize that we must have transmitted this belief to our own Body-Minds, which have then transmitted it to our Higher Self and the Higher Selves of our patients. This facilitates their healing and helps them heal themselves.

This happens because all life is connected. In a sense, the entire Universe is a single organism and all beings are bound together by the substance of the Universe. We, as human beings, belong to this universal organism as much as our blood cells, heart, and other organs belong to us.

Invisible threads connect us to each other just as one heart cell connects to another. Together, we form a bond allowing us to communicate in ways we may have never considered, but which have always existed.

Even though we initially did not know it, this belief empowered the transmission of our beliefs to all those around us, especially to our patients. Now that we understand it, we can do this knowingly and purposefully. This process often coincides with our internal desire to heal our self as well as our desire to find and become our highest, healthiest, and best Selves.

While the first set of beliefs operates through the Body-Mind, the set of beliefs of our interconnectedness is that of the Higher Self. The Higher Self sees everything as connected to itself and the Universe. There is no separation. The Universe and each one of us are one. You and the Universe are one. We are all one.

While our Higher Self is capable of extraordinary feats and powers, it never interferes with the roles of the Body-Mind or Conscious Aware Self unless we call on it to do so. Unlike the Body-Mind, the Higher Self is not directly concerned with personal survival. Life is eternal for the Higher Self. For the Higher Self there is no such thing as death. It therefore does not work in any overt way to promote our individual or group survival. Rather, it works to promote its connection with the Intelligence of the Universe. This is why spiritualists and clergy talk less about mortal life and more about the immortal soul.

The Higher Self is not involved in religion or organized spirituality. Religion is man's Conscious Aware Self's view of what immortality is all about, when filtered through the teachings of a particular leader or group of leaders. The Higher Self has no religion. It sees no color, no nationality, no race, and has no church affiliation. All that the Higher Self knows is that it communicates with the Intelligence of the Universe (God) and that all beings and things are part of this Intelligence, including us.

Our Higher Self acts through us to let us know that our essence – the spirits we think of as the Body-Mind and Conscious Aware Self – never die. It does this through dreams and visions. It acts through the Body-Mind letting us know that our love, and the recognition of ourselves as intelligent beings, ultimately facilitates our health and overall well-being.

To the Higher Self, value and morality, decency and truth are of utmost importance. To the Higher Self, all people are part of the Intelligent Universe and are revered. Life is to be venerated, by living fully, honestly, and understanding that through our three Selves, which make us one, all must work harmoniously together.

Tension is
who you think you should be.

Relaxation is
who you are.

~Chinese Proverb

Chapter Ten

STRESS & DISEASE BELIEF SYSTEMS, STRESS & THE CREATION OF ILLNESS

Up to this point, we have explained some of the important ways the Body-Mind, Conscious Aware Self and Higher Self interaction works. We have discussed in fair detail these three levels of the Self and how they interact with each other. We previously suggested that on the physical level, everything happens in the mind and that we directly interpret the events of our life through our belief systems. We see the Universe and the world around us through our belief systems, as well as through our memories and judgments, or lack of each.

We filter the world to make it look the way we expect. This makes the world less scary and more malleable. We discussed the fact that conflicts created by the difference between the way we want our world to be and the way it actually is, activate and turn on the Stress Mechanism. When the stress created is experienced as negative, we feel negative pressure or tension, physical pain, and emotional discomfort. However, if we experience these same events as a positive situation, we do not experience tension, pain, or discomfort. Instead, we experience these events as challenge, opportunity, and even as joy. Stress can be experienced as a negative or positive depending upon how we interpret the events that trigger it and the affect we believe it is going to have on our lives and us. While we might think of stress as only being negative, this is not true. If you were to win the lottery, the physical changes your body would experience as you jump for joy would be the exact same physical changes as those you would experience if you were running from an enemy. The differences are only in the causes, their outcomes, and what you believe about them. While we think of negative stress as Fight-or-Flight, we can also think of positive stress as challenge and opportunity. The excitement before a trip or the expectation before beginning a project, are created by our sense of challenge and opportunity as we start out enjoy and master our life and what we do with it.

Stress and challenge are the same thing. Yet, like up and down, right and left, or good and bad, they are polar opposites. Through the remainder of this book, we will consider challenge as a positive situation and consider stress as its negative counterpart.

Since we never truly see or experience our entire reality or the entire Universe, what we know about each of them is limited to our belief system about them. Hence, what we know about life is simply what we believe about it. Science is simply a particular set of belief systems about the world and the way it works. What we call "truth" is also a particular set of belief systems to which we assign a certain degree of positive power. When we don't believe something, we assign it no power. When we disbelieve something, we are likely to assign it a negative power. When we believe something, depending on how much we believe in it, we assign it some level of positive power.

**In reality, all beliefs are relative to
what we know about the subject
& the position from which we view it.**

All beliefs are relative to what we know about the subject and how we view it. Love and hate are also belief systems to which we assign positive or negative power. The degree of love or hate we experience is determined by the intensity of the emotions associated with them. The concept of positive and negative is always relative and can abruptly change or last a lifetime. All that we have written in this book represents our own personal belief systems. You may as one of our readers, disagree with us from time to time, maybe even all the time or not at all. Your agreement or disagreement will ultimately depend on your unique point view and the many belief systems you have created over the course of your life. Agreement means that either we have the same belief systems or they are close enough to allow acceptance. Disagreement means that we have different or even opposing beliefs.

What this means is that we all create our lives and the way we see the world around us from what we believe about "our world" and about "the Universe" in which we live. When these beliefs serve us and are consistent with those of other people around us, we have agreement and the world is a pleasant place. When our beliefs are faulty or inconsistent with the reality of the world around us, or significantly conflict with the views of people we like and respect, conflict may be created along with a sense of negativity and negatively powered feelings, emotions, and beliefs. When these unresolved conflicts appear to threaten our life picture and our belief systems about the world in which we live, they create stress. If this stress goes unchallenged or the underlying problems and conflicts are not resolved, they may eventually lead to illness.

> **Faulty beliefs are any belief systems
> which do not make our life better.**

Faulty beliefs are those that misinterpret the world around us. For example, feeling unloved when we do not allow people to love us is a faulty belief. We may not be loved for several reasons. We may not be spending time with loving people. We may be expecting too much from others. We may be choosing people who cannot give love or are not capable of receiving love. We may even create a body of evidence out of our life experience that we interpret as proving that we "can't be loved" or that we are "unlovable." Possibly a more truthful belief might be, "I do not feel love because I do not give or accept love. I do not allow myself to feel loved because of my choices and belief systems." This is only one example of a set of faulty belief systems. Faulty belief systems can be virtually infinite in number and type. Faulty belief systems are any individual or set of belief systems that do not make our life healthier, happier and better.

WELLNESS–STRESS–DISEASE MECHANISM
(also known as the Stress-Illness Mechanism or Continuum)

Wellness → Stress → Dis-Stress → Dis-ease → Disease
→ Chronic Disease → Death

Table:10-1

DISEASE IS NOT NECESSARILY A NEGATIVE PROCESS

Most of us have been taught that disease and illness are negative situations. We hope that you have been able to see by now that this is not necessarily true. In most situations, our lack of understanding of the true meaning of illness leads to a series of beliefs that illness is bad, or that it is a negative or even evil situation. In most cases, the illness or disease process continues and is allowed to progress far farther and much longer than it should have, we assume that they are "real" and that they are "bad" for us. In fact, their negativity is often "proven" by the evidence of how negatively illness affects the people who we consider "ill" or "diseased."

Actually, illness and disease in their earliest stages are simply teachers telling us what our Body-Mind is experiencing and providing clues to the problem and unresolved conflicts which our Body-Mind is telling us require resolution. Often what people think of disease it is the result of a process that when understood and acted upon, leads to challenge and opportunity. When these stresses are recognized early and dealt with effectively, they can lead to prevention and early reversal, improved health and well-being, even enlightenment.

Since illness and disease occur as the result of unresolved conflicts and problems, if we allow these conflicts to persist, we can face increased risk of illness and disease. These conflicts and problems are trying to get our attention to tell us that something is wrong in the only way they can through physical, mental or emotional signs and symptoms. These are the only way our body can talk to us. These signs and symptoms are the language of our Body-Mind. When we listen to our Body-Mind we can learn about and resolve our conflicts. We can do this either on our own or with the help of someone who understands the language of the Body-Mind. If we do not listen, if the message is not heard or the conflicts are not resolved, the process can continue to advance over time, now the signs and symptoms begin to transform as the process moves from a message requesting help, into a process of overwhelming and even breaking down our body's immune, healing and repair systems and eventually advancing into a full disease state, then chronic disease or even death. While it may, when we look back, appear to us as if this illness or disease had simply just occurred out of nowhere, this is an illusion fostered by our lack of understanding the Stress-Illness-Disease process and the Body-Mind interaction. If we use these signs and symptoms for what they are – communications from the Body-Mind – they can become our teacher and help us solve problems and heal ourselves.

HOW DOES A HEALTHY PERSON BECOME ILL?

In the previous sections, we suggested that wellness can turn into illness, and that this process has a definable purpose. In the remainder of this section, we look at this process and discuss how this happens.

To illustrate this process, the transformation of Wellness into Stress-Related Disorders and its ability to progress to chronic disease and even death, we suggest that you take a moment and study Table: 10-1 to see an overview of this Wellness to Disease or Death process.

We refer to the process, as outlined in Table: 10-1, as the Wellness-Stress-Disease Pathway or the Stress-Illness Mechanism or Continuum. To best understand how it works, we present a true story that demonstrates how wellness is subverted when stress is activated and not relieved. We will look at a young couple who developed a number of significant illnesses over a period of several years and see the Stress-Illness Mechanism in action.

Once we review how this process advanced for this young couple, we can then look at the Stress Mechanism itself to see the steps that generally take place when we move from wellness into illness and later on illness back to optimal health.

Peter And Amy's Story:

Peter and Amy met in high school and fell in love. Three months before Peter was to graduate from high school, Amy told him she was pregnant. They were married shortly after Peter graduated. Reluctantly, putting off his dream of becoming an engineer, Peter got a job in a local factory. Amy had no specific direction in mind, so she quit school to care for their baby.

At first, the baby seemed to make everything worthwhile. However, as the years passed, Peter became increasingly bored with his job at the factory and began thinking about his childhood dream of becoming an engineer. After 3 years of marriage, Amy announced that she was pregnant again. From this point on, Peter and Amy began moving into disease.

Peter's income was sufficient when there were only three, but by the time the second baby arrived, they were deeply in debt. Peter worked and Amy controlled the money. Peter took a second job to help make ends meet. Amy, overwhelmed with the two children, began having episodes of anxiety and depression. She started gaining weight and became a compulsive buyer. Starved for companionship, shopping was her only happiness. Although it caused guilt, buying things, whether she needed them or not, made her feel good.

Peter started working overtime on his second job just to make enough money to pay their bills. He was unaware of Amy's compulsive buying and became angry with himself for not being more successful. Because of his feelings of worthlessness, he started drinking and smoking heavily.

By the fourth year of their marriage, Amy was having migraine headaches that were so severe she would go to the local emergency room for painkilling injections. Peter started having a problem with indigestion and heartburn. As Amy's compulsive buying continued and Peter's drinking worsened, they began bitterly arguing. Neither could see a relationship between her compulsive buying, their debt, and his heavy drinking and smoking. Peter's indigestion progressed into full-blown abdominal pain and became a peptic ulcer. He told his doctor that he only occasionally drank alcohol, which was not true. After taking medication, cutting down on his drinking, and going on a bland diet, his condition improved for a while.

During the next few years, the children began having frequent ear infections. The whole family now had medical problems. Each saw different doctors, so no one doctor, was able to put together their entire story.

Four years after the second pregnancy, Amy became pregnant again. While they briefly considered an abortion, they decided against it for religious reasons. By the time the third baby was born, Amy and Peter were hardly talking to each other about anything meaningful. Amy then had her tubes tied to prevent any future pregnancies. Shortly afterward, Amy developed a lump in her breast. A biopsy found the lump to be a benign cyst. Five years later because of fibroid tumors, Amy had a hysterectomy. During this period, the couple began talking about divorce, but their religion forbade it.

Peter was again drinking heavily. Peter fell and hurt his back one evening while coming out of a local bar. He was off work for 10 days and was not able to resume normal activities for several months. He developed severe abdominal pain and a bleeding ulcer and was rushed to the emergency room. All treatments failed to stop the bleeding, and he had emergency surgery to remove part of his stomach.

During the next few years, Peter gave up drinking. He lost weight, had constant back problems, and was taking several medications. Amy gained even more weight after her hysterectomy, had several more breast biopsy surgeries, and continued having migraines. Both became severely depressed.

This story provides an excellent demonstration of how life events, personal beliefs, and faulty decision can and come together to create illness. In this example, problems and disagreements occurred one after another for a period of many years. Because of their lack of clarity, these two young people made many faulty decisions. These decisions created increasing conflict and, since Peter and Amy were unable to resolve their problems, their stress increased. The stress, which was not released, changed to Dis-Stress (negative stress), which further increased the many pressures that already existed. The process persisted unresolved until the next stage, Dis-Ease, was reached. With no help from the outside and no recognition by either of them of what was happening, they entered into the next phase of the process – the Disease Stage. As time passed and nothing changed to reverse or eliminate their conflicts and stresses, they eventually reached the stage of Chronic Disease.

To fully understand this important series of events, let's examine each of these steps as they unfolded. Peter's heartburn and indigestion were early warning signs indicating that he had already entered into the stage of Dis-Stress. Using the concept of Body Symptom Language, we can identify the significance of these symptoms. Amy's anxiety represented her fear of being trapped and feeling of loneliness. Peter's indigestion represented his inability to digest his situations, boredom and hopelessness, as well as many other painful events in his life. Both ate poor quality diets. Both of their diets were high in refined and processed foods, refined sugars, and fats. Heavy drinking and smoking due to fear, anxiety, and extreme tension increased the great internal stress that smoking and drinking could only temporarily relieve. They also represented Peter's hopelessness and inability to face and solve his problems. His lying about his drinking, and inability to reduce drinking and smoking further demonstrated the depth of his problems.

As time passed, their original problems along with new "feeder" problems (that is, any new problem or problems which would feed into the already existing conflicts and complicate them, such as second and third babies, Amy's compulsive buying, Peter's self-denigration), coalesced to form larger and more oppressive problems, more conflict and hence an increased level of stress. As the pressure on the two reached a critical level, the process advanced to the next stage, the state of Dis-Ease. Peter's abdominal pain, Amy's headaches, and their persistent arguing were all indications of advancing stress and the onset of the Dis-Ease stage.

Eventually, both Peter and Amy moved into the next level – the stage of Dis-ease. Their symptoms worsened and became more defined in this stage. This was evidenced by the worsening of Amy's compulsive buying and by her migraine headaches, which required powerful medications, her breast cysts, and finally her fibroid tumors. As Peter reached this stage, he became even more alcohol dependent, developed an ulcer, injured his back and was left with chronic pain and disability. If the original conflicts and the feeder conflicts had been resolved, this suffering could have been avoided.

Unfortunately, the process didn't stop in the disease stage. When Peter's ulcer worsened and began bleeding, in spite of his taking his medication and changing his diet, he ended up having to have surgery. Peter ultimately had part of his stomach removed, which forever changed his anatomy and physiology. Amy's irregular bleeding and breast lumps led to surgeries as well. Once Amy had her hysterectomy, she was also left with an altered anatomy and physiology. Once each had major anatomy and physiology changing surgeries, they each had reached the stage of Chronic Disease and their Stress-Illness process now had caused irreversible injury to each of their bodies.

It is now important to see that there is often a ripple effect with this process. As the pressure of stress affects one person, it also unavoidably affects all the other family members. Peter and Amy's children reacted to their parents' stress, arguing, silent and vocal anger and rage, by developing ear infections and frequent upper respiratory infections. The oldest child developed behavioral problems as well, feeling unloved and unwanted. The Stress-Disease Process is often learned during childhood, acted out in adulthood, and taught to the next generation.

Unlike many other people, Amy and Peter's story did have a happy ending. About six months after Amy's hysterectomy, their relationship reached a crisis. Amy, who had come to our office for hormonal therapy, broke down and cried out, "I can't take it anymore." She proceeded to tell their whole story, at least what she knew of it. We explained how the Stress-Illness process applied to her situation. She was finally able to see the relationship between their stresses and their illnesses. We referred the entire family for family therapy. After several months of intense effort, they were able to resolve most of their conflicts. They set their differences aside and for the first time in their marriage began working together for their relationship. They discovered they truly loved each other. Amy lost 30 pounds and rarely had migraines. Peter completed an alcohol detoxification program, joined AA, and no longer drinks or smokes, and now helps others with addiction problems. Their children have had no more ear infections and are doing well in school. The last we heard, Peter had signed up at a local college to begin courses to get his engineering degree.

THE WELLNESS-STRESS-DISEASE MECHANISM

The connection between stress, illness, and disease is poorly understood by the medical profession. To understand the relationship of stress to the illness and disease process, we must start at the beginning of the process: The creation of stress.

Our built-in Stress Mechanism is triggered whenever we sense a potential danger or threat to our life or to our well-being. It is the body's natural way of reacting to a perceived threat. This threat does not have to be life-threatening. The triggering event, the stressor, needs only be something perceived as threatening to our life or to our well-being. Once the Stress Mechanism is triggered, it takes on a life of its own. Since the Body-Mind may have no way of telling what originally triggered it, it may not be able to judge the real level of the threat. In a sense, it simply reacts and leaves it up to the Conscious Aware Self to determine the threat, whether it is real or imagined, how much of a threat it is, what is actually threatened, and what can be done about it. The stress process acts in much the same manner, no matter the actual cause or degree of the threat. The only difference may be in the intensity of its effect and the depth of its desire to get us to make needed changes.

While the stress response mechanism has been recognized since the dawn of the human species, it was first named and explored by a University of Montreal professor, Hans Selye, MD. While in medical training at the University of Prague in 1925, Selye was deeply impressed by what he later would call the "syndrome of sickness." On one occasion, several very sick patients were brought into a case presentation conference. Selye then observed a common thread within the symptoms in all cases regardless of the presented diagnoses. His instructor emphasized the need to look for characteristic signs of diseases that had been diagnosed, Selye observed, "the many features of disease, which were already manifest, did not interest his teacher very much."

He realized that this was because each of these signs and symptoms were considered nonspecific and that they were therefore considered of no value or use to the physicians in making and proving a diagnosis. It was this group of signs and symptoms, these nonspecific signs and symptoms, which would ultimately, become the basis of Selye's life's work. These nonspecific signs and symptoms would later become the foundation of the Stress Syndrome. Interestingly enough, this same group of signs and symptoms, which define stress, still do not interest most physicians.

Yet, these same nonspecific signs and symptoms are the foundations of the process we are discussing in this book, not in relationship to the diagnosis of any specific illness or disease, but rather as 1) the basis of the Wellness to Chronic Illness Process, and 2) those signs and symptoms that, if recognized early, could allow us to stop the illness process and then allow us to help our patients return to full and complete, optimal, health and wellness, and even prevention.

THE STRESS CASCADE

The Stress Mechanism's purpose, as already stated, is ensuring our survival. We believe this to be a highly Intelligent purpose. The Stress Mechanism's level of complexity demonstrates not only the resolution and purpose behind it, but also the great Intelligence that appears to have designed it.

When we are affected by a stressor, a number of physiologic, neurochemical, and anatomical changes occur. We refer to this complex of events as the Stress Mechanism. Initially, there is a release of hormones and other chemicals in organs throughout the brain and body that trigger specific changes designed for Fight-or-Flight, (See Table: 10-2).

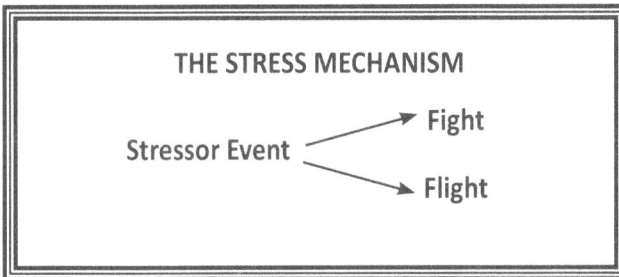

THE STRESS MECHANISM

Stressor Event → Fight
→ Flight

Table: 10-2

Two major stressor types stimulate the Stress Cascade. One type is called "real" in the sense that an actual attack or real life-threatening situation is occurring. This could be an actual life-threatening event, such as someone with a gun; or a smaller physical threat, such as an invasion of your body by microorganisms.

The second type of stressor event could be a perceived or imagined threat. Here, the perceived or imagined stressor acts as a threat even without any real threat or the existence of any past, present, or future physical injury. In this situation, while the threat may not be actually happening now, the response is based on the possibility that an attack or injury could happen now or in the future. Since we create our own reality, anything we believe to be real can become real, whether it is real in fact or not.

In the end, there is only one type of response to this stress event. This response is the same whether the stressor is real or imagined. All types of threats – whether physical, mental, emotional or spiritual – trigger the same physiologic changes, those we call the Stress Mechanism.

(See Tables: 10-3 and 10-4).

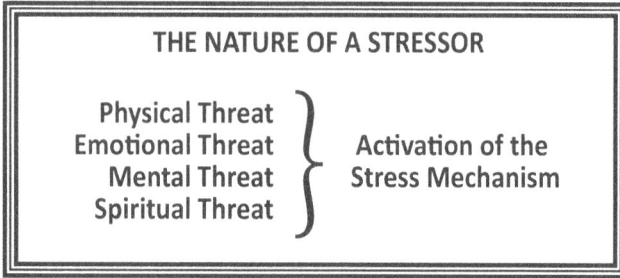

Table: 10-3

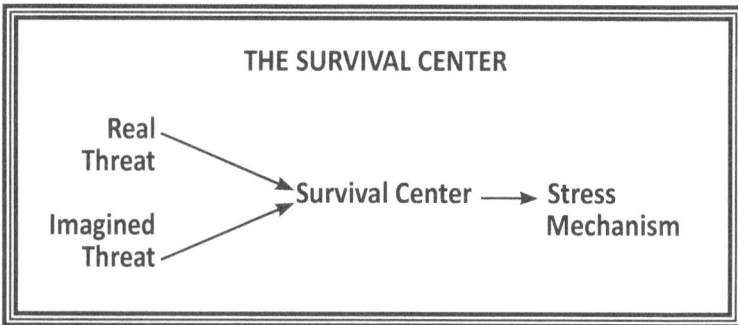

Table: 10-4

We can divide the Stress Mechanism into three parts:

1) The Stress Cascade, 2) the Stress Response, and 3) Resolution Response. Once a person consciously or subconsciously senses a potential threat and the Stress Mechanism is activated (See Table: 10-5).

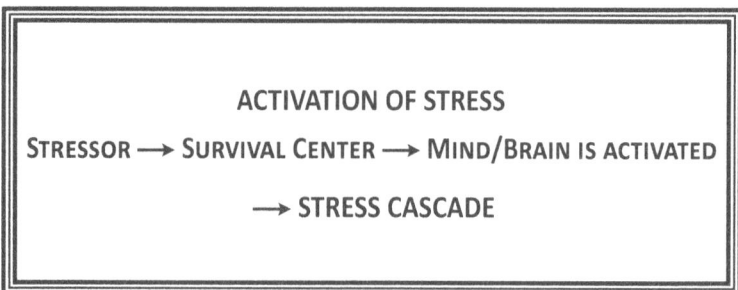

Table: 10-5

This starts the Stress Mechanism's first phase, the Stress Cascade (See Table: 10-6).

The first portion of the Stress Cascade includes the involvement of the brain, pituitary gland, hypothalamus, and the release of a number of stress chemicals, hormones, and neurohormones.

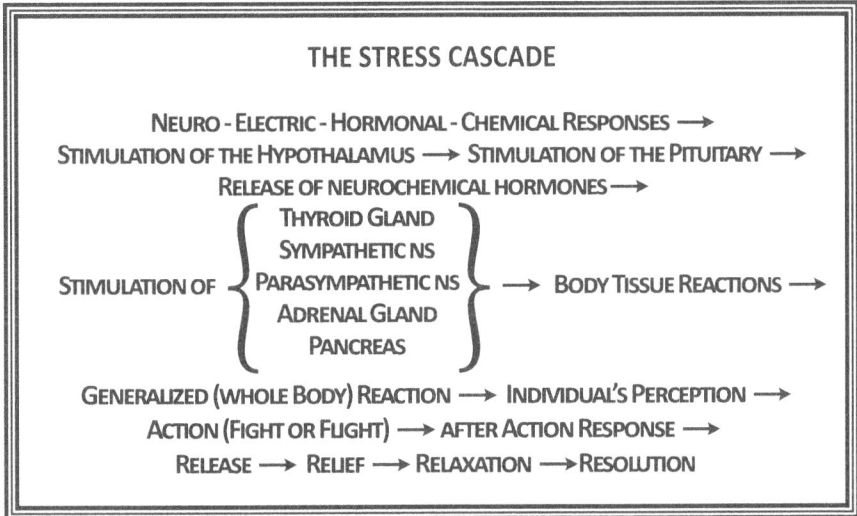

THE STRESS CASCADE

NEURO - ELECTRIC - HORMONAL - CHEMICAL RESPONSES ⟶
STIMULATION OF THE HYPOTHALAMUS ⟶ STIMULATION OF THE PITUITARY ⟶
RELEASE OF NEUROCHEMICAL HORMONES ⟶

STIMULATION OF {
THYROID GLAND
SYMPATHETIC NS
PARASYMPATHETIC NS
ADRENAL GLAND
PANCREAS
} ⟶ BODY TISSUE REACTIONS ⟶

GENERALIZED (WHOLE BODY) REACTION ⟶ INDIVIDUAL'S PERCEPTION ⟶
ACTION (FIGHT OR FLIGHT) ⟶ AFTER ACTION RESPONSE ⟶
RELEASE ⟶ RELIEF ⟶ RELAXATION ⟶ RESOLUTION

Table: 10-6

The second part of the Stress Cascade triggers affects in the rest of the body and is mediated by the Stress Response. This is the total body response caused by the activation of the Stress Cascade and its effect on our body. It is during the triggering of the Stress Cascade portion of the Stress Mechanism where you first (consciously or unconsciously) perceive a sense of threat. The mechanism is triggered, and it is during the Stress Response where you should experience the physical and emotional symptoms associated with stress. (See Table: 10-7).

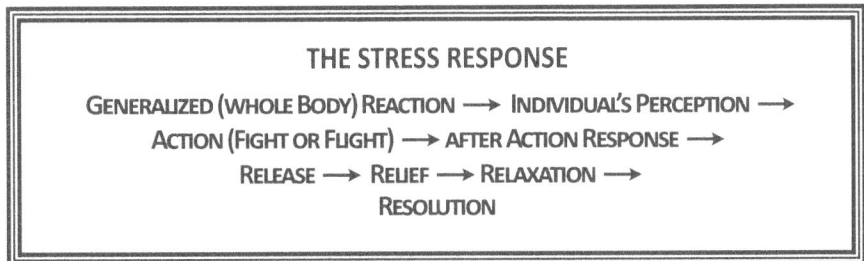

THE STRESS RESPONSE

GENERALIZED (WHOLE BODY) REACTION ⟶ INDIVIDUAL'S PERCEPTION ⟶
ACTION (FIGHT OR FLIGHT) ⟶ AFTER ACTION RESPONSE ⟶
RELEASE ⟶ RELIEF ⟶ RELAXATION ⟶
RESOLUTION

Table: 10-7

The total complexity of the Stress Mechanism is well beyond the scope of this book. We have provided a series of tables in this chapter to provide an overview of the Stress Mechanism's depth and extent. These tables indicate the organs involved, the organs affected, and the symptoms and physiologic changes that occur with either an acute or a chronic stress situation.

In Table: 10-4 and 10-5, we introduced the concept of an area of the brain we call the Survival Center. We believe that the function of this part of the Stress Mechanism determines whether there is a real or perceived threat to our life or well-being, and whether the Stress Mechanism should be invoked. We believe that this area represents all past memories, self-knowledge, instincts, and intuitions. Hence, it is part of the Body-Mind. Whether or not there is an actual physical area within the brain where it is located is yet to be determined. If we hold fears or faulty belief systems about the ensuing event or events, the Stress Reaction may be initiated even when there is no actual threat to our life or well-being. Even though there is no specific part of the brain which is currently referred to as the "Survival Center," the events that stimulate or turn off the Stress Mechanism suggest that some area or part of our brain that acts to direct and control the Stress Mechanism. The Survival Center's activation occurs with the onset of the stress process. The Survival Center acts as a gatekeeper between the stressor event and triggering the Stress Mechanism. It must first "believe" or at least recognize that there is some evidence that there is a threat, real or imagined, before triggering the Stress Mechanism.

The entire Stress Mechanism is diagrammed in Table: 10-6, we call it the Stress Cascade. This is a cooperative function of the Body-Mind working with the brain; endocrine and nervous systems; skeletal muscles; the immune, defensive, offensive, healing, and repair systems and every cell, enzyme, neurochemical, and neuron in the body. It is this interaction of our Mind-Body and our physical body that is the overall mediator of the Fight-or-Flight reaction. The stress response is a total body reaction.

Up to this point, we have discussed what activates the Stress Mechanism. Now, we will discuss what turns it off, and that this requires a second set of stimuli. This second set of impulses is generated through the same mechanism. The shutdown of the Stress Mechanism, rather than being dependent upon a stressor event to initiate it, instead responds to our reaction to the crisis. When the Survival Center perceives that the crisis has been resolved, a message is sent throughout the body to reverse all of the biochemical and neurohormonal activity initiated by the Stress Mechanism's activation. At this point, the Stress Mechanism is slowed down, reversed, and stopped. We refer to this reversal process as the Resolution Response, the third part of the Stress Mechanism.

While all aspects of turning on the Stress Mechanism are important, the Resolution Response is also extremely important. We may have very little control over the events that initiate the Stress Mechanism and the hormonal-biochemical operations that ensue, but we can and do have a significant ability to control and direct the Resolution Response. We have stated many times that Chronic Stress and Stress-Related Disorders exist because of specific recurrent or chronic stresses, yet, the main reason for Chronic Stress and Stress-Related Disorders is that the stress process does not naturally conclude or turn off. Therefore, the release, relief, relaxation, and resolution stages do not or cannot occur. This means that the person is left in a state of chronic neuromuscular and biochemical tension, which magnifies each subsequent stress event. It is this chronic tension plus recurrent stresses that lead to chronic stress, which ultimately leads to the breakdown of the stress mechanism, the immune, defensive, offensive, healing and repair systems of the bodies which then open the door and allow illness, chronic disease and eventually, premature death to occur. In Table: 10-7, above, we see the normal and ideal process in detail. Stressful events occur; they are handled and resolved. In Table: 10-8, below, we see the portion of the Stress Cascade that focuses on the action of the hypothalamus and pituitary, the two glands that regulate most of the endocrine glands and how they respond during stress. Table: 10-8 also demonstrates what happens when the Stress Mechanism is activated, and which hormones are produced and released into the body from the pituitary, thyroid, and adrenal glands.

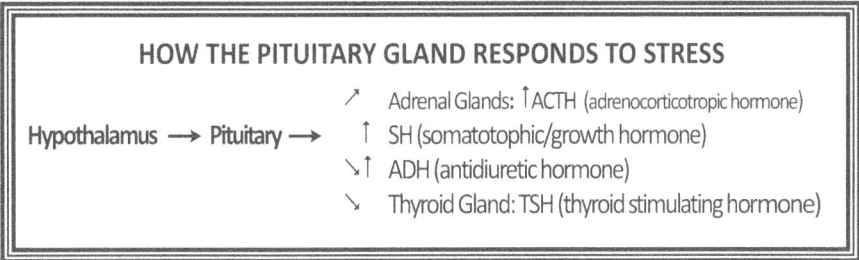

HOW THE PITUITARY GLAND RESPONDS TO STRESS

Hypothalamus ⟶ Pituitary ⟶
- ↗ Adrenal Glands: ↑ACTH (adrenocorticotropic hormone)
- ↑ SH (somatotophic/growth hormone)
- ↘↑ ADH (antidiuretic hormone)
- ↘ Thyroid Gland: TSH (thyroid stimulating hormone)

Table: 10-8

The adrenal glands are most commonly associated with the Stress Mechanism. These two "sister glands" sit on top of each of the kidneys. In turn, each adrenal gland is made up of two parts – an outer shell or cortex, and an area of inner pulp-like tissues called the medulla. Adrenal Cortical Stimulating Hormone (ACTH) made by the pituitary gland stimulates the cortical area of the adrenal gland to produce the adrenal stress hormones' first adrenalin (epinephrine) to start the stress reaction and then cortisol (See Table: 10-9) to slow down, release and finally stop the stress mechanism.

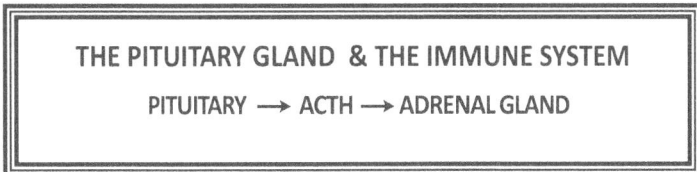

THE PITUITARY GLAND & THE IMMUNE SYSTEM

PITUITARY ⟶ ACTH ⟶ ADRENAL GLAND

Table: 10-9

Adrenalin is released because of the Stress Cascade in response to a stressor event. Adrenalin is not only responsible for the bulk of physical events we attribute to stress, but it also stimulates the onset of the inflammation process, which we discussed earlier in the section on Primary and Secondary Defensive Systems and Tissue Defenses. The second adrenal hormone, Cortisol, reverses the inflammatory process and then activates healing and repair processes throughout the body.

The Stress Mechanism not only plays an important role in the creation of the stress response and affects our ability to create inflammatory reactions throughout the body, it also activates the body's ability to repair and heal tissues injured before and during the Fight-or-Flight period, or because of the inflammatory reactions created by the release of adrenalin. While this is a greatly simplified description, it demonstrates the linkage between the Stress Mechanism and the creation of illness and healing.

THE PHYSICAL SIGNS AND SYMPTOMS OF STRESS

The physiologic changes created by the Stress Mechanism produce a number of significant internal and external physical signs and symptoms. Many of these signs and symptoms are as characteristic of stress. The initial changes prepare us to do battle or escape from an immediate threat – Fight-or-Flight. The initial characteristic of these changes are increases in our level of alertness, respiration, blood pressure, heart rate, and blood flow through the body's organs. All of these are important if we are going to face an enemy in battle. As the Stress Mechanism deepens, blood starts shifting away from the digestive system and is redirected to the larger muscles in the upper and lower extremities, the abdominal muscles, as well as the chest and back muscles in preparation for either doing battle or turning away and running.

THE ADRENAL GLAND PRODUCES ADRENALIN & CORTISOL

The Adrenal Gland ⟶   ↗ Adrenalin (Stimulates Stress Response, Inflammation, Protects Against Injury)
↘ Cortisol (Reduces Inflammation - Promotes Healing & Repair)

Table: 10-10

Table: 10-10, above, lists the events associated with "Primary Stress Response," both the Initial Stress Effects and the "External Signs and Symptoms of the Stress Reaction." This Table allows us to see what is actually going on within the body as well as what the individual is experiencing internally and externally

It provides a road map demonstrating how, where, and even why chronic, persistent stress leads to the breakdown of internal systems, and hence illness and chronic disease and disability.

THE PRIMITIVE BRAINS AND AUTONOMIC NERVOUS SYSTEM

At the center of our Subconscious Mind, our Body-Mind, is the Primitive or Reptilian Brain Complex (the brain stem and the cerebellum and other lower level brain complexes) and Autonomic Nervous System. The purpose of this primitive brain relates to physical survival as well as the maintenance of the body. The cerebellum orchestrates movement. Digestion, reproduction, circulation, breathing, and the execution of the Fight-or-Flight response of the Stress Mechanism are mediated within the brain stem. Because the Reptilian Brain is primarily concerned with physical survival, the behaviors it governs are also associated with overall physical survival behaviors. It plays a crucial role in establishing territorial, reproduction, and social dominance. The most important aspect of these behaviors is that they are automatic. They often have a ritualistic quality and generally, they are highly resistant to change.

The Autonomic Nervous System is made up of two separate and very primitive nervous systems. These two systems, the Sympathetic and Parasympathetic Nervous Systems, work as polar opposites. They maintain harmony and balance by working with and against themselves. Their overall purpose is maintaining the body's automatic functions. They are, in a sense, the Stress Mechanism's nervous system. Table: 10-11 (below) demonstrates that the majority of the physical changes occurring, when the Stress Mechanism is triggered, are caused by activation of the Sympathetic Nervous System. Heart rate increases, blood shifts to the muscular system, constricted fields of vision, decreased intestinal motility are a few of the effects.

Once the Stress Mechanism is completed, the release process is then mediated by the Parasympathetic Nervous System, which then takes over, reversing the Sympathetic Nervous System changes and returning the individual to a state of normalcy. After reviewing Table: 10-11, you will see the wide range of effects the Sympathetic and Parasympathetic Nervous Systems mediate during the stress reaction.

THE ROLE OF THE ENDOCRINE GLANDS

Simultaneously with the onset of stress, the pituitary gland releases ACTH (adrenocorticotropic hormone), which activates the adrenal cortex to produce adrenaline. Adrenaline, also known as epinephrine, not only controls the outward manifestations of the Stress Mechanism but also initiates events that stimulate the body to either Fight-or-Flight. Adrenaline is responsible for increasing blood sugar that acts to provide for the body's increased energy needs. It also activates the Sympathetic Nervous System. These functions, along with others demonstrated in Tables: 10-10, 10-11, and 10-12, are essential for readying the body for whatever ordeal it must face.

THE PRIMARY STRESS RESPONSE

INITIAL STRESS EFFECTS:
1. Alertness increases
2. Respiration increases and deepens; air passages dilate
3. Heart beats faster
4. Blood pressure rises
5. Blood supply increases to the brain and skeletal muscles
6. Numerous chemical changes occur in the body: increases in blood sugar, glycerol, amino acids, fatty acids, cholesterol, elevated HDL, elevated oxygen, decreased CO_2, increased secretion of pituitary hormones, adrenalin (epinephrine) and other corticosteroid hormones.
7. Blood is directed away from the skin and digestive system.
8. The blood becomes more concentrated and thickened.

EXTERNAL SIGNS & SYMPTOMS OF THE STRESS REACTION:
1. Pale and cool skin–blood is directed away from the skin
2. Dry mouth–breathing is rapid
3. Fearful or anxious feelings–release of adrenaline and other hormones
4. Rapid pulse–heart rate increased

Table: 10-11

The thyroid gland is also involved in the Stress Mechanism. The thyroid gland controls the body's metabolism, its capacity to burn food and regulates the body's energy needs. Once the Stress Reaction is initiated, it takes control of the thyroid gland and overrides its inherent capacity for regulating the body's normal metabolism. The Stress Reaction itself can affect heart rate by using the thyroid gland to speed up or slow down the body's metabolism, or changing body temperature. The thyroid secretions work along with the adrenal secretions producing long- and short-term effects involving the body's Immune System, as well as the Healing and Repair Systems. (See Table: 10-12, below).

Another important pituitary hormone is Somatotrophic Hormone, also known as growth hormone. During response to stress, this hormone stimulates the pancreas to produce a substance called glucagon.

Essential to the production of blood sugar, glucagon is important in regulating blood sugar levels, hence the energy supply during the Stress Reaction.

Another important hormone is Antidiuretic Hormone (ADH). ADH plays a significant role in the body's fluid and electrolyte distribution and regulation. This is essential in case of injury since it can help mediate the shock response, should you sustain a severe injury. It also supports fluid retention, which is often necessary to manage bodily fluids during the Stress Response.

STRESS AND THE ENDOCRINE SYSTEM

ACTH STIMULATES ADRENAL HORMONE SECRETION
The Adrenal gland produce Adrenalin (Epinephrine), Cortisol and other corticosteroids. These hormones have the following effects on the human body:
1. They increase blood sugar production
2. They increase energy supply to cells
3. They affect visceral vasoconstriction
4. They prolong Sympathetic NS effects
5. They stimulate or decrease inflammatory effects
6. They increase concentration of the blood amino acids
7. They cause formation of glucose from carbohydrates
8. They increase the release of fatty acids

THYROID HORMONES
Thyroid hormones stimulate many organs within the human body and have some or all of the following effects:
1. They increase the body's metabolism
2. They increase energy release from carbohydrates
3. They stimulate activity of the nervous system
4. They increase rate of protein building
5. They accelerate growth and healing

SOMATOTROPHIC (GROWTH) HORMONE
Somatotrophic hormones stimulate the Pancreas to produce Glucagon which mobilizes:
1. Energy sources - glucose and carbohydrates
2. The uptake of amino acids by cells

ANTIDIURETIC HORMONE (ADH)
Antidiuretic hormone stimulates the retention of sodium (Salt) ions by the kidneys which increases blood volume.

Table: 10-12

THE ANATOMY OF THE STRESS MECHANISM

Earlier, we discussed the basics of the Stress Mechanism, and the physical, neurochemical, biologic, mental, and emotional changes associated with it. This section takes a brief look at the Stress Mechanism's anatomy.

The onset of stress occurs with a threat. Simultaneous to the triggering of the Stress Cascade are changes that rapidly move us from a state of rest and normalcy to a state where the changes noted in Tables: 10-6 and 10-7 begin playing out.

Diagram: 10-1, below illustrates a normal stress response. On the vertical portion of this diagram, we see the intensity of the response and on the horizontal is the time through which this specific "normal stress response" moves.

Diagram 10:1 represents a single stress episode.

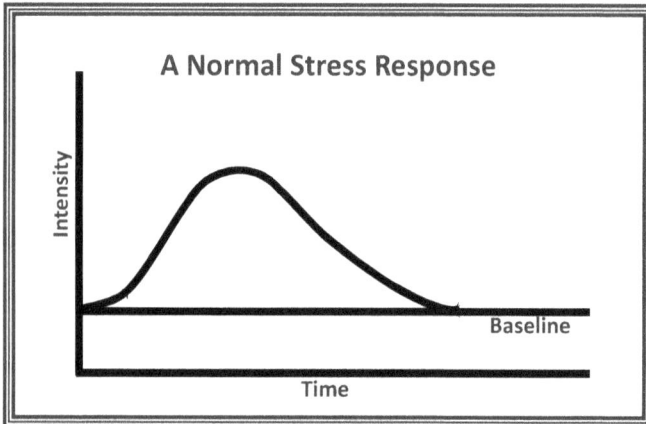

Diagram: 10-1

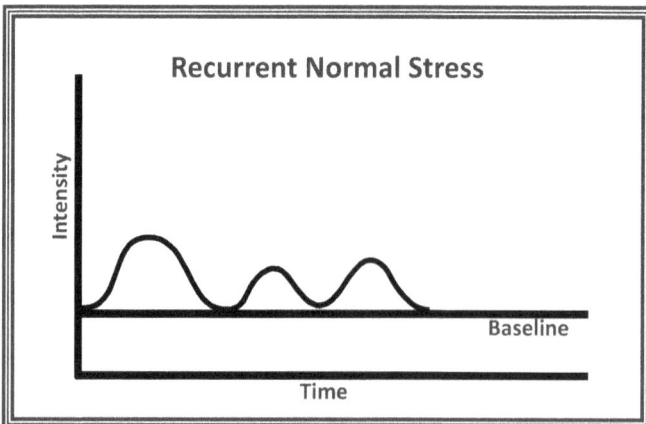

Diagram: 10-2

Diagram: 10-2, above, illustrates multiple, recurrent episodes of stress. Each bump represents a different episode of stress. Diagram: 10-3 gives names to each of the steps or phases of this response cycle.

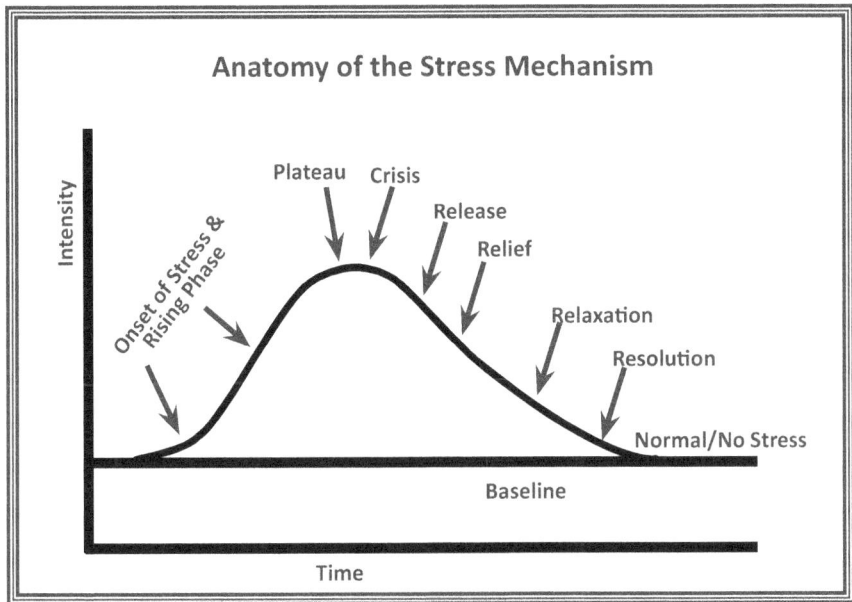

Anatomy of the Stress Mechanism

Intensity

Plateau   Crisis

Release

Relief

Relaxation

Resolution

Onset of Stress & Rising Phase

Normal/No Stress

Baseline

Time

Diagram: 10-3

The first step is the triggering the Stress Mechanism. Next is the Rising or Accelerated Phase as the cascade of events progress. This early response is often represented by increased muscle tension, shifting of blood from the intestinal tract and other organs toward the larger muscles and to the brain in preparing the individual for Fight-or-Flight.

As the process moves forward, you either take action or hold ready to take action – Fight-or-Flight. This slowing down, holding, or leveling of stress tension is called the Plateau Phase. During this phase, you are either holding for action or have already taken action and are waiting for a response from the threat. The next important point is the Crisis. The Crisis is the turning point in the immediate conflict situation when it becomes clear to the Mind-Body that it must either take further action, or step down or recover from the stress response. When taking action, the Body-Mind does one or more of three things: 1) Fight (either attack or respond to an attack), 2) Flight (turn and run, orderly retreat), or 3) Withdraw or Freeze. With withdrawal, a person stops his or her physical response and instead they turn inward. This is clearly a form of internal flight since they do not necessarily physically move away from the enemy.

It is a mental or emotional retreat, similar to a deer caught in a vehicle's headlight, and hence the notion of freezing.

At some point after fight, flight, or withdrawal the stress episode runs its course. The person survives and it is time to cool off and return to a state of normalcy. At this point, release occurs. As the shutting down or reversal of the Stress Process occurs, there are three additional phases: Relief, Relaxation, and Resolution. During these three stages, the physical, neurochemical, and biological changes that just took place undo themselves, and the body returns to its normal non-stressed state of being.

In the next chapter, we show you diagrams of what happens with the Stress Response cycle in each of the following four stages: Distress, Dys-Stress, Dis-Ease, and Disease.

SUMMARY

It should be apparent to you that the Stress Mechanism has an effect on almost every organ and system in the body. Once stimulated, the Stress System takes complete control of the physical body, the Body-Mind, and the Conscious Aware Self. Acting through the mechanisms we have just described, the long-term effects of the stress when associated with unresolved conflicts can lead to the wide variety of illnesses and diseases previously referred to as Stress-Related Disorders. At its extreme boundaries, the stress reaction is hardly noticed by the person. It appears as an exaggerated anxiety attack or even as a panic reaction or panic attack.

This becomes especially meaningful when you consider that by the time most people reach the state of Dis-Stress (as you will soon see) they have already been in a chronic state of stress for many months or even years. The glands, organs, and tissues, as well as the nervous and circulatory systems that connect them, have been overworked and overstimulated, sometimes undernourished and in a chronic state of tension, readiness, and alteration. Many have begun functioning at levels well below the body's optimum requirements.

By the time the state of Dis-Ease is reached, the body has been desperately crying out for a very long time for the conflict to be resolved and Stress Mechanism reversed. It is during this period that symptoms often change from ill-defined to a more defined status. It is also during this stage that the body's Intelligence begins the serious process of informing the person that conflicts exist and that the Body-Mind believes that they must be resolved.

The next chapter defines the Wellness-Stress-Disease Mechanism and takes an in-depth look at the stages of Dis-Stress, Dis-Ease, and Disease. It tells you what is happening to your body when they are present, how you can recognize them, and how this can help you stave off illness and injury to your body.

Chapter Eleven

CONFLICT & STRESS

THE WELLNESS-STRESS-DISEASE MECHANISM & STRESS-RELATED DISORDERS

The Stress Mechanism, initially designed to protect us from life-threatening danger, may be activated whenever we are faced with a conflict that is inconsistent with how we see our world around us. This is especially true when a conflict threatens our lives, or our immediate or future well-being. It is also true when any conflict affects our picture of the way want our life to be. Whether we are aware of it or not, each of us have a series of pictures spelling out how and what we want our life to be like. We often refer to the sum total of these pictures as "our dream," our wish for our future, what we want out of life, the house with the white picket fence, the perfect job, the perfect mate, the perfect children, and so on. When we get "our dream," we feel as if we have everything we ever wanted. When we don't get our dream, we may feel as if something has been taken away from us and we have lost. Our dream has been undermined, destroyed or killed. When a conflict occurs and "our dream" is threatened or even worse, it has been taken away from us, a piece of us is attacked, maybe even destroyed. When there are no life-threatening assaults attacking us, these threats can and do often trigger fear of loss and stress to the same degree, or more, than if we were under attack. When this happens, our stress mechanism may be triggered just as if we had been attacked and our life physically threatened.

When we resolve these conflicts, we move away from the activated Stress Mechanism directly into the Resolution Process. The Stress Mechanism is naturally terminated. Any stress-reaction caused by the specific incident will be released. Subsequently, there is a sense of relief and return to the normal state of relaxation.

If the conflict is not readily resolvable, the Stress Mechanism, likely remains activated. Conflicts can rise and fall, get worse and even be suppressed or reduced to almost no activation of the stress mechanism at all.

Over time, the original conflict may have been forgotten by the Conscious Aware Self, yet the Body-Mind may persist in searching for a solution.

If the conflict is meaningful, that is, important to the Body-Mind, the Body-Mind may empower itself to set in motion communication to the Conscious Aware Self to find a solution. We discussed earlier that during the time that the Body-Mind is searching or working to find or create a solution, the Stress Mechanism may continue to be operating. It may do this as long as the conflict remains unresolved. Since the normal process of resolution – release, relief, and relaxation – does not occur in these situations, the body is left in a state of chronic biochemical and muscular-nervous system tension, or a state of chronic stress (see Tables: 10-6, 10-7 and 10-11 above). This tension is added to the tension from all other unreleased conflicts. With its physical and mental components combined, the added tension may be experienced as physical, mental, and emotional sensations from vague to severe and even incapacitating symptoms. These symptoms can range from intermittent to persistent symptoms such as fatigue difficulty sleeping, confusion, vague sensations of distress, diminished memory, mood swings, depression, anxiety, guilt, feeling unclean, feeling empty, or feeling alone and isolated. In their mild-to-moderate form, we often think of the mental and emotional symptoms as a general state of anxiety. In their extreme form, they become severe anxiety and even burnout.

Many of the symptoms listed above were the same symptoms Dr. Hans Selye recognized as the Syndrome of Sickness which gave rise to his illuminating work on stress and the symptoms and problems it causes.

What we hope to make clear to you is that all of these symptoms (along with many others not listed here), whether mild or severe, are advanced states of communications from the Body-Mind to the Conscious Aware Self that there are unresolved conflicts that the Body-Mind believes need resolution.

When we only think of these symptoms as "anxiety" or "minor illness," this may preclude us from making the connection that these are symptoms of the Stress Mechanism, that they are meaningful and that they need resolution. During the earliest stages of this process, the great majority of these signs or symptoms involve one or more aspects of the muscular, nervous, gastrointestinal or endocrine systems. This again is directly out of Dr. Hans Selye's work on stress and its effect on the human body. In order to stop this process you must recognize that these signs and symptoms are the beginning of Stress-Related Disorders. They also must be considered to be Intelligent communications from the Body-Mind to the Conscious Aware Self that there are unresolved conflicts, and that they are also clues to the conflicts themselves. Ultimately, this turning off the stress mechanism and activating the resolution process is essential to healing.

In Table: 11-1, below, we have outlined the above process and how it works.

This entire process is the basis of the Wellness-Stress-Disease Mechanism (also referred to as the Stress-Illness Mechanism). Here is how it works: The

Body-Mind recognizes the tension and wants to release it, but can't because there is one or more unresolved conflict's that are fomenting the underlying turmoil and maintaining the possibility of a threat to our well-being. As the Body-Mind identifies the unresolved conflict or conflicts, the cause of the stress, the Body-Mind soon recognizes our inability to turn off the Stress Mechanism and to release, relax and enter into its Resolution Phase. Since it cannot resolve these conflicts by itself, it attempts to communicate this information to the Conscious Aware Self. If the Conscious Aware Self is willing and able hear and recognize this communication, it then acts on the conflict by resolving it and making proper conflict resolution. The Stress Mechanism is released and turned off. When this happens the physical, mental, emotional, or spiritual tension is released and eliminated. Along with this relaxation comes the ability to learn from the experience, hence making the entire process valuable to the person. The person then has not only acted from their true nature as a problem solver, but they also grow and evolve from the experience.

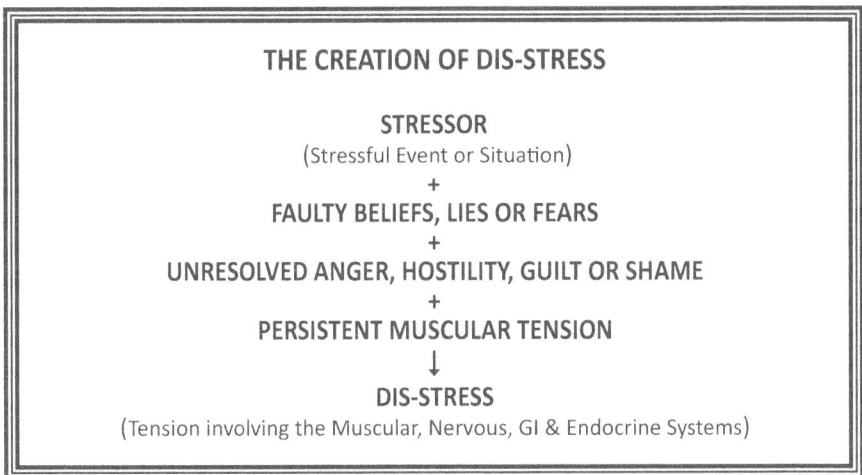

THE CREATION OF DIS-STRESS

STRESSOR
(Stressful Event or Situation)
+
FAULTY BELIEFS, LIES OR FEARS
+
UNRESOLVED ANGER, HOSTILITY, GUILT OR SHAME
+
PERSISTENT MUSCULAR TENSION
↓
DIS-STRESS
(Tension involving the Muscular, Nervous, GI & Endocrine Systems)

Table: 11-1

TO BETTER ILLUSTRATE THIS PICTURE CONSIDER THE FOLLOWING SCENE:

As you are driving away from your home, you suddenly remember (an intelligent communication from your Body-Mind) that you left an electric heater on in your bedroom. You worry that something might catch fire. You turn your car around, go back, and turn off the heater. You feel relieved and much more at ease.

This is a classical type of Body-Mind to Conscious Aware Self interaction with positive problem resolution. What we think of as "worry" is the sudden onset of the Stress Mechanism as you become aware of danger and what could happen because of it. The Conscious Aware Self, recognizing the danger, makes a decision to turn the car around (to solve the conflict and reduce your stress) and check it out. As you return, you may even run (Flight-or-Fight) into your bedroom to see if the heater is on. When you find nothing on fire, you take a deep breath (the onset of the relief, release and relaxation, the Resolution Mechanism). You turn off the heater and you suddenly feel almost powerful (you have won this battle). All of the elements of the Stress Cascade, and the Stress Mechanism, including resolution, are present in this example.

What happens if we give this scenery a slightly different ending? You have left your home and gone away for the weekend. You are many miles away from your home. Soon after you check into your hotel, you have the same thought, "Did I turn off my wall heater?" The problem now is that you are many hours away from your home. Driving back to check the heater will take hours and then driving back to the hotel will take most of the night and you will be exhausted and unable to function at your business meeting tomorrow morning. There is no one to call and you are left worrying as to whether the heater was left on or had been turned off. That night, you have difficulty sleeping. You toss and turn. The next morning you are tired but you have a very important meeting so you must go. During the meeting, your mind turns back to thinking about the heater repeatedly. By the time the meeting ends you are exhausted, you may feel that you did poorly in the meeting and you may even be more worried than before. You try to sooth your worries but you can't. Two days later, exhausted and almost in a state of panic, you drive home to find your home still intact and no evidence of any fire. You now take that deep breath, sigh and release all of the tension you built up over the past three days.

We have all experienced situations like this, worry, anxiety, tension and stress created by an unresolved conflict. Consider what happens when one or more conflicts have been present for many years. The cause has been suppressed or pushed down into your subconscious mind (Body-Mind) and left unresolved. It is this mechanism that is usually responsible for two of the earliest SRD symptoms – tension and fatigue. This is the root of Stress-Related Disorders.

If your Conscious Aware Self was either unable to acknowledge and recognize the conflict and act on the Body-Mind's communication, there would be no release, relief or relaxation. There may actually be an increase of tension as the Body-Mind would identify two conflicts. First issue is the initial unresolved conflict. The second conflict occurs from our increased need to resolve the original conflict. This creates a spiraling cycle. The Body-Mind, knows that these conflicts require resolution and begins diverting energy from other areas toward creating a solution (see Chapter 14, Creating Wellness Through Harmony and Balance). Now the energy that was to be used by the body for other needs becomes tied up during the process of dealing with this conflict. Because of this energy loss, the areas that were in the process of solving their own problems by building, healing, and evolving, became undermined, constricted, and even misdirected. An analogy would be by diverting energy from one job to another; we lose momentum in the original project. If the problems are not easily or quickly resolved, we may either lose control of our lives or end up moving in a negative direction moving toward illness, as we are about to describe.

Since we are not able to either fully relax or fully grow and evolve until our conflicts are resolved, this process can rapidly become costly. Once illness occurs, we may lose time from our jobs and possibly go into debt. Businesses are sometimes lost, relationships negatively affected, valuable time and life experiences are lost. In the end, people suffer.

If the conflict is resolved, this energy blockage is released and the previously blocked energy is now used in positive areas that are more appropriate. Growth and personal evolution can resume. If the conflict is not resolved in a reasonable period, the process often takes on a life of its own. The Body-Mind begins directing these vague symptoms to an area of the body that is most symbolic of the conflict. This is an Intelligent act on the part of the Body-Mind. It is a direct attempt to communicate to the Conscious Aware Self to acknowledge that a conflict exists and that it must be resolved.

If the conflict persists, the process may escalate and more energy is drawn from other areas of the body. Eventually, two things begin happening. First of all, the symptoms you experience begin and then they increase and change as they move forward along the Stress-Illness Continuum (see Table: 10-1). At the same time the Body-Mind increases its efforts to communicate the conflict to the Conscious Aware Self, and the symbolic areas become negatively affected. The local immune system may become weakened, allowing foreign invaders to enter. At this point the Healing Mechanism may become impaired by the hormonal/biochemical exhaustion created by the unresolved crises and healing becomes impaired. Regular maintenance and healing may be disrupted, blocked, or even ignored. The message given to the Conscious Aware Self at this point is that the conflict is causing harm. The Body-Mind now, more than ever, wants to step up its efforts to communicate to the Conscious Aware Self to do something, to find a solution. If nothing is done, no solution is found, the illness process usually does advance. The Body-Mind wants the problem to be resolved and in order to make this happen, it increases its efforts and pressure on us. If no resolution takes place and the stress process persists, eventually body tissues and organs become irreversibly injured.

While all of this is happening, the drain of energy from additional areas begins impairing the ability of these drained areas and even the entire body from protection and healing. If the process persists, more and more areas of the body become affected. Eventually, the body's overall ability to defend and repair itself becomes impaired. Now distant, uninvolved areas begin breaking down and the person becomes increasingly vulnerable to invasion and serious illness. In some cases, a kind of civil war may break out where the body, trying to solve its own problem, attacks itself and may lead to and cause autoimmune diseases.

From a single small unresolved conflict, many potential disasters and life-threatening problems can result.

Remember the verse, "For want of a nail, the shoe was lost. For want of a shoe, the horse was lost. For want of a horse, the rider was lost. For want of a rider, the battle was lost. For want of the battle, the kingdom was lost. And all for the want of a horseshoe nail[14]." From small conflicts, such as lack of self-confidence, inability to solve problems, lies, fear, or pain, we can lose our health, our well-being, and even our lives.

THE DIS-STRESS AND DYS-STRESS STAGE

At one time or another, all of us have felt the effects of stress. For most of us, an occasional episode of stress causes little harm. Why then are we concerned about stress?

The truth is that we are not concerned with occasional, harmless stress episodes. What we are concerned with are those distortions of the stress process which lead to or create persistent unresolved conflicts. This leads the stress reaction to become potentially excessive, recurrent, persistent, or chronic stress. Once the process reaches a level where it becomes a significant problem, we refer to it as Dis-Stress. This is the abnormal or pathologic situation, which is often confused with what is commonly thought of as stress.

Dis-Stress is the earliest stage of the stress reaction that leads to the earliest form of discomfort and lowest levels of illness. This often occurs when a stressor inappropriately interacts with our conscious or subconscious anger, guilt, hostility, or shame. It then causes us to feel anxiety and secondary muscular tension.

Dis-Stress may also be created when we hold one or more unresolved, faulty belief systems, lies, fear, or other conflicts. These conflicts, along with the muscle tension they create, act as a threat to our well-being and ultimately lead to more stress. This stress is maintained if we are unable to resolve the conflict that creates it. It can also become an issue when we lose control over our life to any degree and when we can't stop this loss or regain control. This happens when we have false beliefs creating increasing levels of conflict.

Remember Peter and his wife Amy in an earlier section? Peter got Amy pregnant while in High School. When he found out, he decided that he had to marry her. Once married with children, Peter decided he could no longer become an engineer. He soon began to believe that he was a failure. He was always in debt, even though he worked hard desperately trying to support his growing family.

He believed early on that he had lost complete control of his life that he was controlled by what Amy and his children needed and not what he wanted or needed.

---

14   An Old English proverb. The earliest reference to this full proverb appears to refer to the death of Richard III of England at the Battle of Bosworth Field. Its author is unknown.

There may have been many possible ways of thinking and many potential solutions, Peter persisted in feeling like a failure for many years. Since in fact he was not a failure, this was a faulty belief system. Peter often experienced anger at himself because Amy had become pregnant and because he believed he "had" to marry her. These faulty belief systems and the conflicts they created within him lead him into a state of chronic stress. His belief that he had totally lost control over his life led to even more anger and hostility which were ultimately directed against himself, his wife, his children, and his work. During the first years after his marriage he suffered from a persistent negative mental state, episodes of anger at Amy and his children, hostility toward himself and Amy, episodes of anxiety, muscle tension, inability to sleep and chronic fatigue. We now know that these were caused by his many unresolved conflicts and faulty beliefs, he simply felt that he was losing control over his life and himself.

Ultimately, this state of mind led him into the Dis-Stress Stage and the slow but steady undermining of his will to live, his immune system, as well as his healing, and repair Systems. The initial indication that Peter entered into the Dis-Stress Stage was clearly demonstrated by his increased anxiety, negative thinking, and fear of failure. This, along with his feelings of helplessness, anger, loss of temper, and self-contempt, added to the process. Together, these out-of-control emotions pushed him toward smoking to relieve anxiety and tension and alcohol to "drown" his negative feelings. The very symptoms his Body-Mind used to warn him that he needed to solve his problems ultimately triggered these negative symptoms and problems as well as the stress process.

As Peter's condition progressed, he experienced first heartburn and then indigestion as secondary symptoms and additional reminders from his Body-Mind that was trying to get him to change, solve problems, and eliminate his conflicts. Because he did not listen to his body, the process continued to progress. It eventually began to undermine his feeling of normalcy and brought about a state of depression. The symptoms went unheeded; he was left in a clearly Dis-Stressed State of existence.

During the Dis-Stress Phase, our physical, mental, and emotional symptoms are generally vague. The symptoms of Dis-Stress are often not considered to be related to illness and are often easily rationalized away as do to "a bad diet," "stress," "not sleeping very well," "a change in the weather," "seasonal changes," "injury" or even, "bad luck." Examples of Dis-Stress behaviors, signs, and symptoms are moderate to heavy alcohol use; use of illegal drugs; abuse of prescription drugs; gambling; loss of temper; nervousness; anxiety; loneliness; mood swings; headaches; difficulty getting to sleep or staying asleep; indigestion; constipation; stomach and abdominal discomfort; nausea; vomiting; back, neck and aches and pains; fatigue; lowered resistance to influenza and colds; mild infections; low-grade fevers; intermittent diarrhea; post-nasal drip; increase allergies to foods and substances; rashes; itching; accidents; and minor injuries. These are just a few of the many symptoms that occur during the Dis-Stress Stage.

People experiencing the signs and symptoms of Dis-Stress often use home remedies to self-treat. They use many different over-the-counter medications, sometimes in large amounts, and for long periods, attempting to control their Dis-Stress symptoms. As the process progresses, some may come to the point of abusing these medications. They may develop side effects or complications from the medications. They often tell others that they "don't feel well," or they may tell their family and friends that they feel "run down," or "out-of-sorts." They may think or talk about feeling sick. Children miss school or act out more than usual. They may have nightmares or bad dreams. They may even suffer either loss of appetite or an increased appetite. Anxiety, tension, muscle aches, and generalized "bone or joint pains" are quite common.

In general, these symptoms are rarely severe enough to cause the sufferer to seek medical attention. When and if they do see a doctor, no specific diagnosis is made. In fact, the doctor may even say that there is nothing wrong or he might suggest that it is just stress and to take a vacation. These are clearly clues that these people are experiencing Dis-Stress.

When a physical examination is performed on people suffering Dis-Stress symptoms, there are rarely, if ever, any abnormal findings. When any abnormalities are found, they generally relate to the immediate illness that brought them in for the examination such as a cold, flu, or allergies. Laboratory or other diagnostic testing are also normal and if positive, reveal only minimal abnormalities related to the present illness. When any laboratory test or part of the physical examination is abnormal, these usually return to normal when the acute illness is resolved. As this condition progresses and moves toward Dis-Ease, the symptoms' frequency and severity begin to increase and worsen. As the symptoms worsen, they become more annoying and frustrating. The affected individual is more likely to seek medical attention once they have reached the Dis-Ease Stage.

The later part of the Dis-Stress Stage is referred to as the Dys-Stress Stage. This signals that the signs and symptoms and how they affect the individual are more advanced and problematic than during the earlier part of the Dis-Stress Stage. This is usually characterized by frequent small illnesses, as well as mild-to-moderate recurrent or chronic health problems. Anxiety may worsen and chronic low-level depression becomes a greater problem. Chronic muscle and joint pains, nervous tension and neck pains, as well as backaches and headaches are common.

The person seems to get ill more, but the symptoms are still quite vague and generally easily treated by over-the-counter medications. They may seem to recover from one illness only to fall victim to another illness within weeks or days. The triggering cause of the Dis-Stress Stage, the patients "stress," is usually missed, and the physician rarely feels that their problems are meaningful. In time, both patient and doctor, and even the entire family may become involved, frustrated, and confused. Nothing seems to work to cure the person's problems.

Eventually, a label of hypochondriac is used both by the doctor and even family members. The complaints are taken less seriously and the person soon begins to feel alone and may even doubt their own sanity. Everyone, including the person himself, may begin doubting the truthfulness regarding their illness. They may even hide their illnesses and symptoms from family, coworkers, and friends. This increases the stresses in their life and moves the process forward to the Dis-Ease Stage.

THE DIS-EASE STAGE

As the Body-Mind begins to see that the Conscious Aware Self is not making course corrections or resolving the conflicts that need resolution, it increases the pressure on the Conscious Aware Self. It increases the process to the next level, the Dis-Ease Stage. This next level often means an increase in physical, mental or emotional pressure, physical signs and symptoms as the Body-Mind goes from whispering that there is a problem to shouting loudly about it. This moves the process from the Dis-Stress to Dys-Stress to the Dis-Ease Stage.

Dis-Ease is the stage before the onset of any actual disease or organized illness, the Disease Stage. While there is a continuum from the stage of simple stress, to Dis-Stress, Dys-Stress, Dis-Ease and Disease up to the Chronic Disease Stage, the only difference between Dis-Stress, Dys-Stress, and Dis-Ease is that the physical, emotional, mental, or spiritual symptoms of the Dis-Ease Stage are now occurring more frequently and they are somewhat more defined.

The symptoms most commonly associated with this early phase are fatigue, depression, anxiety, and recurrent small illnesses. As the process progresses, these recurrent small illnesses appear increasingly problematic and even more severe. The symptoms become more specific, more clearly defined and localized. They are less arbitrary and more likely to occur in specific areas of the body and even specific organs. The Body-Mind is now creating a strategy using specific signs, symptoms, and illnesses involving specific areas of the body, specific organs, and specific tissues to communicate its message. As the Body-Mind becomes more emphatic in its need to get its message across, the body code becomes more specific and clear. The individual's conflicts need resolution, the Body-Mind now is providing us more information if we simply understand the code it uses to tell us what the conflicts are and how problematic they will become if they are not resolved.

The Dis-Ease Stage is the earliest aspect of the Disease Stage. During this stage, the physical symptoms are more clearly defined and fit more closely into existing established disease patterns.

The physical examination, laboratory, and diagnostic testing however, remain either normal or inconclusive, hence we have not yet reached the Disease Stage where they will start becoming abnormal.

As Peter passed from the Dis-Stress Stage into the Dis-Ease Stage, his digestive system problems advanced from episodes of simple indigestion into episodes of pronounced abdominal pain. He began seeing several doctors and specialists. All the tests done were entirely normal. The only diagnosis that could be made was related to his indigestion and the onset of gastritis. While two of his doctors suspected that he might have a peptic ulcer, the tests did not show this. Other doctors suspected that his symptoms were related to stress. None of his doctors asked any questions about his alcoholism or his relationship with Amy, or about what was going on in his life. Once it was found that his tests were normal, all the doctors simply dropped their concern about the possibility of a peptic ulcer, although he was given a diet by one of the doctors and prescription medication by another to treat his pain and other symptoms, none of the doctors appeared to care or become involved with his personal problems.

This is typical for the Dis-Ease Stage. When no answers or diagnosis can be established based on the patient's medical history, laboratory, or diagnostic testing, most physicians simply prescribe medications directed at treating their patients' symptoms. Rarely is the underlying cause of stress examined, dealt with, or treated, other than with prescription medications. During this phase, it is common for most patients to be treated with over-the-counter and simple basic prescription medications. These basic medications are relatively low-level prescription medications. However, many do offer a significant risk because of their negative side effects or adverse reactions. If and when there may be any indication or signs of infection, antibiotics are commonly prescribed. Pain relievers, tranquilizers, mood elevators, antidepressants and sleeping aids are frequently prescribed as well. It is common to see patients in the later phases of the Dis-Ease Stage taking anywhere from two to six different medications on a daily basis, even though no real diagnosis has been made and no abnormal findings have been recognized.

The Dis-Ease Stage may also be marked by progressively worsening symptoms. With no answers and feeling ill, the patient often increases the frequency of medical visits to the doctor. Not getting answers from their old doctors, new ones are sought out. Unfortunately, this does not seem to help as they still get few real results or answers, even after seeing specialists. While the person's symptoms may be better defined than in earlier stages, a diagnosis is still not established. Multiple vague or very general diagnoses maybe made, yet nothing really helps to resolve the patient's situation. In most cases, even when a diagnosis is made, it is most likely that it has been given to increase the doctor's ability to bill the patient's insurance rather than because it is a real or meaningful diagnosis. The diagnoses sent onto the patient's insurance companies are usually simply a list of the patients' symptoms or a listing of minor illnesses the patient has presented with such as allergy, upper respiratory syndrome, abdominal pain, fatigue, sleeplessness,joint pain, and so on, to facilitate reimbursement.

After awhile, most of these doctors become fed up with these patients. This occurs because either they are not getting better, often because they are not responding to prescribed medications or not following instructions, or because

they cannot be cured. Often many of these patients are accused of either not taking the medications prescribed for them correctly or of being malingerers. The
physician may suspect the patient of having ulterior motives to fool the medical
establishment, for example to get out of working or that they are addicted to
drugs, especially pain medications, tranquilizers, and such.

Likewise, many of these patients become frustrated with their doctors because they are not providing a cure. In addition, it is common during this stage
that some doctors will end up telling these patients that their symptoms are,
"all in your head." The doctor now may label these patients as hypochondriacs,
medical system abusers, or even on occasion as "crazy!"

Since most doctors are not trained to recognize these various stages of
Stress-Related Disorders, and because they are not able to successfully treat
these vague and elusive symptoms, the patient is often brushed off or referred to
another doctor, a specialist, or a psychiatrist.

If a specialist is consulted, he will generally repeat all of the same diagnostic
and laboratory tests. Higher levels of medication are most likely going to be prescribed. Often, the consultation report sent back to the primary doctor provides
no meaningful or new information.

Eventually, the patient, who is not getting better, tires of what they now believe is a "runaround" and sees yet another doctor. Each doctor usually repeats
laboratory and diagnostic testing, discontinues the medication prescribed by the
last doctor and tries a series of new medications. Soon, these individuals have
medicine cabinets filled with half-used and useless medications. Still no one is
dealing with the real problems that underlie this process.

Occasionally, however, a physician or a psychologist will tap into the base
problems and actually help the patient. However, this is usually a rare occurrence. It is more common for months and even years to go by. The person is
generally put on one or more anti-anxiety or antidepressant medications as well
as a host of other medications that act to either control or make their symptoms
tolerable, but have no long-term effect on the overall occurrence or progress of
their symptoms. They have likely experienced one or more adverse side effects
from the medication that were prescribed. They have lost time from their job,
their family and friends are worried, and they may now feel hopeless, helpless
and abandoned. However, since no single doctor is aware of the patient's total situation, this is not usually recognized or factored into the diagnostic or treatment
process. Overall, the patient's condition stays the same or it gradually worsens.
Somewhere along the way, the condition progresses into the Stage of Disease.

THE DISEASE STAGE

When Peter's ulcer was finally seen on an upper gastrointestinal X-ray study,
his condition became elevated to that of a true disease. The Disease Stage begins,
according to most doctors, when they have some physical evidence and when one
or more pathologic changes are diagnosed by physical examination, laboratory,

or diagnostic testing. This can be in the form of physical signs, such as a bleeding ulcer or weight loss, or it may be upon finding a positive laboratory test, such as abnormal white cell count, a positive x-ray procedure, or an abnormal electrocardiogram. In Peter's case, it was the diagnosis of a peptic ulcer on an upper GI test.

Many physicians simply ignore the early symptoms of the Dis-Stress and Dis-Ease Stages. Illness and disease only become a serious process when there are positive physical findings, diagnostic testing, and/or laboratory tests. There is no clear-cut differentiation of the stages previously defined within the medical profession. Instead, most medical doctors have no clear idea of what is really going on with their patients before the Disease Stage. Only when a disease is finally found are the patient's symptoms taken seriously. The early stages are often overlooked or treated only symptomatically. For our purposes, we define disease as the state that occurs when there are symptoms along with positive laboratory and/or positive diagnostic testing that specifically define a pathologic condition. Whether what is found fits exactly with the textbook definition of the particular disease process or not is unimportant. Since textbooks often require multiple criteria, which are usually not all seen in any one patient, the physician's experience is frequently the best guide for making a diagnosis.

In addition, for the purposes of defining the effects of the Stress Mechanism, we consider the Disease Stage beginning at that point where there is demonstrable damage occurring to the body. While damage may have been occurring in the previous stages, it could neither be seen nor tested. In the Disease Stage, it is now clearly recognized. This is not only recognized by the findings from a physical examination, laboratory and diagnostic testing, but in the effect it has on the individual's life and well-being. The patient now has a specific or generalized loss of well-being and wellness. This may involve their physical, mental, emotional, or spiritual aspects.

In the stages previously mentioned – Conflict, Stress, Dis-Stress, Dis-Ease and the early parts of this Disease Stage – the symptoms are fully reversible. All that is necessary is solving the problem and resolving the conflict. However, once a person reaches the later parts of the Disease Stage, the illness process may no longer be fully responsive to simple treatments. There are only two directions this process can go – toward chronic disease and disability, or toward death. While the process is still reversible prior to the onset of the Disease Stage, the longer this process exists and the more severe the process becomes, the less likely the chances are of reversal. Once the process reaches the point of becoming a Chronic Disease, complete reversal is much less likely, and often no longer possible.

THE CHRONIC DISEASE STAGE

Clearly, the chronic disease stage is a natural continuation of the Stress-Disease Process. Once disease is allowed to occur, the likelihood of the process advancing to become a chronic disease is extremely high. In Peter's case, the lack of resolution of his conflicts and his not loving himself pushed the process until he developed a peptic ulcer. Once the ulcer began bleeding, Peter had few choices other than surgery. This transformed his condition from an Acute Disease to a Chronic Disease. After Peter's surgery, his condition became fixed in the state of Chronic Disease. Part of his stomach was removed, producing irreversible tissue damage, not to mention his emotional, physiological, mental, and spiritual injuries.

In the context of this book, Chronic Disease begins when the process creates irreversible tissue injury or when the process reaches a point of no return and is no longer fully reversible. This does not mean that the process can't be stopped, or that the original problems shouldn't be resolved. It simply means that the person can never be returned to their original state of normalcy.

We still believe that miracles can occur when people create a vivid picture of what they want. Seeing themselves as healthy and giving their Conscious Aware Self and Higher Self specific orders to create this picture of health is the basis of the healing process. Even at the stage of Chronic Disease some conditions can be reversed when a person is capable of creating a clear enough picture and then doing whatever is necessary to make it work. In the earlier stages of the illness process, people may attain relief for reasons other than resolving the causing conflicts. The specific symptoms may even spontaneously reverse or disappear. If the conflicts persist, they may either return as before or worse, or show up in an entirely different form.

Even after someone reaches the Chronic Disease Stage, resolving underlying conflicts is still important. Many of the old conflicts are no longer meaningful, but they still are acting negatively and need resolution. Without resolution, these unresolved conflicts can cause a worsening of the Chronic Disease process. This can eventually lead to new illnesses or even death. Since any conflict can create multiple levels of problems, multiple levels of unresolved conflicts can lead to one or more Stress-Related Disorders, profound Dis-Stress, Dis-Ease, or more severe Diseases. Finally, without resolution, the person remains blocked from reaching their highest, healthiest, and best Self.

In Table: 11-2, below, we offer a summary of the six primary Stress-Related-Disorders Stages. Previously we have discussed the primary stages involved within the Wellness —> Stress —> Illness Continuum. These stages are Stress, Dis-Stress, Dys-Stress, Dis-Ease, Disease and Chronic Disease. These are summaries of the important defining criteria and how each of these stages can affect us either moving toward illness and chronic disease or healing when moving from Disease back to total and complete Wellness.

SUMMARY OF SRD STAGES (STATES OR PHASES) - 1

Symptoms	Signs	Examples	Outcome
Optimal Health & Well Being			
None	None	Full complete vibrant health and wellness	Long healthy life
Stress			
Mild to moderate generalized anxiety, depression gastrointestinal disturbances, fatigue. Emotional and behavioral acting our fears, changes in eating habits including overeating, loss of enthusiasm or energy, and mood changes.	Mild to moderate muscle tension, difficulty sleeping, headaches, nervousness, anxiety, not many physical signs. More than usual use or abuse of alcohol and drugs, cigarette smoking	Fear before taking a test, job insecurity, relationship problems. Frequent small illnesses, as well as mild to moderate recurrent or chronic health problems.	All symptoms, signs and illnesses are fully reversible.
Dis-Stress			
Moderate to severe anxiety, vague physical, emotional and mental symptoms such as: mood swings, nausea, nervousness, fatigue, loneliness, loss of temper, Excessive eating or loss of appetite, gambling, sex, fear. Children: miss school, they often act out more than usual. Adults may miss work often or more than in the past; bad dreams or even nightmares. The individual tries to handle symptoms on his or her own, generally does not see medical doctor, primarily uses and depends upon over-the-counter medications or illegal drugs. See Appendices A and B, below.	Moderate to heavy use of alcohol, smoking, over-the-counter medications, more likely to use of illegal drugs, sometimes abuse of prescription drugs. Has headaches, difficulty getting to sleep or staying asleep, indigestion, stomach and abdominal discomfort or pains, vomiting, back, neck and aches and pains, lowered resistance to flus and colds, mild infections, low grade fevers, intermittent diarrhea, post-nasal drip, increase allergies to foods, and other substances, rashes, itching, accidents and minor injuries. See Appendices A and B, below.	Everything above only more exaggerated and frequent. More colds, flu, allergies, stomach aches, headaches, episodes of nausea and vomiting, clearly more nervous and tense than had been in the past, sometimes even argumentative. Parents, relatives, friends, co-workers often recognize a difference in attention span, work ethic and overall personality. When any lab testing is done, it is either negative or specific for acute illness of the moment. See Appendix C, below.	All symptoms, signs and illnesses are fully reversible.

Table: 11-2 (1)

SUMMARY OF SRD STAGES (STATES OR PHASES) - 2

Symptoms	Signs	Examples	Outcome
Dys-Stress			
Severe anxiety. Same as above only more exaggerated.	Same as above only more exaggerated. Often labeled as a hypochondriac by family, friends or co-workers	Same as above only more exaggerated. When any lab testing is done it is either negative or specific for acute illness of the moment.	All symptoms, signs and illnesses are fully reversible.
See Appendices A and B, below.	See Appendices A and B, below.	See Appendix C, below.	
Dis-Ease			
Anxiety and/or panic attacks, all of the above persists but appear to be more of a problem. Signs are now more specific, more defined and often better localized. The individual is now seeking to get help from one or more medical doctor(s), chiropractor(s), naturopath(s), herbalist(s), alternative medicine practitioners. Diet, job, co-workers, children, spouse or partners are being blamed for symptoms and problems.	All of the above persists but appear to be more of a problem and they are now more specific, more defined and more localized.	Acid indigestion, frequent colds, sore throats, ear aches, abdominal or stomach pains, hemorrhoids, headaches When any lab testing is done, it is still either negative or specific for acute illness of the moment. When this individual sees his or her doctor other than the acute illness of the moment, nothing is found to be wrong. Patient believes the doctor is missing his or her problem. The doctor often believes patients problems are due to stress, anxiety or they are all in the patient's head. Patient is often labeled a hypochondriac by the doctor.	All symptoms, signs and illnesses are fully reversible.
See Appendices A and B, below.	See Appendices A and B, below.	See Appendix C, below.	

Table: 11-2 (2)

SUMMARY OF SRD STAGES (STATES OR PHASES) - 3

Symptoms	Signs	Examples	Outcome
DISEASE			
Symptoms are more focus and localized. The individual now has one or more bona fide medical conditions. Now the doctor can accept and deal with the patients as a sick person. This makes the doctor's job much easier, concurrently the patient even feels better, "See, I am not (or was not) crazy!"	Signs are consistent with specific medical condition generated by the body-mind. Abdominal pain now may mean peptic ulcer, irritable bowel syndrome, gastritis, etc. Laboratory and diagnostic tests are now demonstrating medical condition and verifying illness. In the beginning, both patient and doctor are happier as a "real illness" exists both feel vindicated and better. Later on conflict unresolved, new dis-stress, dys-stress and/or dis-ease signs and symptoms will arise and this will complicate everything for both of them and everyone else involved family, friends, job.	Migraine headaches, peptic ulcer, irritable bowel syndrome, gastritis, and a host of other simple easy to diagnose medical conditions appear only to simply show up.	Generally these medical problems and their signs and symptoms, intercurrent illnesses are still fully reversible. They will be resolved when the underlying conflict that is causing them is found and eliminated. When this happens, the Illness process is transformed into a Wellness process.
See Appendices A and B, below.	See Appendices A and B, below.	See Appendix C, below.	
CHRONIC DISEASE			
Symptoms may vary greatly depending on the specific chronic condition as well as persisting unresolved conflicts, new dis-stress, dys-stress and/or dis-ease symptoms.	Signs may vary greatly depending on the specific chronic condition as well as persisting unresolved conflicts, new dis-stress, dys-stress and/or dis-ease signs.	Post heart attack, surgery, stroke.	Illnesses have transformed into chronic disease, surgery may have been done in the past. Damage and physiologic changes to the body and bodily tissues have occurred. At this point the illness process is no longer reversible
See Appendices A and B, below.	See Appendices A and B, below.	See Appendix C, below.	

Table: 11-2 (3)

Chapter Twelve

RETURNING TO WELLNESS

WHAT IS WELLNESS?

Up until this point, we discussed the process of how stress leads to illness, specifically Stress-Related Diseases. It is now time to find out how we can "undo" this process and return to good health. Before starting this discussion, some important questions must first be asked and answered: First, "What is Wellness?" "What do I have to do to create wellness?" "Will it be difficult to find my way back to wellness?" "What could keep me from recreating wellness again?" And finally, "How, where and when do I start this return to the wellness process?"

There is no single accepted definition for wellness. When anyone asks us how we define wellness, we suggest that wellness is the total physical, mental, emotional, and spiritual sense of well-being and good health, along with the absence of all illness. For someone who has reached the Chronic Disease Stage and already has permanent tissue or organ damage, wellness is often still possible. However, you must now take into consideration any permanent damage already done, as well as limitations and restrictions this illness created. For those parts and aspects of this person not affected by Chronic Disease, wellness applies as just stated.

The concept of wellness also implies being in complete harmony with our three Selves, our Body-Mind (our Subconscious Self), our Conscious Aware Self and our Higher (spiritual) Self. We generally must also be in reasonable harmony and balance with the world around us. There is no ongoing or acute sickness, illness, or disease. When we are fully well, most people also experience a substantial degree of self-love, self-worth, and self-value. We are capable of accepting the Universe and ourselves as we are.

A well person is a person who feels good about them self. A well person has no significant physical, mental, emotional, or spiritual problems. If there are problems, the well person works on them. He grows and evolves, and he constantly works on improving himself. He constantly works at resolving his problems and is generally able to live a healthy and adventurous life because of his efforts and work resolving these conflicts and problems. A well person loves day to day work and often picks what he works at, not only because it feels good doing it, but also because it makes him feel better about himself. A well person solves problems before they become too big to be resolved. A well person learns not only to listen to, but understand his body, his inner thoughts, and the Intelligent communications from his Body-Mind and what it means to him. A well person recognizes his stresses and uses them to learn more about himself and then uses them as a tool to help him grow, evolve and thrive. A well person lives life fully; he understands that life will sometimes cause pain and suffering, friends will die, loved ones will move on. He understands that life and the world around him are dynamic and always changing and that he has the power to make these changes positive or negative in regards to his life and his needs. However, he also knows that the pain he experiences is part of life and will pass, and that it is always a tool he can use to grow, evolve and thrive.

Using this definition of wellness, how many people do we each actually know who are completely well? Some, but not many!

It is often easier to define what wellness isn't, rather than what it is. Wellness is not simply the absence of illness. It is experienced as a positive. It does not require us to like the way things are. It does not require that we believe everything we see or hear. It does not suggest that everything in our Universe is perfect. However, it does require that we have a sufficiently clear view of ourselves and our Universe, allowing us to be flexible, and capable of surviving, growing, and evolving in an imperfect world which is often complicated and frequently hostile.

Wellness and well-being are not fear, anxiety, conflict, disagreement, power, control, stress, rigidity, or illness. It should be obvious by now that wellness is not about dishonesty, lying, cheating, or diminishing others or ourselves.

Wellness is definitely not about being perfect. Without mistakes, we would lose creativity and some of life's most important lessons. The fully well person is not perfect. Rather, they are always a work in progress.

Within the concept of wellness, it is not important if someone is physically or mentally impaired, or whether the impairment was caused by illness, genetic deformities, or injury. What is important is that the disabled or impaired individual is working toward throwing off their negative beliefs about illness, maximizing their potential, abilities, and capacities in the most positive way possible.

Wellness is also not about intelligence, but using our capacities, positively or negatively. Handicaps are only handicaps if seen or used as handicaps.

> **Handicaps are really only handicaps**
> **if they are seen as handicaps.**

I, Allen, once met a wonderful young man with no left leg. He came to me with a medical disability evaluation form, which he wanted me to fill out and sign. Since he had no left leg from the hip down, I instantly concluded that he was disabled, but asked him what other limitations or disabilities he had. In response to this question he replied, "None. I am not disabled. I have no disabilities!"

I was of course confused because he was here in my office for a disability evaluation. This usually meant, for most of the patients who came for disability evaluations, that they either wanted a statement to prove that they were disabled or they wanted to obtain a disability rating of how disabled they were. Being confused, I then had to ask him, "What do you want me to say on your Disability Evaluation Form?"

He looked directly into my eyes and said, "I want you to say that I am not disabled." He then added, "I have applied for a job and I was told that I must have a statement regarding my 'disability,' but I do not consider myself to be disabled and I do not believe that there is any reason why they should see me as disabled."

I performed a careful exam, talking to him during the process. At the end of the examination, I wrote on the form, "This patient is fully able. He is just missing his left leg. He can do any kind of work which does not specifically require a left leg."

I learned while talking to him that he lost his left leg at 18 months of age and had lived since then without it. He had been a straight-A student in high school and college and he had lettered in several sports. He could drive, swim, ride horses, ski, and he raced cars. He told me that he was a gymnast and then demonstrated to me his ability to flip from standing perfectly on his right leg to standing on his hands, doing handstand push-ups, one-handed handstand push-ups and one-handed handstand push-ups on the tips of his fingers and alternating from his right hand to his left hand and then back again to the right hand. He was clearly able to do more than me. While watching him show me what he could do, I was left asking myself, "Which one of us is more disabled, him or me?"

I personally could not do any of the things he was easily capable of doing. He had proved to me that he was not disabled, even though he did not have a left leg.

Wellness is our NATURAL STATE OF BEING.

We do not have to DO anything specific to create it,
beyond living healthfully, solving problems
& thinking healthy thoughts.

Finally, wellness is as much a state of mind as a physical reality. It is about people seeing themselves as healthy, living a healthy life, doing healthy things, and acting healthy. The healthy and well individuals continually challenge themselves and the Universe, meeting challenges and experiencing the world presented to them. Those people are fully well and feel good. They are healthy, emotionally stable, and spiritually secure. They invariably have a positive physical, mental, emotional, and spiritual attitude and practices, both in their personal and professional lives. They are in harmony and balance within their life and the Universe. Wellness is an active, dynamic positive state of being.

IS THERE A NATURAL PROGRESSION FROM DISEASE TO HEALTH?

In the initial chapters, we explained that there was a pathway from wellness to illness and from stress to stress-related illnesses. For many of us, this path is all too familiar. Nevertheless, you may next ask, is there also a natural progression from disease, specifically stress-related illnesses, to health? The answer to this question is "Yes. Once we become ill and are caught in this process, the return journey to wellness often looks long and hard." While many people just want their doctor to give them a pill that makes all their illnesses and problems go away, this rarely happens. On occasion, a pill or medication may work, but most of the time when it does it is only a temporary solution, one that works for an already self-limiting illness. Most medications, while they may help control symptoms, do not usually return most people to full and complete wellness.

All too often, people who are sick and believe that their doctor or his medication will make them well become angry, disillusioned, frustrated, and depressed when they realize that this not only doesn't happen, but that their condition may even worsen, moving them closer toward a Chronic Disease State. Many of these same people find themselves feeling trapped in a web they unknowingly created for themselves. Initially hopeful that wellness is just around the next corner, they may try all kinds of cures, but nothing works consistently or permanently, and they end up falling deeper into helplessness and despair. Some people may feel hopeless and lost in the Illness-Disease Mechanism. Not knowing what is happening to them nor how to get out of the vicious negative cycle in which they find themselves, they often suffer longer and needlessly.

In the beginning, people looked to their medical doctors for help. When this failed, they may have then turned to alternative medicine. When this didn't work, they may even have turned to anyone who offered them even the slightest ray of hope. In the end, they resolved themselves to being ill, they allowed their symptoms to be treated, and they gave up hope of ever being fully well and healthy again. We see many people exactly like this on a daily basis. Every doctor does.

Is this the end? Could there possibly still be hope? Is full and complete wellness available to even the sickest and most hopelessly ill person?

Experience tells us yes. Spontaneous healing does occur. People with se-rious, even life-threatening illnesses can and do suddenly recover against all odds. Cancers can and do heal and go away. Acute autoimmune diseases do re-solve themselves and disappear. People who have been given death sentences by their doctors may not only survive, but also may even outlive their doctors, returning to full and complete health and wellness. Every doctor has seen doz-ens of people with stories of having survived at least one "fatal" illness.

Are these simply flukes or possible reproducible miracles? The answer here is maybe "yes," but most likely "no." This process is reproducible. It hap-pens every day all over the world. Miracles are miracles only because we have not yet figured out why these healings have happened. Once we understand why they have happened, it becomes science and fact, and each of us may well be able to reproduce this ourselves.

Can total healing happen for anyone? The answer again is "yes." When we look closely, we can see that this primarily happens when the person has first met certain tests. First, they or someone very close to them must believe in wellness. Second, they must be ready or at least willing to let go of their illness, as well as let go of their negative thoughts and belief in their illness, possibly even their belief in the reality of illness itself. They must take away as much as is possible of the negative power their illness holds over them. Finally, they must be willing to do whatever is necessary to heal themselves.

True wellness exists within us all the time. Remember: Wellness is man-kind's natural state of being. We must also continually work however, to main-tain our optimal health and wellness. True wellness occurs when we allow our-selves to feel healthy, full of life, and live creative and vital lives. We also must be willing to solve problems so that we move ourselves off the Wellness-Stress-Ill-ness Continuum and onto the Illness-Stress-Wellness Continuum, the return path to Optimal Health and Wellness.

Unfortunately, with optimal wellness being our supreme goal, many peo-ple take this wellness state for granted. They are content simply to be feeling good in the moment and have no immediate illness. They are not able or will-ing to watch over their wellness and protect it, to do everything necessary to guard it. They get lazy. Negative beliefs such as fear, guilt, and shame, can end up blocking them from doing "everything necessary" to preserve and protect their health and wellness. All too often, only when they are in trouble or when their health and wellness are already undermined or completely gone, do they think about it and want it back.

Others may become so absorbed with their illnesses or fears of becoming ill, or their subconscious desire for a kind of relief, even suicide, to help them end their misery and the anguish created by the conflicts and problems they and others have created for them, that they ultimately bring illness upon them-selves or they block healing from occurring. We do not lose our wellness sim-ply because of bad genes, injury or external factors, but rather as a result of ignoring the factors that create illness – stress, poor diet, unhealthy lifestyle, drugs, lack of problem solving, faulty beliefs, guilt, and fear. We lose wellness because we take the easy way out of situations. We cover up our pain and suffering. We do not deal with and resolve the issues that are causing them. We sell out for ending or limiting our pain and in doing so we lose our peace of mind and very often our health and well-being too.

Just as there is a natural progression from wellness to sickness, there is also a natural progression from sickness to wellness. (See Table: 12-1.) The wellness process lies deep inside us. It exists simultaneously with the illness process. In fact, they are one in the same. In an earlier section we described the many layers of defensive systems. These layers not only protect us, but they also mediate and initiate our personal healing processes.

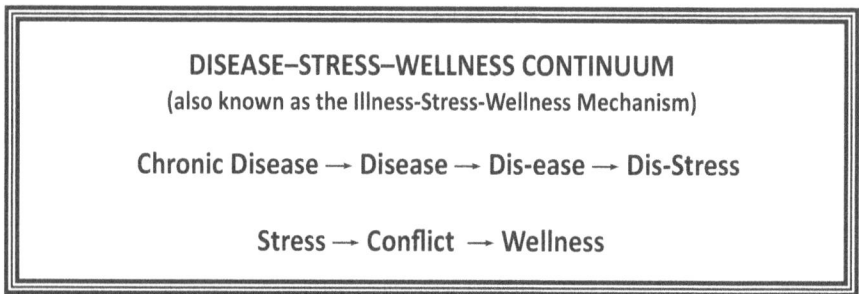

DISEASE–STRESS–WELLNESS CONTINUUM
(also known as the Illness-Stress-Wellness Mechanism)

Chronic Disease → Disease → Dis-ease → Dis-Stress

Stress → Conflict → Wellness

Table: 12-1

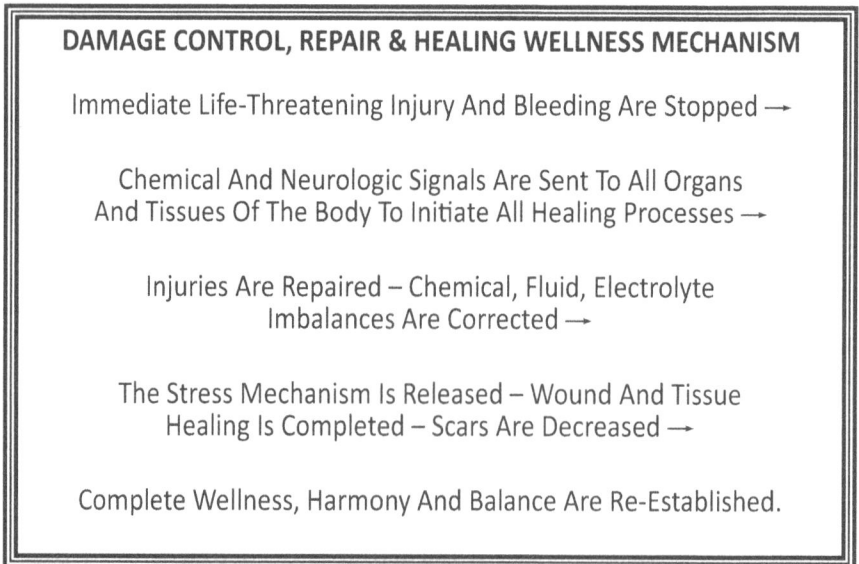

DAMAGE CONTROL, REPAIR & HEALING WELLNESS MECHANISM

Immediate Life-Threatening Injury And Bleeding Are Stopped →

Chemical And Neurologic Signals Are Sent To All Organs
And Tissues Of The Body To Initiate All Healing Processes →

Injuries Are Repaired – Chemical, Fluid, Electrolyte
Imbalances Are Corrected →

The Stress Mechanism Is Released – Wound And Tissue
Healing Is Completed – Scars Are Decreased →

Complete Wellness, Harmony And Balance Are Re-Established.

Table: 12-2

As soon as these defensive processes are activated, the repair and healing processes are also initiated. As stated earlier, the Stress (Fight-or-Flight) Mechanism also regulates the repair and healing mechanism and processes in our body. Both the defense and healing processes are mediated by a similar series of chemical and hormonal reactions that are also controlled by our hypothalamus and our adrenal glands. These hormones counterbalance each other so that the degree of healing corresponds to the degree of injury. All injuries associated with body tissues, cuts, bruises, fractures, internal and external wounds, as well as illnesses caused by Stress-Related Diseases, can be repaired by stimulating the healing portion of our Defensive, Repair and Healing Systems. When an injury occurs, the body responds in three ways. 1) The Offensive Mechanisms are initiated for immediate protection and to guard against further injury or invasion, and 2) simultaneously with this, the immediate Repair Mechanisms are initiated to deal with life-threatening conditions such as stopping active bleeding, plugging holes, and the emergency repair of damage created by the ongoing injury, 3) next, the long-term Healing Systems are initiated and begin all necessary repairs needed to save our life and help us to return to long-term health and wellness.

When an injury is sustained, our body immediately seals off the bleeding areas, now with bleeding controlled the wound entrance will need to be repaired. This will eventually be done either by our built in repair systems or we go to the hospital where a doctor now sutures the wound.

Once the immediate crisis is contained, signals are sent notifying the Body-Mind that the immediate danger is over and that immediate repairs and long-term healing are required. We could call this process "damage control," "repair of injury" or better still, "healing." We will not go into the details of the many hormonal and chemical reactions that are required to make this happen (See Table: 12-1 and 12-2). Instead, we will give you a brief overview of this process demonstrating that our body knows exactly what it needs to do and how to do it to reverse illness and heal itself.

This Intelligent process acts in the following way: Bleeding, if present, must always be stopped first. Very specific cells and chemicals in the bloodstream create clotting and constriction of the injured blood vessels accomplishes this. Next, the white blood cells and lymphocytes are drawn to the area for defensive action to fight infection and clean up the debris related to the injury and repair. The tissues around the wound create a cellular and fibrous barricade that prevents the invasion of any foreign organisms or substances. Bridges of fibrous connective tissue are constructed across the wound and tissue repairs are initiated. The body acts rapidly, aggressively, and effectively to return itself to normal.

Think about a time when you cut yourself. The wound bled for a while but stopped on its own. You may have helped by putting pressure on the wound with your finger, using an ice cube, or applying a bandage, but it really stopped on its own. Eventually, the wound will form a scab and then completely heal. Once healed, all you might experience of the injury is a scar commemorating the injury. While some injuries may be large enough to require medical attention, in most cases we would survive without it. The body and its repair systems heal most wounds without help. Medical help, such as sutures or surgical intervention, can speed up healing and prevent complications, but natural healing occurs in any case.

Significant life-threatening wounds, invasion by lethal foreign organisms, exposure to toxic or caustic substances, or major chemical imbalances can limit, slow down or even prevent spontaneous healing. However, whether or not these occur, our Body-Mind knows exactly what to do and how to heal itself, and other than in severe, life-threatening wounds needs little or no help to do what it must do to heal us. When life-threatening wounds, an invasion by lethal foreign organisms, exposures to toxic or caustic substances, or major chemical imbalances do not exist, healing is usually faster, more effective and more complete.

If we can identify the causative problems or unresolved conflicts, which have lead us down the Wellness-Stress-Illness pathway toward illness. We can begin our process of eliminating these illnesses and diseases through resolving these conflicts. Whether you suffer from an autoimmune disease, anemia, nutrition deficiency syndrome, cancer, depression, anxiety, or almost any other illness, find or identify what triggered it and those unresolved problems and conflicts that feed it. Then, you can immediately start working on them, stimulating your healing systems to heal all existing damage and repair all but the non-reversible damage that has been done to your body, mind, emotions, or spirit. We can then return to optimal health and wellness. Obviously, the earlier we start this process, the better the result.

With more significant injury where tissue is irreparably damaged, when it is too late, dangerous, or lethal foreign organisms or substances have entered into the body, the body's ability to heal is steadily or even greatly diminished. In such cases, medical treatment is often necessary. Even with the best medical treatment, however, the ultimate result in such cases may still be incomplete healing and either chronic disease or death.

The power of the human body and mind to heal itself is great. Nearly any disease or injury can be healed when clear intention and conflict resolution are applied.

We will look at the process and steps for creating healing and wellness in considerably more detail, along with exercises and processes to help you heal yourself in our sequel to When Your Body Talks, Listen!, When Your Body Talks, Heal It!

Chapter Thirteen

CREATING BLOCKS TO WELLNESS & HEALING

HEALING IS EASY

Our ability to heal ourselves is divided between two parts. The first and possibly least accessible to us are our automatic healing processes, which are all under the control of our Body-Mind. We do not have to think or do much about this aspect of healing. As the name implies, automatic healing processes do everything they need to do on their own without any conscious help. These healing mechanisms are inborn and Intelligent. Our Body-Mind and body systems know exactly what to do to activate and manage the body's automatic healing mechanisms. While the Body-Mind requires little assistance from us in managing these automatic systems, it might from time-to-time ask us to do certain things to maximize its ability to heal correctly. It may require that we do commonsense things – wash and clean the wound, protect the wound from the elements, or rest to facilitate the recovery process.

The Body-Mind might stimulate cravings for certain foods or herbs, foods that it might require to provide essential nutrients needed to support the healing process.

It might project certain symptoms designed to let us know that we have certain types of illnesses that require specific types of help, and that we have one or more unresolved conflicts, faulty beliefs, blocks or complexes that must be resolved.

The second part of the healing mechanism is the Conscious Aware Self. It is not always essential that the Conscious Aware Self do anything specific for the healing process, it can either obstruct or support the Body-Mind in using healing energies or seeking specific kinds of support. The Conscious Aware Self can also create a very clear intention to accomplish healing and do whatever is necessary to facilitate the overall process of healing our body, mind, and spirit. The Conscious Aware Self can also help by seeking, finding, and implementing solutions to resolve those conflicts which have been causing illness.

It can also help by finding and eliminating blocks and complexes which are actively or passively blocking the healing process.

We may not be consciously aware that our Body-Mind is working to heal us. We may however be aware from time to time that it is communicating vital information about healing to us. This is why we must learn to listen to and hear it when it is communicating with us. This information tells us what the Body-Mind needs to facilitate healing. If we simply accept these symptoms and signs and do what they ask of us, then healing seems to occur automatically and spontaneously. For example, when the body becomes dehydrated, our Body-Mind communicates this by saying that it is thirsty and needs water. When we get this message, and move to get water, it will assist us in drinking as much water as needed to "heal" and resolve our dehydration. Drinking water is exactly what our Body-Mind wants us to do. When we recognize this and do what is needed to quench the thirst, this facilitates our healing process. Hence, the Body-Mind and Conscious Aware Self work together as a "healing team."

Both the Body-Mind and Conscious Aware Self are formidable, individual resources for creating healing. However, when they work together their total capacity for healing is significantly greater than when working alone.

As we suggested earlier, this book's main goal is to help you understand how to activate and maintain all the healing resources that can be directed and mediated by your Conscious Aware Self. This does not mean to imply that the Body-Mind cannot do what is needed on its own. Rather by working together, the Body-Mind and Conscious Aware Self can speed up, direct, focus, and unblock our ability to heal ourselves.

Your freedom and ability to do this is not always easy or simple. It is often based on how well you understand what is needed, and how and why your Body-Mind works. To make this work optimally you will first need to know and understand:

1. The Body-Mind is fully capable of working and accomplishing its goals on its own, but it can only solve simple problems. To solve complex problems, it must have access to the inductive reasoning powers of the Conscious Aware Self.

2. The Body-Mind's deductive capacities only allow absolute right or wrong actions, and not much else in the way of suggestions or choices. The Conscious Aware Self operates using both deductive and inductive logic. Its capacity for using inductive logic is driven by observations sent to it from the Body-Mind. Using these observations and the information from the sensory systems, past experiences, and projections of what it expects in the future, requires that the Conscious Aware Self is always testing the world around it. The Conscious Aware Self can also work with right and wrong, black and white, as well as many shades of gray in between. It can also sort through and make some clarity out of gray and muddy situations. The development of the scientific method

and our capacity to solve problems often involves a blending of these two types of logical approaches.

3. Our Body-Mind's deductive logic may require absolute proofs, clear answers, and direct responses. It can never work fully and completely in the real world where there are shades of gray. The Body-Mind has no capacity for using what it observes, other than for Fight-or-Flight. It has no capacity for experimentation or testing the validity of a plan of action. It cannot create a plan, premise, or theory to help us solve our problems. In a sense, the Body-Mind simply does what seems logical in the now-moment. If this works, terrific. If not, it turns to the Conscious Aware Self for help. They are both limited when working separately, but by pooling their efforts and working together, they are a problem-solving, healing machine.

4. The Body-Mind is built to take instruction from the Conscious Aware Self. Only in situations where there are immediate threats to our survival or a potentially life-threatening emergency is our Body-Mind able to operate without the help of the Conscious Aware Self. At all other times, our Body-Mind works best under the guidance of our Conscious Aware Self, even when it is capable of operating on its own.

5. Unfortunately, our fears, faulty belief systems, lies, and unresolved conflicts can often get in the way of solving problems and healing ourselves. People become frightened. Blocks and complexes may occur and they may not only get in the way, but they may also stop or derail some or all efforts being made to create healing by both the Body-Mind and the Conscious Aware Self. We may question what our Body-Mind requires. We may be too frightened or confused to act. We may even rebel against what our Body-Mind wants if we feel that it is too much effort. We may entirely misread what it is asking us for, or simply be shocked and not be able to respond to its needs.

While the healing process itself may appear easy or difficult, the Body-Mind knows exactly what to do. It may not always be able to do what is necessary. This may occur because one of the greatest dilemmas we face to full and complete healing and wellness, are the many faulty belief systems, lies, guilt, and fears created through the years and stored within the Body-Mind. These blocks and complexes can slow, stop, or even reverse healing efforts.

Since the mind and our physical body work together as the Body-Mind, we must always be aware that we can sabotage our Healing and Repair Systems by worrying and imagining the worst. We can also help it by trusting our Healing and Repair Systems and by visualizing ourselves completely healed and well. We must accept that our Maintenance, Repair, Healing, and Defense Systems are intimately tied to our Conscious Aware Self and its self-image. The instructions given to the Body-Mind are important in the healing outcome. If either our Body-Mind or Conscious Aware Self has a negative "illness mentality," or we have too many unresolved conflicts, then our ability to maintain, repair, defend, and heal maybe significantly impaired.

In order to heal, we must first believe that we can and will heal. We must help the Body-Mind by creating a clear and uncomplicated plan of what we will look like when fully healed and functioning optimally. This is what we accomplish, when we reach for and find our highest, healthiest, best Self-image. We will give you more details as we proceed to outline those things that can block us from reaching for and finding our highest, healthiest, best Self and those things we can do and that will help us promote our own healing and optimal wellness.

KNOWING THE ENEMY – WHAT BLOCKS US FROM HEALING?

If we really can control our ability to get sick or to stay healthy, then why do we allow ourselves to get sick in the first place? The answer is not easy. We do not believe that most people consciously choose to get sick. Most illnesses and diseases are Intelligent acts of the Body-Mind and are neither random nor purposeless. As we have repeatedly suggested, they represent a form of communication by the Body-Mind to the Conscious Aware Self, which is offered to us to let us know that there are unresolved conflicts requiring immediate solution and resolution. As part of this process, the Body-Mind intentionally or unintentionally may direct energy and attention away from the Healing, Repair, Defensive, and Offensive Systems, which then can open us up to becoming ill.

Even though our Body-Mind only wants to attract our attention, much of the energy it uses to do this is needlessly expended as nonspecific stress, anxiety, addictions, compulsions, insecurity, fear, and managing the effects of these unresolved conflicts. In our earlier discussion of Peter and Amy, we noted that it not only took the form of anxiety, but also of alcoholism, drug addiction, smoking, arguing, compulsive buying, self-hatred, partner- and self-abuse, and more. These actions misdirected their life-force energies and took the attention of the Body-Mind away from finding and solving the very problems that created all these symptoms. Ultimately, this misdirection and drain of energy led to tissue injury and contributed to inhibiting their natural healing processes.

Because the significant stress response's Peter and Amy experienced were negatively directed, their self-images and self-esteems were damaged in the process. This contributed to their feelings of failure, worthlessness, and vulnerability.

When the Body-Mind receives messages, thoughts, and feelings of worthlessness and low self-esteem from the Conscious Aware Self, it assumes that these are commands. It then gives power to any situations that validate these belief systems. Through production and release of specific neurochemicals, the entire body, including the immune system, is exposed to these messages of unworthiness. The Defensive and Healing Systems may then interpret these messages as if the Self is unworthy and therefore does not deserve to be defended and protected. The now-misdirected Body-Mind begins processing all information, and hence all of its present and future actions through this new set of instructions. If repeated enough times and given enough power by the Conscious Aware Self and Body-Mind, these false beliefs begin acting as filters through which everything said, thought, and believed is interpreted. This then may lead to a downward spiral. The ultimate degree of impairment generally depends upon the intensity of the negative beliefs created by these faulty belief systems. The more power given to our negative beliefs, the greater the degree our difficulties will negatively affect us, the more likely healing will be undermined, and illness will occur.

At this point you may wonder how so many people allow negative beliefs to encroach on their life and undermine them. The answer is simple, they don't know that this is happening to them. Most people just live from day to day, never realizing how or what they think about themselves or others, or what power their thoughts have over them, their lives, health, and wellness.

It usually happens that the first time people suffering from SRDs become aware of their faulty belief systems and that these faulty belief systems are at the root of their illnesses is only after they become ill and are working on healing themselves. Unfortunately, most people never make this connection. Their ultimate fate then is to end up suffering from serious chronic illness or disease, or premature death.

When I, Allen, first became aware of how my faulty beliefs had created and intensified my own illnesses, I, too, was surprised. It was not a happy revelation, since I had no idea how to deal with it at the time. It was however, instructive and because I recognized it, and chose to understand this process I was able to give birth to everything I am now writing.

SECONDARY GAINS

We allow illness to happen to us for many reasons. There are hundreds, if not millions, of reasons people give as to why they have become ill, most of these reasons can be broken down into just a few categories.

For example, there are secondary gains. When secondary gains are operating, this occurs because people will trade what might often at first appears to be a greater conflict for a lesser conflict. Take for example a child who doesn't want to go to school because he feels like a failure. In order to not feel like a failure, he may trade his future education for relief of his immediate feelings of being a failure. If the child's fear of being a failure in school bothers him a lot, then isn't it only a very small price, being ill, for getting out of going to school? While he may not think that his being sick was related to his fear of school, getting this "very small illness" does allow him to get out of going to class. The illness gives him a "legitimate reason" for this. If he can't go to school, it is not his fault; it is the fault of the cold that is keeping him from going to school. His being sick is not his failure; it is something over which he had no control. Now he no longer has to feel as if he is a failure. It was the illness that kept him out of school, not his doing.

We can interpret this process through the language of the Body-Mind. If we do, it might go something like this:

"If I go to class, I won't understand the work. I'll feel stupid, and the teacher won't like me. When that happens, I will feel like a failure. When I feel like a failure, I don't like myself. If I fail, people will laugh at me. If they laugh at me, I will be so embarrassed that I am liable to die."

Therefore, "If I go to school, I will die."

On the other hand, "If I don't go to school, I won't die."

"If I am sick then I have absolutely no control over this, so I do not have to feel like a failure (right now), and I won't die!"

It may seem to make no difference to the Body-Mind that this logic is riddled with faulty assumptions and beliefs. The Body-Mind knows differently. The Body-Mind will know and soon recall that it reacted to a set of plausible but faulty beliefs. This action may later trigger a request for resolution of this unresolved conflict, guilt for what the Body-Mind knows really occurred–his avoidance of school and not wanting to confront his fears of failure. Once triggered, as we have repeatedly stated, it may end up being the cause of guilt, unhappiness, fear, and future illness.

We may learn these types of processes as a child, but we carry them into adulthood. We often repeat this pattern many times each day. Two common examples are not speaking up to a bullying boss or not telling our spouse how we really feel because we are afraid of rejection or loss of love. While we may tell ourselves at the time that it really doesn't matter because we do not need to confront these issues or people, it will likely leave us feeling conflicted since we did not tell the truth. The problem is that the choices we made were designed to reduce our immediate anxiety, not to reduce future problems.

Secondary gains are generally powered by our conscious or subconscious needs of the moment. When we take this path, we often set ourselves up to continue with similar actions and make other "bad" decisions in the future. This may occur in spite of our knowing they are wrong and will not work at that time or in the future. The main problem here is that if the individual tries to do anything differently, he may experience a significant increase in anxiety and tension.

We may know intellectually that if we had only handled the situation differently, or had "done the right thing," we would ultimately experience less stress and feel safer in the future. Either way we still have to deal with the present and any anxieties which are occurring in the now-moment.

These faulty patterns become so deeply ingrained that not acting them out can cause great discomfort, stress, and anxiety in the now-moment, so we give up future comfort for feeling less stress in the now-moment.

It may seem absurd that a person could believe that he would die if he went to school or stood up for himself against his boss; the truth is we do things like this all the time. We lie to ourselves, we deny the truth, we ignore our feelings, and accept less than we deserve. The problem is that whenever these things happen, we end up creating one or more conflicts in our Body-Mind, and a door to potential illness in the future is invariably opened.

The Body-Mind always does what it is told, however, it always knows what is true and what is not true. On the other hand, the Conscious Aware Self may not want to know the consequences of its actions. It may only want to get what it wants in the now-moment, no matter the cost. It can and does lie to and mislead the Body-Mind. The Body-Mind, because it is a robotic servant, faithfully does whatever it is told, even though it may be aware of the consequences. The Body-Mind may continue to accept and even help the Conscious Aware Self in this deception, until it ultimately recognizes the danger and decides that this behavior must stop.

Possibly the single most important pieces of information we can give people about preserving their health is to be careful of what you think and say to yourself and others. Remember, the Body-Mind will always give you what you ask for, even if what you ask is not in your overall best interest. If you don't want to suffer from illness in the future or you are already ill, stop this process now. Be careful of what you "ask" for and listen to your body when it conveys risk and danger to you. The more positive you train yourself to think and be, the happier and healthier you will be.

Returning now to our earlier example of the child who fears "dying" if he goes to school, what he really fears is failing, being laughed at and ultimately "dying of shame." His Body-Mind takes these fears literally, and triggers the Stress Mechanism (remember, the Stress Mechanism can be turned on by any real or imagined threat to our well-being), which suddenly creates a full-fledged Fight-or-Flight stress reaction. We may interpret this as an anxiety or panic attack. When this happens over and over again, one of two things is likely to happen:

Over time the child may gradually change from experiencing acute anxiety attacks to more generalized and less dramatic episodes, of nonspecific anxiety, which give no clue to what caused them. Secondly, his anxiety attacks may worsen or transform into panic attacks or possibly eventually into some sort of phobia, such as agoraphobia or claustrophobia, etc. His physical and emotional symptoms are initially based on his fear as well as his negative thoughts and feelings. In time, they may trigger greater physical and emotional upset. The child may cry, become erratic, even throw tantrums to avoid going to school. These are all signs of his acute distress and his emotional conflict. They are not necessarily the solution, and they may or may not work. If they don't work, his anxiety may increase. At some point, he may say or think to himself, "If I were only sick, then I wouldn't have to go to school." Implied in this is the belief,

"Therefore, I won't have to feel like I am going to die."

Under such circumstances, getting sick may initially seem to him like a simple, less problematic, and inexpensive way to protect himself from fear, failure, anxiety, and possible "death." Soon after he thinks this, he may actually get sick. He may accept the illness as a trade for not having to go to school and therefore not having to experience the many negative feelings, beliefs, and emotions that he now associates with going to school. For those individuals who either repeatedly voice these types of options or believe them deeply enough, the Body-Mind will allow illness to occur and in the process it will train itself to do this again and again in response to the "certain" threats, that he fears facing , whether real or imagined.

These thoughts can set a series of acute and later chronic illnesses into motion. Some may be small, while others may be large or even life-threatening. All of these initially may work to help him attain his short term goals. This eventually may lead to his belief in illness and loss of power over his healing and other maintenance, repair, defensive and protection systems. The process then leads to more illnesses and then even more serious illnesses.

What then happens to this child when he becomes an adult? It is likely that his periodic illnesses have worked and created short-term relief from his anxieties. Because they worked, he probably never solved the original conflict. It is also quite likely that because they did work, he has generated a number of new conflicts created because of his illnesses and how he has not solved other problems along the way. Furthermore he may feel like a failure at work and/or in family affairs or other interpersonal areas. The more he trades illness for preventing immediate anxiety and suffering, the more ingrained this process becomes until it becomes so much a part of his being. He inevitably becomes sick whenever he even thinks about failing. Once his Body-Mind realizes that being sick can protect him, it may create illness whenever it believes something is even about to threaten him. Illness may become a way of life.

One of the most common secondary gains occurs when illness is used to get out of work. Illness is one of the few acceptable reasons for taking time off from work without being censured.

SECONDARY GAINS CAN BE POSITIVE OR NEGATIVE

When we go to the market and spend money for food, we get positive secondary gains. By trading of money for food, we get the nourishment and the good taste of the foods we purchase. Sometimes, secondary gains are minimal or even nonexistent, and sometimes they are tangible and substantial. Sometimes they are a win-win, while at other times they may be lose-lose situations. The result of secondary gain trades can vary depending upon what is traded and received.

The result of some specific secondary gain trades may be negative, even destructive, such as in the case of a person who gets cancer after years of wishing for "a way out," or "I wish I were dead," as an escape from their life problems. Secondary gains can also provide positive benefits, even valuable lessons, if and when we recognize them and learn from them.

Sometimes, people find that suffering from an illness is a great way to get special attention, approval, or love. Consciously or subconsciously, they may believe they cannot fulfill these needs in any other way. With illness comes sympathy, help, care, and support, which they may subconsciously believe they cannot get any other way. Much like a house of cards, these types of secondary gains are unsustainable and will eventually lead to even more complicated problems, as well as new conflicts.

Positive secondary gains generally support us and make our life broader and more pleasurable, negative secondary gains often have the opposite effect. They may reduce anxiety, pain, and suffering in the short run, but they rarely leave us better off, healthier, or happier in the end.

Positive secondary gains usually result from doing positive, good acts to help others and heal problems. They often benefit from doing the right thing, helping others, solving problems and taking care of business. For example, consider the individual who receives an unexpected bonus because of measures he implemented to save money or increasing production at his company.

LACK OF SELF-LOVE

Another reason for illness is lack of self-love. Lack of self-love takes many forms, illness is just one. Lack of self-love is another concept that operates on a continuum. While one person might experience only a minimal degree of self-doubt or loss of self-love, another might despise or even loathe them self. When we dislike or hate ourselves, we are indirectly encouraging our Body-Mind to malfunction. "I hate myself!" could be telling the Body-Mind, "I am not worthy of being protected or defended."

Those people who experience self-anger usually blame themselves for the "bad" or "wrong" things they believe they have done to themselves or others in the past, present, or may do in the future. They may then believe that because of these real or imagined deeds, beliefs, or negative thoughts that they are unworthy or even unlovable. Sometimes, these individuals feel unloved by others, by one or both parents, or by some other significant person in their life. These faulty beliefs systems may ultimately lead to illnesses, such as autoimmune diseases where the Body-Mind attacks itself and in the process injures the physical body. This process can create a special kind of hell for the Conscious Aware Self, which may have no concrete idea why these illnesses are attacking "it."

Where one person might live a healthful and joyous life, another might live life with constant negative thoughts, being self-destructive and nurturing death wishes. This negative-thinking person may want to believe that all of his problems are real, or even that they are created by others who are "out to get them." Those who experience self-anger and self-rage often end up using their anger and rage against themselves. They may do this through their conscious or unconscious actions. Illness is generated because of destructive negative thoughts and belief systems placed into the Body-Mind based on this unresolved anger and rage. The negative person may act to protect himself by displacing self-anger outwardly displaying antisocial or even criminal behavior. Others may turn self-anger inward and ultimately develop illnesses such as cancer, auto-immune disease, ulcers, arthritis or even chronic, potentially lethal illnesses.

Self-hatred and self-anger will likely trigger the Stress Mechanism, setting the person up for what comes later on from the SRDs this process ultimately creates. We always look for these negative thoughts and beliefs when dealing with people who have these kinds of illness or disease processes. They are always there, no matter how deeply the individual has buried them and no matter how effectively they deny their existence.

A lesser degree of self-dislike, self-resentment or resenting or disliking others –may take an entirely different form. It might appear as not taking responsibility for one's self. It might also take the form of guilt about prior deeds or experiences, guilt or anger from not choosing appropriate partners, relationships, or career. At its least, it might only take the form of self-criticism, or an inability to accept criticism, lack of self control, difficulty controlling anger, creating grudges, or even as bigotry. In all of these situations, the individual may lack the self-love needed in order to get on with living life fully and healthfully, take responsibility for his or her decisions or for providing a healthy, caring, positive self-image to their Body-Mind.

THE POWER OF OUR BELIEFS

There will always be people who will dispute their role in creating their illnesses. They may not be willing or are unable to believe that they are responsible for everything that happens to them in their life. They may not believe that self-respect and self-love are meaningful and when absent or interfered with can play a meaningful role in creating their own illnesses. Many will choose to blame infinitesimally tiny bacteria or viruses, their own genetics working against them, or simply bad luck, for causing their illnesses. Many people will simply not consider that what they currently think or have thought in the past, what they believe now or in the past, can and will undermine them and lead to illness and problems in the future.

When illness does occur, it is important that we understand the role and power of our own positive and negative beliefs and thoughts, not only about illness, but also about what we think of ourselves and our life, and that these beliefs and thoughts play an important role in our health and overall well-being. The idea that we have any kind of "personal responsibility" in our becoming ill is often a foreign concept to many people. They would rather believe that their illness has just happened to them, rather than that they personally may have contributed to making it happen. The fact is that we do play an important role in creating our own illnesses and the illnesses of others around us. We do this because of how we see ourself, how we talk to ourself how and what we think and believe about ourself and others. We do this by how and what we communicate to our Body-Mind and what we allow ourself to believe. All of these are crucial to our ability to both create and prevent illness now, and in the future. Our personal self-image, positive or negative, is always important to us and to our overall health and well-being.

Illness can also be created when we feel a lack of power in the world. This is especially true when we feel defenseless, overwhelmed, or defeated. During these periods, we are more than likely to "catch something."

People can also assume too much power. They may believe that the world somehow rotates around them and that they affect people and events that occur around them more than they actually do. Guilt may cause people to believe that what they think or do can cause negative things to happen.

One woman we worked with many years ago believed that her son-in-law died of alcoholism because of her. Because he had been making her daughter's life a living hell, she told him one day that he was a "worthless, no-good loser." Soon after that he started drinking and became an alcoholic. Several years later, he died of alcohol poisoning. She felt very guilty and she was grief stricken when she heard he had died. Because of her self-anger and guilt, she ultimately created herself to become sick. She wanted to believe that he became an alcoholic because of her. She believed that if she had she tried harder and got him into counseling instead of criticizing him, he would not have become an alcoholic. She believed that she could and should have done more to prevent her son-in-law's death. The problem here was that she assumed she had power over his beliefs and his behaviors. She assumed that she could have changed him. Her guilt arose from the faulty belief that she caused him to become an alcoholic, when she did nothing of the kind. True, maybe she had said something hurtful, something that she should not have said, but it was he who began drinking and would not stop. It was he who killed himself, because he would not stop drinking. She did not kill him and had no reason for becoming sick over his death.

Another extreme example of this occurs where people believe that they have power or "rights" over the lives and the well-being of others. Criminals, tyrants, dictatorial bosses, or overly critical parents are examples. Consider how much "disease" Hitler and Stalin created and how the consequences of their actions affect us even today.

This all-consuming assumption of power, when it is not for the good of all involved, can and often does lead to negative results. This type of extreme behavior usually causes injury or disease to themselves and others.

DEATH WISHES

At the extreme of self-anger and hatred is the individual who has a death wish. This can be so overt that it leads to suicide. It can also be very subtle, such as smoking, excessive alcohol drinking, driving carelessly, using dangerous drugs, overeating, severe thrill seeking, or even pathologic lying, and cheating. Anything that is dangerous can lead to injury, illness, divorce, and the alienation of loved ones or even death. We have all known people like this and maybe we have even said to ourselves, "What could he possibly be thinking?" or "He must be trying to kill himself."

In extreme cases, people with death wishes seem to either be willing to or even trying to, take others with them. While most people with death wishes are not overtly trying to kill themselves, many live their life on the edge, toying with and teasing death, or destruction. Their actions are not wholesome, loving, or caring toward themselves or others. While there can be a host of psychological reasons for this type behavior, these individuals often invite risk and illness into their lives. People with this underlying dynamic are often more subject to accidents and are more likely to end up dying of a fatal process such as cancer or heart disease. In addition, they are frequently responsible for creating illness, pain and suffering in the people who love and care for them.

Anger at others often leads to illness. Some people project their anger onto others. When someone lives with anger, whether projected internally or externally, stress is created and illness eventually occurs either within him or within the people around him. Their anger can take many forms, such as prejudices, hostility, or abuse of spouses, children, employees, or friends. The hostility may even be directed against total strangers. When internally projected, it can lead to nearly any illness, but especially rashes, allergies, autoimmune disorders, high blood pressure, cancer, or heart disease. Whether internally or externally directed, the angry person often ends up with virtually the exact same type problems; often only the target is different. Always, whatever the cause, the target organ, or external targets are clues to the anger's cause and effect. No matter the specific cause, at its core this anger is generally generated because of faulty logic or belief systems. Resolve these faulty belief systems and the anger, no matter how deep or how long it has been present, can be resolved, and healing and good health can return.

ACCEPTING AND LEGITIMIZING ILLNESS

Illness is generally accepted because it has clearly been legitimized in our society. Everyone knows what illness is and when we do things that we should not. It is often an expected outcome. It is also clearly legitimized by both the medical and advertising industries.

When someone goes to his doctor feeling ill and the doctor gives the illness a name, prescribes medication, and then charges for it, it clearly must be real. This undisputed "proof" in the reality of illness is cultivated by the medical establishment for many reasons. Illness is the stock and trade of the medical profession; doctors, nurses, and administrators make their livings from it. They have a stake in maintaining the myth of illness. We sincerely hope that one day our society will be able to let go of illness-oriented medicine as a business, and turn their capabilities into becoming full-fledged illness preventers and healers.

In recent years with the acceptance of drug advertising, the population is bombarded with ads for one or another drug that is supposedly qualified (regardless of their risks and side effects) to treat illness. The underlying message is clear, "Illness is real, and we have a drug to treat just about every illness you could possibly get or suffer from!" Then the ads usually add, "If you have questions, ask your doctor ..." this now tells the viewer that even the doctors are fully behind them, hence verifying to the viewer that "all" doctors fully believe in illness.

Illness is also often legitimized by non-medical people. It is frequently legitimized by people in our lives, such as parents, friends, family, and those who play significant roles in shaping our beliefs as we grow up. Many mothers clearly believe in illness. We hope after reading this book, most will change their viewpoint about illness and tell their children to solve problems hence learn, grow and evolve rather than get sick.

Possibly the most frequent reason for illness in our own lives is our personal belief in illness. If we end up becoming ill from SRD's this is most likely because of the power we give to our own negative beliefs that illness exists, that it is real and that it is caused by forces outside of us rather than by our own faulty belief systems. Illness has likely been an important part of your life in the past. We personally experienced and survived childhood illnesses. We all remember family members becoming ill. We have experienced deaths of siblings, friends, grandparents, parents and other family members from one or another illness. Who has not read or seen on TV news stories about famous people getting sick and dying? With all of this, it is difficult, and in some cases impossible, to extinguish the influence of illness upon us.

In the future, we hope that the role of the medical profession will become vested in educating people about the forces that create and maintain illness such as SRDs, but more importantly how we can create wellness and optimal health and well-being.

We hope the profession will tell how we can learn and grow from any illness we do experience and how we can transform potential illness into full and complete wellness, and even into enlightenment.

CHOICES OVER ILLNESS

Should you recognize that you are becoming ill, your next thought should be to ask yourself whether or not you want to be ill and then whether or not you will want to stay ill. Next, ask if you have any unresolved conflicts that may be moving you toward becoming ill. If so, then stop and ask what you can do to resolve these issues and in so doing, stop the illness in its tracks. By using your positive power of belief, your ability to search yourself, and understand who you are, you can shorten or cure virtually any illness. You can start doing this now, even before you actually become ill and hence prevent all future illness.

The first and most important step is to recognize that illness does not have to occur. That it does not occur because your body is a failure in doing its work. It is only an intelligent communication from your Body-Mind directed to your Conscious Aware Self, letting you know that you have one or more conflicts that require resolution. By accepting and acting on this, we activate the immune system and bodily defenses to stop the illness process and instead ensure wellness.

If belief in illness occurs in any person because they believe that they have no other choice, then you can help them by teaching them that they can learn to change their "programming." They can give up their illness beliefs and choose a healthier set of beliefs, referred to as their "wellness mentality." Since belief in illness is often learned as a defensive mechanism against the pain of life, it can also be unlearned, and healthier, more appropriate wellness-creating mechanisms can be introduced in their place. When we do this, we protect ourselves from the many negative forces that may be working within or outside of us that are steadily pushing us toward illness. We can substitute healthy mechanisms for unhealthy ones.

Using this information as a framework, we can make positive changes, create new healthier decisions and beliefs that protect you from future illness and add happy, healthy years to your lives. In order to create good health, you must take responsibility for your own health and well-being. You must do this because it is too important to relinquish this power to anyone else. Ultimately, you must be responsible to yourself, not just to survive, but also to thrive. Whether or not you accept this great responsibility is up to you. If you don't, you may end up compromising your quality of life, health, happiness and success.

TAKING TOTAL RESPONSIBILITY

People tell us that they don't believe they have any choice over whether or not they get sick. One man once told us, "I didn't choose to get sick. It just happened." On the surface, this seems reasonable and plausible. However, by believing this, he avoided all personal responsibility for himself and his overall well-being. When you don't accept full and total responsibility for your health, your Body-Mind will be given the message that you really don't care, that your health and well-being are not up to you and it will ultimately be helpless to do anything for you in order to help you stay healthy, maintain wellness and flourish rather than simply survive. You will also give a message of helplessness to the rest of your being, to your Conscious Aware Self, your body and to your Higher Self. Without taking total responsibility for your own life and well-being, you cannot fully love or trust yourself or others. Thus, you are at the mercy of any and all negative forces operating within or around you. While we are children, we should have learned to be fully responsible for ourselves. As adults, we should have already known this and if not already done, we should set out to accomplish this. Certainly as adults, we should have already been sufficiently exposed to life's realities to know that we should learn that we are responsible for everything in our life. If we have not learned this already, then we might already be paying some price for not knowing it. We could end up paying a much higher price than we would want to pay.

Taking full and total responsibility for everything we do, think or say, and everything that happens to us is an act of caring and self-love. Self-responsibility is extremely important in both preventing illness and in creating healing.

HOW WE SUPPORT AND MAINTAIN ILLNESS

So far, we have discussed the creation of Stress-Related Disorders. Now we must ask, what about the maintenance of already-existing illness or disease? We discussed factors earlier, such as secondary gains, lack of education, faulty belief systems, and external pressures to believe in illness. It should be clear by now that if the factors that originally caused the illness are not resolved, there is nothing acting against the illness process. How then can your illness go away? With no force operating to heal your illness, other than your body's natural protective mechanisms, and with your stressors and stress undermining the healing process, how can we get better? Let's say you can improve your illness by using relaxation and stress reduction procedures, or you are being treated with medications, surgery, or other standard medical procedures. How then can you keep your illness from coming back?

If no attempts are made to resolve your underlying conflicts, you will never be safe from becoming sick again or having an illness progress into a Chronic Disease State. Yet, for most people who are sick, the illness process itself, especially the belief in its reality, is one of the most important factors in determining whether it can be limited or reversed. Even with medical treatment and medications, most illnesses are only at best controlled and not cured. The symptoms are made tolerable or even acceptable, but the illness itself is not cured. Since many illnesses are self-healing, we are often spared long-term problems. However, this is not protection against becoming sick again unless the underlying causes are found and resolved.

For many people who are already sick, illness often robs them of the best parts of their lives. Why should they allow their illnesses to continue? Why should they tolerate symptom reduction instead of total cure?

The answers to these questions are complex. It would take volumes to explain. Simply stated, once created, each illness develops a life of its own. If the sick person does everything possible and the illness is still not cured, then the initial underlying causative process was likely missed and after awhile the illness begins to chart its own course. It will take on a life and destiny of its own since your body's defensive and protective mechanisms are undermined.

THE LAW OF SURVIVAL - MAINTAINING ILLNESS

Since the Law of Survival applies to every aspect of life, everything that has life, even thoughts and ideas; then illnesses, as well as the organisms that might cause them, will also be working to survive. Illnesses and diseases want to survive, especially when bacteria and virus are allowed in. Some illnesses are self-limiting, they run a specific course, and then they resolve themselves and simply "go away." Other illnesses will do whatever they need to do to survive. This may even include killing the host organism. This may seem like a strange concept at first, but think about it for a moment. We want to survive and will fight for our beliefs. Many people have fought for liberty, others have fought equally as hard to keep totalitarianism alive.

Viruses adapt and mutate to stay alive. The child within fights in every way it can to ensure its survival. Why not our illnesses and diseases and all the organisms and ideas that cause them? If this wasn't true, why are some illnesses so hard to "cure"?

Almost all diseases and illnesses have some sort of built-in ability to persist, mutate, adapt, evolve, and learn from their circumstances. Frequently, the sick part of us, the part that benefits from the primary and secondary gains, fights to get and keep what it wants. In so doing, it will also keep the illness process alive. Our Body-Mind clearly wants to hold onto those belief systems that empowered it, even faulty ones. We have all seen how hard it can be to change some one's mind "once they have made it up." We have all seen how hard it is for some people to give up addictions, bad habits, or bad relationships. This is just as often true with faulty belief systems. Even though they may create and maintain illnesses, it is often hard for our Body-Mind or Conscious Aware Self to give them up and simply walk away from them. If our Conscious Aware Self is unwilling to let go of a certain bad or faulty belief system that causes stress and leads to disease, what happens to the stress that is caused?

It grows! Negative physical and chemical changes progress through the Wellness-Stress-Illness Mechanism. These illnesses often appear to be resistant to medical treatment or alternative care. Ultimately, they may worsen, even lead to chronic disease or death, and we as well as the medical profession, can do little to stop this from happening.

Many people with entirely curable illnesses, people who are unaware of or refuse to look for the underlying faulty belief system, can worsen and die in spite of everything medicine has to offer. In some cases, this is because the information we are discussing has not been available to them. In other cases, they may have been provided this information but instead of embracing and using this information, they refused to consider it and hence refused to accept the very concepts that could heal or cure them.

In fact, we see healing all around us. For example, what about those people who cure illnesses such as high blood pressure, diabetes, high cholesterol, simply by changing their lifestyle and their diet or by losing weight? Does this not demonstrate that changing one's behavior and belief systems can have positive benefits?

Yes, it does!

On the other hand, what about people who continually "forget" to take their medications or don't follow directions? What about the woman who goes to her doctor year after year and never gets better? What about those people who continue smoking even after being told that it is killing them? What about women who refuse to have breast examinations because the doctor might find cancer? Aren't these people refusing to take responsibility for themselves? In their behavior can't we see faulty belief systems and ongoing conflicts that are not being resolved? Can we see how they are either protecting or maintaining their illnesses, or even worse, setting themselves up for increased future problems?

We see how our lack of knowledge, lack of taking responsibility, self-anger, self-hatred, and our unwillingness to give up faulty belief systems, insufficient self-love, fear, death wishes, and anger at others can and do play roles in our illnesses. No matter what the specific cause, the bottom line is that lies exist and responsibilities are not assumed. We allow illness because we empower these lies. We maintain illness because we do not take the responsibility for ourselves and for solving the problems that are causing them. We don't do what is needed to prevent or reverse these illnesses and their underlying faulty beliefs and conflicts. Can you see that the ill or diseased person is caught up in a life-and-death struggle between their lies and the truths that can save them? Once we accept it, we can move forward toward finding our highest, healthiest, and best Self.

Once we recognize our need to be responsible and solve previously unresolved conflicts, then all Stress-Related Disorders and the symptoms and problems they create can begin resolving themselves.

When we accept faulty belief systems, we expose ourselves to internal and external conflict. Our Body-Mind can and does interpret this lack of action in resolving our conflicts as clear threats to our survival. This invokes the Stress Mechanism and ultimately leads to advancement of the illness process. If we can find and eliminate these conflicts, then the Stress Mechanism is eased and even turned off. As it is reversed, there will be release, relief, and relaxation. The struggle ends, wellness is reestablished and the natural protective mechanisms of the body are reactivated and better utilized.

THE HEALING PROCESS

There are two main steps involved with the healing process. First, we must identify whether the conflict is real or imaginary, and therefore whether our life and well-being are actually threatened. If so, we must act accordingly to accept the Intelligent communications the Body-Mind sends us and immediately do everything that is necessary to protect and heal ourselves. If our immediate survival is not threatened, all we have to do is to know this and communicate this to our Body-Mind by taking appropriate actions and making appropriate acknowledgments. For example, you can say something like the following to yourself, *"Alright, this is not an immediate threat to "our" (the Conscious Aware Self and Body-Mind's) life or well-being. We now need to begin thinking about finding and solving our problems. In the meantime, let's make ourselves aware of what is happening and then initiate the process of solving all of our problems and conflicts as best as we can".*

Second, we must take all necessary actions based on the promises just made to Body-Minds and ourselves. We must open ourselves by listening to and watching for what the Body-Mind has to tell us. Finally, we must start working on and resolving all of the problems our Body-Mind communicates to us and those we identify from our life experiences. In so doing, we not only prevent future illnesses, but also begin healing the existing illnesses and imbalances. The elimination of Stress-Related Disorders and illnesses requires this process.

LET'S LOOK AT ANOTHER CASE HISTORY:

Consider the example of Cindy W. Cindy a 25-year-old waitress suffering from anxiety attacks, recurrent illnesses, fatigue, and chronic depression. Cindy hated her job, but she was unwilling to look for another. As a child, her father repeatedly told her, "Women are only good for two things–waiting on men and having babies."

At one point Cindy told us, "My father must have said that hundreds of times, if he said it once!"

Cindy started working as a waitress shortly after she graduated high school. She had tried two other non-waitressing jobs, but did so poorly that she was fired both times. Even though she hated waiting on tables, she had such anxiety about looking for any other job that every time she even considered it, she got sick. When we first met Cindy, she said that she had two reasons for working where she worked, first to pay her rent, and next to meet someone with whom she could fall in love and have children. When asked who she was supposed to meet, she said, "someone who would take me away from my misery."

During the course of working with her, we pointed out that she had internalized her father's faulty belief systems about women only being good if they wait on men or have babies. We pointed out to her that by being a waitress, she was waiting on men and by waiting for someone to take her out of her misery, she was most likely, whether she liked it or not looking for someone to give her lots of babies. By continuing to do what she was doing, fully accepting and internalizing her father's beliefs. She never really created any workable belief system of her own that would allow her to be the woman she really wanted to be.

Cindy was eventually able to see that she was operating entirely through her father's belief systems and that she really didn't agree with them. Cindy was able to free herself up almost immediately afterward. She decided to create her own personal belief systems about working and relationships. Cindy also realized that she spent a great deal of her time dating the "wrong" men. She then decided to put off dating for a while.

Cindy told us that, "deep inside", she had always wanted to work in the medical profession, and so began training as a medical assistant. At the end of her training, Cindy had graduated as a certified medical assistant. She began working in a doctor's office and eventually worked herself up to managing the office. She now loves what she is doing. She has grown stronger, healthier, and happier. She no longer has anxiety attacks, she is rarely fatigued and never depressed and, best of all, she is rarely ill.

The process of healing, much like the fabled "journey of a thousand miles," always starts with the first step. The first step, in this case, is making the decision to heal yourself. This is often one of the loneliest decisions we human beings can make.

The next chapter looks at the healing process and what it takes for people to make the decision to change their lives and heal their illnesses.

*In order
to change
we must be
sick and tired
of being
sick and tired.*

~Author Unknown

Chapter Fourteen

RETURNING TO WELLNESS — THE JOURNEY

MAKING THE DECISION TO HEAL

By now you should have a good idea as to how and why stress leads to or causes Stress-Related Disorders. It is likely that if you are currently suffering from a Stress-Related Disorder, you want to find out how you can heal yourself. It is also likely that you now understand that to create healing, you must make a decision and plan to start the healing process. You will also see that once you make any decision to heal, healing requires that you must be willing to do whatever is needed to undo your stress, solve your unresolved conflicts and those conflicts which initially triggered the onset of your Stress-Related Disorders. This must be done in order to help you not only heal yourself, but also maintain your wellness for the rest of your life. In this chapter, we will look at the factors involved in making these decisions and what likely happens once you do.

For several years, I, Allen, worked as a locum tenens physician, "Have Stethoscope, Will Travel." I moved from practice to practice, from one group of patients to another. What I found was both reassuring and depressing at the same time.

I learned that people are the same. People who are ill generally want to get better. Most are willing to do everything they can to get well. Unfortunately, since they often did not know what to do, they rely on their physician and the medical system to tell them what to do and how to do it. This is an unfortunate situation for most people. While the standard Western-trained physician can remove a ruptured appendix, save a baby's life with an emergency cesarean section, set a broken bone, or save a life after a catastrophic emergency, they usually cannot and do not heal SRDs. In fact, they rarely heal any non-traumatic disorder. What the great majority of the medical profession does, is treat symptoms and wait until the Body-Mind and the body heals themselves.

This is great if the Body-Mind and body can actually heal themselves, but this process of treating symptoms and not finding or resolving the conflicts or problems that have created and are still maintaining the illness, may not be so great for the person who is ill and wants to be cured.

There is also a large number of people who do little or nothing to heal themselves. There are also many people who resist making changes in their lives. I have seen many patients who elected to have surgery rather than do regular exercise. I have seen people resist losing weight to lower their high blood pressure, opting instead to take medication. I have seen women come near death simply because they were unwilling to touch their own body and perform regular breast self-examinations. I have seen people show up at their doctor's office with lists of symptoms clearly consistent with SRDs, and yet they were entirely unwilling and unable to deal with the stresses of their lives. I could and did understand all of this, because I too had resisted dealing with my own stresses and illnesses for a long time.

More than might be imagined, the problems and stresses people suffer are similar. While the exact faulty beliefs or potential threats may differ from person to person, the SRD patterns repeat themselves. A knowledgeable physician can often predict in advance which SRDs will occur in certain patients. The patient's physical appearance, lifestyle, the stresses he or she endures, the signs and symptoms created by the patient's stress, are all clues that the patient will become ill, and they even provide clues as to the illnesses they will most likely experience.

Too often, the quality of medical care most people experience is generally inadequate. Some physicians know exactly how to help their patients, especially when they suffer acute short-term, self resolving illnesses, or even after major injuries. The problem is that the vast majority of physicians are unaware of what is really happening to their patients and the role stress plays in their ultimately becoming ill. Even worse, most physicians do not recognize that their patients are steadily progressing from wellness into illness. Because of this, many physicians miss crucial opportunities to help prevent their patients from becoming ill during the early part of the illness process.

Years earlier, I was so resistant to my own problems that I allowed myself to become depressed and burned out. I recognize now that I had been aware of the answers to my own problems, yet I was unable and unprepared to make the appropriate decisions to resolve these problems, nor act on them. While I knew that I needed to learn more about helping and healing people than was available through practicing standard Western medicine, I used rationalization after rationalization to resist doing this.

What kept me from doing what I needed to do in order to heal myself was my fear of success and possibly its mirror image, fear of failing. I was afraid of changing my life into what I wanted rather than what everyone expected of me. The decision was and always had been mine. I knew that I hurt, but I was unable to make a commitment to myself. What held me back was the same thing that created my problems–faulty belief systems. My fears and inertia kept me from doing what I know would ultimately heal me.

Looking back now, I realized that I had to go through this crisis. Ultimately it allowed me to understand not only why I resisted healing myself, but why others also resist. It allowed me to better understand the insecurities, fears, and frustrations of the people with whom I was working. It taught me compassion for others and for myself. In the end, it permitted me to accept that each of us can only decide and take action when we are ready. I ultimately recognized that my role was to educate people, and not to force anyone to change.

HEALING OURSELVES AND REVERSING OUR STRESSES

It is time to begin our discussion of how you can reverse your Stress-Related Disorders and heal yourself. We have outlined this process in Table: 14-1, The Healing-Wellness Process.

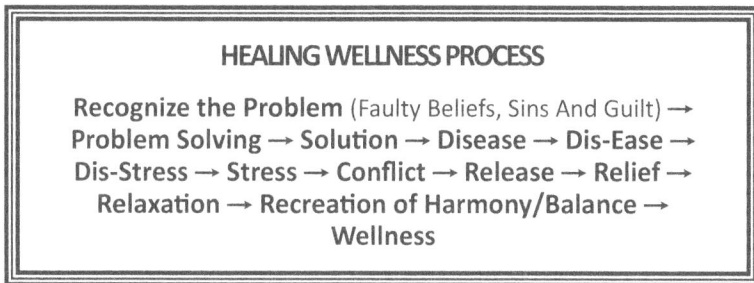

HEALING WELLNESS PROCESS

Recognize the Problem (Faulty Beliefs, Sins And Guilt) →
Problem Solving → **Solution** → **Disease** → **Dis-Ease** →
Dis-Stress → **Stress** → **Conflict** → **Release** → **Relief** →
Relaxation → **Recreation of Harmony/Balance** →
Wellness

Table: 14-1

We will look at each of step of this process and learn to recognize them, what they mean to you and the criteria you and your physician or alternative healer can use to apply them. We will also look at many of the most common pitfalls and how we can make each of these pitfalls work for you.

Before we go further, let's look at another case history – one which can help us better understand the process of making the decision to heal one's self.

THIS IS THE STORY OF MARTIN L., AGE 57

Martin's story demonstrates a good portion of what we are going to be talking about. Martin L. suffered from abdominal pain for several months. He belonged to an HMO, and every time he called for an appointment, he saw a different doctor. In fact, Martin saw a total of seven medical doctors before he came to see me. The last doctor Martin saw diagnosed him as having a gastric ulcer. When this doctor asked Martin what was going on at work, Martin told him that everything was fine, work was okay he had no problems. However, he did tell the doctor that he had not been thinking very clearly for the past few months. At this point, the doctor told him that he believed that the ulcer was probably related to his work as an accountant.

When I first saw Martin, he was only looking for a second opinion. He was disappointed with his lack of improvement and felt that after seeing so many doctors that his HMO did not have the wherewithal to help him. I had asked him to bring in with him a copy of his HMO's medical records. When I saw Martin, he came in with a chart that was at least four or more inches thick, as well as a stack of x-rays, which had been taken during the past year.

Upon reviewing Martin's medical records, I noted that he had been perfectly healthy until a little more than eighteen months earlier. About that time, he started seeing his HMO doctor relatively regularly. He was being seen for a number of complaints which included recurrent headaches, recurrent viral infections and chest colds. As time passed, the number, frequency, and severity of the symptoms appeared to increase dramatically. Eventually, Martin began suffering from indigestion, had difficulty sleeping, and then had recurrent upper abdominal pain. Martin had been seen many times at his HMO for these complaints, and each time he was given one or another prescription medication to calm his symptoms. During the first year of his complaints, two x-ray series of his stomach and small intestine were performed. Both of these x-rays were negative for ulcers and any other pathology.

Approximately six months before my seeing him, Martin's pain had significantly increased and a third set of x-rays finally revealed a fresh gastric (stomach) ulcer. Under his doctor's instructions – and because of increasing abdominal pain and discomfort – Martin took two weeks off from his job. During his time off work, the pain became even more of a problem, causing him to become even more fearful and dissatisfied with his care at his HMO. Suddenly, after ten days of rest, Martin experienced what he later described to me as, *"... the worst pain I had ever experienced in my life!"* He vomited up nearly a cup full of bright-red blood. His wife called 911 and he was transported to his HMO's hospital.

After only a brief exam, he was told that his ulcer was bleeding and that he might need surgery. After a few days of "conservative treatment," he was told that he was going to be scheduled later that day for surgery to remove the part of his stomach that was bleeding. Fortunately for Martin, the operating room was unavailable because of a multi-car crash, and by the time they were ready to take him into surgery the next day, his bleeding had stopped. He was discharged a few days later and told that if bleeding were to recur, surgery would be needed.

Martin's history clearly suggested that something had happened about eighteen months to two years earlier and that something then happened to escalate the process about six months earlier when his symptoms suddenly worsened and the gastric ulcer was subsequently found.

Whatever it was that happened six months earlier, it had created enough change and stress to move Martin from the Dis-Ease Stage to the Disease Stage. When I finished my review of Martin's records, I asked him if he was experiencing any stress. His reply was startling, but not unexpected.

"I have no stress in my life," he replied.

"None?" I asked.

"No, I really don't have any stress in my life."

Next, I asked him what had been going on in his life in the past two years.

Martin thought for a minute or two and then responded, "Eighteen months ago, my mother was diagnosed with breast cancer. She had to have a radical mastectomy. At the time of her surgery, the doctors also found tumors in several of her lymph glands. When the doctors told this to my father, he had a heart attack. The doctors decided that they couldn't start Mother on chemotherapy until he was stable and she was more relaxed. Once Mother was out of the hospital, we had no one to take care of her or my father. My wife had to take a leave of absence from her job so that she could watch over my mother and father. Mother needed someone to take her to the hospital for her chemotherapy and radiation treatments and Dad needed someone to take him to his doctors for follow-up care."

"What happened six months ago?" I asked.

Martin looked down at the floor and his lips tensed as he was clearly fighting off tears. "My younger brother, Mark, was arrested for possession and sale of cocaine. He's not an addict or anything, but he fell in with the wrong crowd. After Dad had his heart attack, Mark just lost control of himself, and well, I guess he wanted to help them financially so he began to sell cocaine."

"How did this affect you?" I queried.

"Well," Martin replied, "when I first found out, I was very angry. I begged him to stop, but he felt that he owed our parents something and he just wouldn't listen."

"How did this affect you?" I asked again.

"I was so frustrated and angry that I would think about it all day and all night. I couldn't sleep at all."

"Did you tell any of this to your doctor?"

"Well, sort of. One of the doctors asked if I was having any problems and I told him that I was having problems keeping my mind on my work."

"Did you tell him about the rest of what was happening?"

"No."

"Why not?"

"Well, he was busy and he really didn't seem to be very interested. As soon as I told him that I was having difficulty concentrating, he told me that I must have been working too hard."

"Why didn't you tell him the rest?"

"Well, he's the doctor so I thought he must be right. I was having difficulty at work; I wasn't functioning very well. Besides, I really didn't want to tell him that I was worried about my brother going to jail for being a drug pusher."

"What happened then?"

"Mark was ultimately sentenced to five years in jail. He had nothing in the bank and he had made no provisions for his family. He has a wife and two young children. Someone had to take care of them, so I started sending his wife money to live on."

"How did that affect you?"

"Well I could afford it, but I had to take money from my savings. With my wife not working and taking care of my mother and father, Linda, my wife, and I had very little time together or with our children."

"Earlier you told me that you had no problem with stress. After all you told me, do you still believe that you have no stress in your life?"

"Well, I guess that I just thought that everyone goes through things like that. It's just life, isn't it?"

Martin and I talked for another hour. Gradually, we both realized that the real problem was not Martin's mother having breast cancer or his father's heart attack. It wasn't even his brother Mark's arrest and prison sentence. He could deal with all of these problems. What we finally discovered was that Martin hated being an accountant, and for many years he had been planning to retire when he was sixty years of age. To accomplish this, Martin had been counting on a steady income based not only on his earnings, but also on his wife's earnings and no new expenses. With his wife having to take time off of her job, his having to help his parents financially, and finally his brother's arrest and now taking care of his brother's wife and children, he subconsciously saw that he would have to put his retirement off for many more years. This is what actually triggered his stress and the ulcer. He was not going to be able to retire at age sixty and he hated what he was doing. After talking for a while more, Martin began to understand how these stressors were affecting him and how he had developed a series of Stress-Related Disorders, which ultimately ended up causing his ulcer.

I asked why he gave his sister-in-law money rather than giving her a job. He said that he had not thought about giving her job where she could earn the money and help take some of his work burdens off him. He said he would talk to her about what she could do and how it might work for both of them. During the next few weeks, Martin's ulcer pain significantly decreased. He made some substantial changes in his life. He offered his sister-in-law a job in his office so that she could earn her living, and she accepted. It turned out that his sister-in-law was great on the phone, so he set her to work collecting monies from clients who had stopped paying him. Within two weeks, what she was collecting not only paid her salary but also created a profit for Martin. His sister-in-law was now doing a wonderful job for him, and she was happy to earn her own way.

Martin also changed his life style to allow himself more time with his wife and children. Finally, he found a first-class retirement home and moved both his parents into it. They had qualified nurses and staff to watch over them and get them to their doctors' appointments. This took a huge burden off Linda. Linda was able to go back to work, which improved their financial situation. Linda felt better and much more productive.

Martin ultimately came to terms with the problems in his life. He looked for and found solutions for each of his problems. Because of this, he was finally able set his life back on his long-desired track. Six weeks later, his ulcer was entirely healed and he was wiser and stronger for the experience.

THE POWER TO HEAL

The power to heal resides within each of us. We must love and care for ourselves enough to go beyond simply treating our symptoms to finding solutions for our problems and the unresolved conflicts that cause them. This process may dredge up many of the old anxieties and fears from the past. These fears and anxieties must go, so that we will be able to resolve all of the unresolved conflicts and problems which have brought on our illness. Resolving them is the only way that we can cure ourselves. Only then can we make the important decisions regarding what needs to be done to resolve these negative beliefs and the circumstances that block us and create illness. Unfortunately, we often have to do this alone, unless we are able to find competent professional help, and can, when it is appropriate, enlist emotionally healthy family members, friends or neighbors to help support us.

We must come to this place of healing on our own. No one can make the decision to begin our healing process except us. While others can suggest and encourage us, the final decision of what to do and how to do it must be ours. When we are ready, we must do all that is necessary to heal ourselves. So we ask, "How do we make the decision to heal ourselves?"

The answer is simple. We must first recognize the price that we and those we love pay for our <u>not</u> solving these problems. We must agree that this price is much higher than we are willing to pay. Then we must finally decide whether or not we are willing to pay it and if so, for how long. If we are not willing to pay what it costs to allow our illness and the pain and suffering associated with it to persist, we must then decide that we are ready to do something about it. Only then can we initiate the healing process and know that it will work.

Once the decision is made, you must do whatever is needed to heal yourself, as long as it causes NO harm to yourself or to others. You must look at all sides and all issues, considering all possible scenarios. You must be willing to take responsibility for your problems and for their resolution. Then you can make the decisions you know you must make.

Decisions alone are not always enough. To get what you want in life, you must act on your decisions. When you finally do act, be willing to correct your course of action whenever necessary. In the end, all healing is simply problem solving, finding and telling the truth, trial and error, making decisions, making mistakes, learning from them, and growing from what you have learned. This is what we mean by taking responsibility.

Once you are willing to take responsibility for your problems and for their solutions, you must give up all of your lies, make the decisions you need to make and act on them. Now you are ready to reach out for life and make it work every day. Remember, in order to heal yourself of whatever problems or illnesses you suffer, you must be willing to do everything in your power to make the healing process work for you. This is what you will need to do to heal yourself.

ELIMINATING STRESS

Healing and wellness are dependent upon two main conditions. First, how long the process has been in operation and second, how much we desire to reverse it. The length of time any process has been in operation is meaningful in different ways. While the Stress Process is entirely reversible at any point along the Illness-Disease Continuum until it reached the stages of Chronic Disease and/or Death, it is important to start eliminating stress as early as possible. The longer the Stress-Illness Process works against us, the more difficult it can be to heal.

Working on reversing stress and undoing all injuries is already difficult, so the longer the disease process has been operating, the more deeply it will likely be entrenched. The longer you are sick or feeling sick, the more power you will have likely given to your illness and to believing that being ill is who you are. In addition, the longer the Stress-Illness Process is in play, the more likely there will be strong secondary gains and the more likely you will find yourself relying upon and needing these secondary gains. The more you depend on these secondary gains, the greater the possibility of developing resistance to healing and ultimately sabotaging yourself. The longer all of this happens, the greater the number of negative belief systems that may likely be in play, which can now work against you.

Another important factor is how fast you have progressed through the Stress-Illness Mechanism from Normal to Stressed, from Stressed to Dis-Stress, from Dis-Stress to Dis-Ease, from Dis-Ease to Disease and eventually to the official diagnosis that a disease exists. The speed and depth of this process will in the end determine whether or not and how much tissue injury has or will occur. The longer this process is allowed to operate, the greater the potential for injury and damage to take place. In many cases, the amount of injury having occurred can be substantial, even before the individual has reached the Chronic Disease Stage. The more damage, the more unlikely there can be full and complete healing and total return to normalcy. Finally, you must determine how much work must be done – not only to reverse the illness process – but also to return all injured tissues to their most normal state of being, as well as maximum physical, mental, emotional, and spiritual healing.

To activate the healing process, you must find and eliminate most if not all faulty beliefs and negative seed thoughts that were implanted in your Body-Mind through the years and then triggered. You must also be concerned regarding the number of layers of protective defense mechanisms you created to shield and protect yourself from the conflicts you have not been able to resolve and are responsible for initiating your Stress-Illness Process.

You may ultimately have to eradicate many layers of non-illness-related stresses which added to your stress load, even when they have been completely unrelated to triggering the original conflict. This is important, since unresolved conflicts are cumulative. Two, three or more unrelated conflicts can all coalesce to trigger the Stress-Illness Mechanism. The more unresolved conflicts you have, the faster and further the Stress-Illness Mechanism is pushed. At the same time, it may be necessary to seek medical treatment for tissue or organ damage that the Stress-Illness Mechanism created.

Doing all this is critical, but it is also essential that you determine as early as possible how motivated you really are to heal yourself. Even more important is whether the reasons you are operating under to heal yourself, are actually the right reasons to create healing.

Often in the past we have known people who profess that they wanted to heal themselves, but clearly sabotaged themselves. As stated earlier, each illness process takes on its own life, and it soon wants to survive as if it were a living, breathing being. Often, these unresolved conflicts and negative personality fragments live in our Child Within. Here, they may be in constant fear that your resolving your conflicts will ultimately destroy them. Now they ask of themselves, *"If we allow you to "fix" yourself, what will happen to us?"* These fears may not only create a belligerent resistance, but they may ultimately undermine our resolve and sabotage even the healthiest parts of our self. Because of the fear of pain that is often associated with the elimination of existing conflicts, our actions and life changes might actually create more stress, even as we are trying to heal ourselves. Possibly it has best been said as follows, *"It is better to accept the devil we know, than fear the devil we don't know."*

HOW WE DEFINE STRESS IS THE KEY TO ENDING IT

In an earlier chapter, we defined stress as, *"the difference between the way we want our world to be and the way it actually is."* It is through this definition that we can find the best way to eliminate stress.

Initially, the stress resolution process is accomplished on two levels. The first level occurs when we work on the stress process directly. The second level occurs when the problems causing the destructive conflicts and the stress they cause are finally resolved.

In order to work on the stress process directly, it can help greatly to enter into a stress-reduction program. Most stress-reduction programs include regular exercise, improved diet, meditation, and behavior modification. While many stress-reduction programs are valuable, few deal with or teach resolving the problems that caused the stress in the first place. When used alone without solving the problems that originally caused your stress, any stress-reduction program is of limited value.

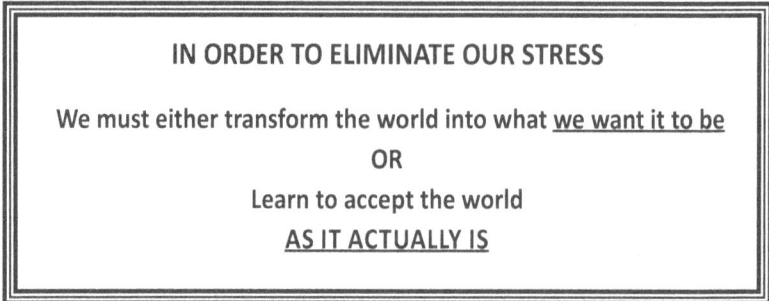

```
┌─────────────────────────────────────────────────────────┐
│                                                           │
│            IN ORDER TO ELIMINATE OUR STRESS               │
│                                                           │
│   We must either transform the world into what we want    │
│                          it to be                         │
│                            OR                             │
│                  Learn to accept the world                │
│                      AS IT ACTUALLY IS                    │
│                                                           │
└─────────────────────────────────────────────────────────┘
```

The next most important issue is how to eliminate stress once you've identified the faulty belief systems and conflicts that triggered your stress reaction.

Stress is created by the conscious or unconscious desire to have the world be the way we want it to be. Therefore, to eliminate your stress you must either transform the world into what you want it to be or learn to accept the world as it actually is. Many people think that accepting the world the way it is ultimately means giving up control of their lives. Others fear that if they try to change the world around them, they only end up increasing their stress levels.

These two points of view are both true and false at the same time. These beliefs are simply faulty belief systems when they block us from dealing with our stresses and leave us stuck and unable to take the appropriate actions that can help us eliminate our stress and better survive and thrive. They are meaningful belief systems when they help us make better, more meaningful decisions which help us rapidly and effectively eliminate our stresses.

There is another way of thinking about these problems. We can allow ourselves to fully accept the world as it is, faults and all, and then create a new clear picture of a better world the way we would like it to be. We do this by creating an internal picture of this new world, which is more like what we want and what we need. When we do this, we also account for the way things actually are in the real world. We can create this new world while working with reality so that it allows our lives and the lives of all others around us to become better.

This new world we now create is likely to be a world that is more realistic for us, for who we are, where we are, and where we wish to be in the future.

From this new position, we can then transform ourselves and the world around us to bring about what we truly desire. This is the way most of the great people of history changed their worlds. People like Washington, Jefferson, Ford, Susan B. Anthony, Florence Nightingale, Gandhi, Madam Curie, and Jonas Salk changed the world they lived in – generally not through force – but by creating positive workable visions of they wanted to bring to life. These men and women saw life as it was, accepted it, and then set out to change it. They also clearly saw what was wrong and what could be created from what already existed.

We are not telling you that what you need to do must be done on the same scale as these people. Changing your life by making it match your picture basically requires a similar, scaled-down approach. This is not always done without creating some new stress. However, the clearer your picture of what is and what can be created, the more determined you are to have it, the more you see it in its finished state, the less stress you will create.

It is extremely important to remember that making mistakes must always be expected, even anticipated. It helps to always keep your overall goals in mind. Much like the Intelligent Universe in which we live, this action is always part of our own personal evolution. We must constantly learn and grow from everything we do and everything that happens to us.

To bring about transformation, we must first observe the people around us, as well as the world in which we live, and the way both operate. A full understanding of the world requires recognizing that the world is always changing, and that most change is natural and necessary. While it may appear to us that massive expenditures of energy are required to accomplish any meaningful change, this is not always the case.

Major changes in our life can occur easily, often simply by changing our approach, asking for different results, and expecting them to take place.

Many people believe that life is difficult and is stress unavoidable. This is an illusion. This is just one of the many lies and faulty belief systems created by misunderstanding the true nature of the world around us. Often because many changes are made in such small increments during long periods, they are difficult to see and so they are ignored. Big changes can occur in just seconds or over millennia. Small changes are often easier to create and can accomplish similar results. This is especially true if we want things to change right now. Immediate changes often require major efforts, and the likelihood of getting exactly what you want under these circumstances is often very limited. On the other hand, small changes made during long periods can bring about significant results.

CREATING CHALLENGES AND OPPORTUNITIES

Once unresolved conflicts are identified, set goals to resolve them and create movement in a positive direction. Your ultimate goal must be to transform all negative situations into positive, and more productive "challenges and opportunities." If we think of stress as a negative process, then challenge and opportunity are its positive counterparts. If you want to change either yourself or the world around you, you can best do this by transforming unresolved conflicts and problems into challenges and opportunities. Transforming conflicts and problems into challenges and opportunities reduces negative stress, and turns off or tones down the Stress-Illness Mechanism. This also allows you to create a positive way to solve problems, learn and grow from them, and ultimately create what you desire using positive, productive life-force energies. Changing problems into challenges and opportunities will bring you to where you want and need to be in your life. Thinking positively and creating a workable plan can help you get where you want to be going with less work and less stress. Accepting and working with your unresolved conflicts as challenges and opportunities will reduce stress in your life and facilitate healing.

CREATING GOALS

To be most successful in life, it helps to establish a series of well-selected, small, but meaningful and progressive goals. Each goal must be chosen because it will not only help you get where you want to go, but because it will help you get there with the least possible effort and the best possible results. Each goal must be practical and reasonably easy to attain in the time allotted to accomplish it. The first step in this process is to create a clear picture of what we ultimately want and what it will eventually look and feel like. This could be considered the primary goal. Its job is to point the way so that we know where we are going, in which direction to start, and what we expect to have when we get there.

Our next job is to then set up a series of mini-goals to get you where you want to go. This process has two advantages. First: less energy is required to reach each mini-goal than going all the way to the primary goal. Second: we can periodically alter our mini-goals as we determine whether they are still taking us in the right direction. When working toward very large goals, it is not always possible to put in all of the energy needed at one time to reach this larger goal. When using mini-goals, you can move in an orderly fashion, putting in just the right amount of energy needed to accomplish each one of these baby-steps. Remember, we must still save a good deal of energy for day-to-day living.

If you try to rearrange all your priorities and needs at the same time, you may miss the fact that your priorities may change with time. Remember, these mini-goals should never be a final resting place. Instead, they should be opportunities, challenges, and incentives that you now use to achieve your overall purpose of evolving yourself and accomplishing your overall and greater goals.

Creating mini-goals allows you to periodically re-evaluate progress, change direction, learn, grow, and steadily mature as you reduce your stresses. Mini-goals are installment solutions that permit you to attain what you want at your own pace. They reaffirm that you are on your way to where you want to go and that this is really what you want, where you want to go, and that it is worth the time and effort you are expending.

Through this self-evaluation process and trial and error, you can allow yourself to better define who you are and what you really want out of life. By using mini-goals, you can best determine what you want to do with your life and what you want to work at without moving too far, too fast and without losing sight of your ultimate goals.

The key value of mini-goals is that they can allow you to solve problems along the way. In so doing, you can use them to resolve specific conflicts and to help you heal your Child Within. You can use them to create ongoing harmony and balance in your life, and you can direct them in such a way as to help you become the person you want to be. Using them appropriately can also help you enhance your capacity for self-love while you are becoming stress free.

Stress-free people usually have a clear picture of themselves. They do not live with lies or unresolved conflicts. They know who they are, what they like and dislike. They also know what they value and desire. Their goals are generally firm, but flexible. They have a specific direction and a general path to get there.

The stress-free person understands that there can be deviations, detours, roadblocks, and setbacks during the process of getting where they want and need to go. They not only expect these obstacles, but often look forward to them because they know that these challenges are their teachers and that the opportunities they create provides them the chance to grow and evolve, as well as helps them create or look for and find their highest, healthiest, and best Self.

Stress-free people are willing to learn and grow. They have the ability to transform apparently insolvable problems into creative solutions.

Stress-free people love, respect, and value themselves and what they do. They respect and care for others. They never work against anyone. They may be competitive, but are not destructive or selfish. They often help others around them succeed, grow, and move toward finding their highest, healthiest, and best Selves.

Stress-free people live life fully, without fear and regret. They make mistakes. They may make bad decisions, but they use what they learn from these to constantly grow and evolve and better themselves.

MAKING MISTAKES

People who fear making mistakes are blocked from getting what they want out of life. As noted earlier, mistakes are teachers; they educate us about life. They help define who we are and what we really want and need. Whenever a mistake is made, we should celebrate ourselves for having tried, for without trying, progress is impossible.

> Without Trying,
>
> No Progress Can Be Made.

Many people are unable to accept their mistakes and forgive themselves for making them. They may turn these mistakes against themselves instead. They may criticize, blame, and belittle themselves. Because of the fear and anger created, they resist moving forward. This leads to increased stress that not only further limits their growth, but also undermines their ability to evolve. Perhaps the most important thing to learn from this process is being more tolerant of yourself and your abilities. Creating mini-goals is one way to help you become stress free. Mini-goals facilitate your finding and reaching your overall life goals. Your mini-goals should always be realistic and attainable. Once a goal is established, look for the most natural steps to attain it.

An example of this for me, Allen, was my desire to become a medical doctor. It required that I graduate high school with a certain grade point average. Then, I had to attend a good university and graduate with an overall superior record. A high score on the Medical College Aptitude Tests (MCAT) was needed. Finally, I had to make a good presentation when interviewed by the various medical schools that were on my short list.

Rather than worry about the MCAT and the interviews for years, I decided while in high school to set a number of mini-goals that would address challenges before they became problems. I learned what was needed to pass these hurdles and then prepared for them during the years. I learned how to take tests and did as much public speaking as I could.

Rather than simply wanting to get into medical school, I took the steps necessary to accomplish this goal and to do it well. I also used positive, visual imagery to see myself being successful. I then applied these principles in all relationships and situations that required problem solving along the way.

PROBLEM SOLVING

As we move through life, it is important to reduce our stress occurrences. Nothing accomplishes this better than solving difficult situations before they become bigger and more complex problems. We must also create a sense of who we are and what we want at each level of our lives. It is important to have both short and long-term mini-goals.

Having a clear sense of one's self is imperative to problem solving. How can you solve any problem if you have no clear idea of who you are, what you want out of life, and the many potential solutions to problem solving?

This requires a clear set of life goals and a basic self-understanding of who you are and what you want out of your life, your personal life-image. Who you are, or want to be, may well change many times during your life. It is always based on how you live your life and how you experience your life, the decisions you make, the decisions you don't make, the paths you choose and those you do not choose.

At each level of your life, you must either create a new life-image or revise it accordingly so that your life-image and subsequent lifestyle work for you.

Usually, your life-image is based on your immediate needs and future goals. However, these are influenced by how you handled life in the past. For example, if someone wants to own her own business, she must not only live a lifestyle that allows her to operate this business, she must also live a lifestyle that allows her to save or raise the capital for starting this business. She must have a life-style that keeps her from getting into debt. She must live within her means and pay her bills. Her business plan will likely be a combination of ideas and beliefs she has stored from her past, ideas of how the present and the future will look, beliefs and projections of how her business will look and be in the future. She can get competent financial advice and other help when she needs it. Avoiding money problems and other unexpected problems, which are among the most common reasons for stress and failure in business ventures, is essential. She can prevent stress and failure by thoughtful planning, help from experts, and having a clear and flexible business and life plan.

Always make decisions from strength. Decisions made from weakness eventually work against us, because we will usually accept or take less than we actually need to accomplish our goals. Decisions made from strength require clarity of purpose, knowledge of the appropriate facts, and understanding of the alternatives and consequences. By working this way, we ultimately emerge stronger and healthier.

Once we make a decision, we must take full and total responsibility for all the consequences associated with it. In order to lessen stress and conflicts in our life, we must remain fully responsible for every decision we make. Avoiding responsibility invites conflict and problems, and creates more lies. Ultimately, our decision or indecision to avoid taking responsibility can and will get us into trouble.

Working toward reaching our highest, healthiest and best Self, who we really are inside, can prevent and eliminate stress because we are working within our personal truth[15]. Strong healthy personal truths eliminate lies and conflicts. They also help us resolve our problems.

At first, this may seem scary. However, living a more truthful life ultimately reduces stress and helps us grow, find, reach for, and become our highest, healthiest and best Self.

---

15   *This means that your beliefs, decisions, and actions act to empower you and make you healthier. They help you solve your conflicts and support your personal growth, which will allow you to become and be the best person you can be. Moreover, they help you to evolve as a person and grow spiritual-ly, and support becoming and being your highest, healthiest and best Self.*

SOLVING CONFLICTS WITH FORGIVENESS

Clearing up old problems and conflicts in our lives as well as in our relationships is important for reducing conflict and stress. When working with conflicts involving other people in our lives, always negotiate solutions until all parties are satisfied.

When others are unwilling to be involved or are no longer available to solve unresolved conflict then you have the opportunity to solve the conflict on your own. First, forgive all others in your life for any and all hurt they may have caused you or your loved ones. You do this not to free them from what they have done, but rather to release you from anger, pain, and stressing over what was done. Remember that your giving forgiveness has less to do with them and much more to do with you releasing yourself from the negative forces that have been working against you.

There are several ways available for you to forgive others and thereby release yourself. You can do it face-to-face, by letter, telegram, email, Twitter, by audio or videotape. These processes can release you from the negative feelings and conflicts that caused you injury in the past. Your goal here is to release all of the anger and stress you hold and have held on to in the past.

If you do, then you may want to tell those who have caused your anger and stress that you are from this point on, forgiving them and letting go of any grudges, anger, or any ill will that you may have held against them in the past. It is entirely up to you to do what feels right.

What is most important is that whether you write it and never send it, or you actually do tell them, you must include everything you need to say in order to fully release yourself, forgive them, and finally, forgive yourself for all of the negative feelings you have harbored against anyone in your life.

Once this message is complete and as detailed as needed, you can send it to them, burn it, or bury it (here you only need to put their name on the outside of the envelope that contains your letter before burning or burying it). Whatever you do is best done in a symbolic or ritual procedure, as a gesture for sending it off to them and burning or burying it so that it reaches them through their Higher Selves. Burning or burying your message requires that you acknowledge that you are doing this with the knowledge that the Universe is Intelligent and that because of your ritual – in a sense your prayer your message will reach whomever it is intended for.

If the person or people you are forgiving are unavailable or dead, your message is best presented by making your statement to the world at large, or by writing down everything you need to say to them and then burying it superficially at their grave site or burning it as a symbolic act of sending it out into the Universe and to their Higher Self. Since the Universe is Intelligent and we are all connected, the message will get to them. How it gets to them is really unimportant; just trust that it will find them. Do what needs doing, and then let it go, so that you are complete with this process. It is now in the past and should never negatively affect you again.

You have now released all anger, hostility, and stress against everyone you ever held anger or a grudge against. What is next? Now, all of your anger and hostility no longer have to get in your way. If they still do, repeat the exercise until they are completely gone and you are entirely free.

DON'T LIVE IN THE PAST

It is important to remember that the past is the past. Here in the present, we should only have positive recollections and remembrances. Our negative grudges, anger and hostility are really only our memories of the events or situation from our past. They are not real in the present. They happened in the past, a long time ago.

Very often, our memories cause us to be unhappy and unhealthy in the present by forcing us to live in or relive the past. Old, negative memories can alter our vision of the future and the decisions we make in the present. Negative memories act as negative filters. They distort our current reality. They cause us to live in a false world of lies. This is destructive and stress inducing.

Happy memories do the opposite. They make us feel good, lighten our mood, generate happiness, and promote our overall well-being. By letting go of unhappy memories and enjoying our happy memories, we begin to better focus on the present, solving problems and creating a healthier and happier future.

ACTING TOWARD OTHERS

In the past, you may have held grudges or anger toward people who wronged you. It is important, as we stated earlier, to forgive these people. The energy used in maintaining your negative emotions ultimately acts much like blocks and prevents you from getting what you want in your life. These blocks then drain your life force energy. They drain your power to obtain what you need and want. They also block your ability to create what you want for your loved ones. They create stress and this can lead to illness and disease. These negative belief systems and emotions diminish you. They decrease your ability to feel love and to give love. They make it difficult for others to give you the love. They block and undermine your ability to reach for and find your highest, healthiest, and best Self.

Always act to help others around you who are working toward attaining their highest, healthiest, and best Self. Appreciate and support their efforts, as well as your own. This creates ongoing truth and goodness. It makes up for your past sins and for guilt from the past, and balances the scales in your favor. It will make you feel good about yourself, and good feelings go a long way toward removing stress and creating happiness.

KNOW YOURSELF

Lastly and of utmost importance, take time to know yourself. Make peace with yourself and constantly work toward creating a positive balance and harmony in your life. Visualize yourself as complete right now and getting better every day. Stress elimination is possible in the integrated self because the integrated self comes from strength, healthy goals, and positive self-worth.

Chapter Fifteen

PROBLEM SOLVING AND WELLNESS

PROBLEM SOLVING TO HELP WITH HEALING STRESS-RELATED DISORDERS — THE PREPARATIONS

For those who suffer from Stress-Related Disorders, the most import-ant question is, *"How can I heal myself and return myself to full and complete wellness?"*

The answer is simple yet difficult at the same time. You need to activate your body's Healing, Repair, and Maintenance Systems. To do this, you will need to find and resolve as many of your existing conflicts as is possible, hopefully all of them. As you resolve them, you can create total physical, mental, emotion-al and spiritual health and wellness. In order to do this, it will help if you can follow a process called, "Problem Solving." Below is an outline of one helpful approach to problem solving.

1. IDENTIFY AS MANY PROBLEMS AND CONFLICTS AS YOU CAN & RECOGNIZE THE RELATIONSHIP BETWEEN THEM & YOUR ILLNESS(ES)

It is virtually impossible to heal any problem or illness unless you first recognize that you have a problem or are ill. In order to heal your illness, you must also accept that one or more problems, conflicts, or lies exist that are at the base of your illness or illnesses.

Once you accept this, begin looking for those problems and conflicts that feel unresolved and have negative energy associated with them. There are three major types of problems.

Small, Every-Day Problems

The first group of problems and conflicts are those small ones we live with every day. We know them well. They range from problems with little effect on us to problems that have significant short or even long-term effects on our lives and overall well-being. A few examples of small everyday problems with little effect may be making breakfast, keeping on schedule on a busy day, getting to work on time, fitting what you want and need to do into your daily schedule, remembering your anniversary, etc. While these problems may be small, they are still meaningful and important. They are rarely important enough to affect our health or overall well-being. If they do affect our health, it is often in the form of feeling "over-stressed" or being in some mild to moderate distress, such as having recurrent heartburn or indigestion or catching colds easily. They rarely lead to significant illness. However, they can add to the overall force of negative stress upon us when added to other more significant types of problems.

Before moving onto the next group, it is also important to restate that stress is an additive phenomenon. That is, while one small stressful situation might not on its own be significant or capable of leading to illness, each unresolved stressor event can add additional power to all of the other stress in your life. Ultimately, it is the total weight of all of the stressful events in your life that leads to illness. Therefore, when many small, unresolved stresses pile upon larger unresolved stress, the total effect may outweigh the sum of each individually and can then lead to illness faster than any single small or moderate stressor event alone.

Significant, Yet Ignored or Suppressed Problems

The second group of potential problems is those that are significant, but that we either ignore or suppress. This group includes problems such as disliking your job; hating your boss; working too many hours; marital problems; problems between you and your children; problems with in-laws, co-workers, friends, or neighbors; being seriously in debt or about to become homeless. To most people, these types of problems often seem natural, even normal, as if everyone around us has similar problems. Yet, they are affecting you and not everyone else. These problems can create internal reactions, which can range from minor annoyances to serious illness-causing distress.

Often, the people experiencing problems within this group may know that something is wrong. They may even see clues such as frequent illness, difficulty sleeping, rapid heart rate, anxiety, and even panic reactions.

However, the exact nature of the conflict or its cause may be consciously unrecognized, ignored, or suppressed[16].

---

16   *This means that your beliefs, decisions, and actions act to empower you and make you healthier. They help you solve your conflicts and support your personal growth, which will allow you to become and be the best person you can be. Moreover, they help you to evolve as a person and grow spiritually, and support becoming and being your highest, healthiest and best Self.*

An example of this might be the man who hates his job, but since he needs the money, he simply ignores his feelings and "pretends" to be happy. He knows he is unhappy, but will not experience his unhappiness or be concerned by how this makes him feel. He may ignore or suppress his feelings of anger, helpless, frustration or even his hopelessness, so that he will not have to act on them and somehow lose his job or quit. To understand the overall affect on him we must first consider the messages he is sending to his Body-Mind. *"I will not act because I am afraid." "I am worthless since I will not even solve my own problems." I neither respect nor care about myself."* This situation is fraught with danger for him. If he is not already experiencing symptoms of Dis-Stress, frequent minor or recurrent illness, or if this has gone on for a longtime, than it is likely he is undermining his immune system and that he will sooner or later experience a more severe, even potentially life-threatening, illness. Over time, any illness he does experience will likely increase in severity. This individual may require more than over-the-counter medications or multiple over-the-counter medications, to control his symptoms and his eventual illness or illnesses.

The problem is that while he knows something is wrong, he may have buried it so deeply that he is not able to put his finger on exactly what is happening to him. Co-workers, family, and friends may see what is happening, but they are usually not skilled enough to help or counsel him. Admitting to himself or others that a problem exists might mean having to take some sort of corrective action, such as telling his boss off or quitting his job. If he did any of these, he would lose his job, and this would create an entirely new set of "much worse" or even "more threatening" problems for him. Ignoring or suppressing his feelings may well be perceived, consciously or subconsciously, as a safer alternative for him. Yet, his Body-Mind knows that what he is doing is a lie and this creates more conflict regarding his survival.

We are usually aware of the problems and conflicts causing what we are experiencing. However, at the same time, we may totally be unaware of their connection to how and what we are feeling and our overall state of health and well-being. In most cases, even if we do know how these conflicts are affecting us, we still might not want or be able to deal with them. This is especially true if we perceive that the consequences of dealing with them may be significantly worse than what we feel will happen to us when we ignore them. Obviously, from what you already must know about what happens in these types of situations, this is a long shot.

As with the first group, most people in this group simply accept how they are feeling as normal, *"The way everyone else feels"* or as we are frequently told in the office, *"Doesn't everyone feel this way?"* Most people do not connect their unresolved problems and conflicts with their health or lack of it. The earlier example of young Peter fits this category and demonstrates what happens when we ignore resolving important, stress-producing issues.

Deep Suppression

This third group is considerably more complex than the first two. The people belonging to this group are often already experiencing Dis-Stress, Dys-Stress, or Dis-Ease. They are already experiencing illness and especially, SRDs. Generally, these people have little or no conscious awareness or memory of these events or situations, or what is at the root of their health problems. The triggering events may have occurred very early in life when they were very young, or the triggering events were extremely traumatic and painful, leaving what is often referred to as, "a lasting scar." The memories of these events are deeply suppressed within their subconscious by the Body-Mind in order to protect them.

The conflict-producing situations in this group occur when people experienced a major trauma during childhood, as a youth, or adult. Some examples of this may be the traumatic death of a parent; a person who has been raped, molested, or abused; children of alcoholics or drug addicts; or people who have been injured at some point in their life but are unable to deal with the specific event, its causes, or consequences. This can also occur when a lesser trauma has occurred and has created sufficient fear or altered state of consciousness causing the Body-Mind to submerge some part of itself deeply into what we often think of as our subconscious mind.

One of the most common examples of this type of response is where a person was molested during childhood. The memories associated with this experience – which may have gone on for hours, day, weeks or years – may be so painful and terrifying that the Body-Mind buried it deep inside of its Subconscious Aware Self. Sometime later, it may act as a significant block to this person's ability to function normally and stay healthy. This person may be affected on multiple levels: physical, emotional, mental, or spiritual. The effect created by this trauma can leave the person in a state of apathy or in a state of anger. They may hate themselves. They may hate the person who molested them. They may even have suicidal feelings. Yet, they still may have little or no memory of the actual events. They may not even be consciously aware that any sort of trauma ever happened to them. Imagine how frustrating it might be to experience waves of negative feelings and have no memory or ability to recognize why any of this is happening.

As suggested, this group differs from the previous two groups in that these individuals have little or no conscious remembrance. Those in group two are often aware of what happened, but they do not want to face remembering the event nor their feelings about what happened, nor the negative emotions they previously experienced when they did bring any memories of their traumatic events to the surface. They often feel there is little they can do anyway, so why think about it or act on their feelings, as this will most likely only get them into trouble. In this third group, all or most of the memories associated with these events are deeply suppressed. Since they are often so painful their Body-Mind will not let them surface in the awake state, at least until some sort of crisis or therapeutic experience brings them to the surface. The individual may experience sleep problems as the Body-Mind communicates its need for resolution in the form of "bad dreams" or "nightmares."

In this third group, there is no clear or firm conscious memory of the events, only at most very indistinct or vague feelings that something happened in the past. They may even have split off the part of their personality that has any memories of these events, hence developing two or more personalities (the so-called split or multiple personalities). Because these conflicts are buried so deeply that there is no conscious memory, these people may actually live without any evidence of conflict related to what happened to them. Then something might occur, another trauma, or some portion of their memory about these events may rise into their consciousness. At this point, the Body-Mind begins to require a process of healing, which may create a crisis, with or without a physical, mental, emotional, or spiritual, or illness. The Body-Mind wants the conflict uncovered, resolved, and healed.

None of these groups is better or worse than any other. They are simply different ways in which our Body-Mind handles unresolved conflicts. More importantly, it is the degree of the problem they ultimately create for the individual that is meaningful. While the small, everyday conflicts rarely cause serious illness, conflicts that are ignored, superficially or deeply suppressed can create a wide range or problems for the individual. They are more likely to lead to illness. The Body-Mind is more likely to see them as meaningful, even serious, or major conflicts requiring resolution. It may work hard to resolve them. It may see them as life-threatening, inviting greater reactions to them, which can more likely lead to activating the Wellness-Stress-Illness Mechanism.

A (very) few of the people who have deeply suppressed, extremely traumatic, conflicts may be successful in resolving these deeply embedded traumas. A few ultimately may commit suicide because they are in such great emotional pain and they see no other way out. Generally however, most people find outlets for dealing with their pain, including use of alcohol, drugs (legal and illegal), smoking, gambling, all aimed at suppressing and ignoring those issues that cause them pain.

Accessing, Understanding, And Dealing With Our Conflicts

Even when consciously aware of unresolved conflicts or problems, people still may experience distress. This distress may be equal to or even greater than any distress they might have experienced if they were totally unaware of the conflicts and problems they have suppressed.

The difference is only in our ability to access, understand, and deal with these conflicts and problems. If/when suppressed, we can't deal with them because we are unaware that they exist. But even when we know they exist and are fully aware of them and what they are, we still may not be able to deal with them if we consciously or subconsciously choose not to do so. Only when we know them and choose to act will we get the best results.

Therefore, the main problem with creating healing is our ability to access, discover, understand, and resolve these conflicts. Healing almost always takes time, work, and effort and frequently requires making changes in our lives. Hence, it requires hard work and focused intention to create healing.

Healing usually is broken down into a series of reasonably complicated steps. These include recognition that a conflict exists, awareness and recognition of the many parts of the conflict(s), creating a healing plan, problem solving, and finally healing ourselves of all of our guilt, anger, hate, hostility, and other negative emotions in order to create total healing. Only when we have fully returned to or found health for the first time, will we know that we have identified and resolved all the important conflicts of our lives.

At the beginning of this chapter, we said that to heal ourselves, it is important to first identify that we have a problem or problems, and second that we consciously or unconsciously allowed these unresolved conflicts and problems to negatively affect us.

People often experience fear when they first recognize that they are ill. Since in the beginning, their Stress-Related Disorder symptoms are vague and appear unconnected, they may not be sure of what is happening to them. This may generate apprehension, anxiety, and fear. We may delay for months or even years before taking any action at all. Some people end up waiting until the problems are almost insoluble, while others may take action almost immediately.

No matter how or when we recognize that our unresolved problems led us to illness, it is up to us to decide whether we wish to do anything about this or not. Before we go to the next step, we must accept our role in creating our illnesses. It is also helpful if we can forgive ourselves and decide that we not only want to solve our problems, but that we are willing to do everything we must to accomplish this goal. We must be ready and willing to learn from our actions and conflicts and allow ourselves to grow and evolve in order to fully heal. We must also be able to convince ourselves–both our Body-Mind and our Conscious Selves–that we are not only ready, but also, that we deserve to be fully well and healthy again.

Journaling

One technique to accomplish these goals is journaling. Journaling allows us to write down our thoughts and feelings; what we know and even what we do not know regarding how our illness is affecting us. We can also write down other thoughts, ideas, dreams, fantasies, or beliefs as to what happening or has happened to bring us to the point of illness. The information we are giving you right now can make journaling significantly easier for you. This information allows you to recognize what is important to know. It also allows you to begin the process of listing all conflicts of which you are consciously aware. Journaling can do even more. It can help you begin a process of communicating with your Body-Mind, letting it know that you mean business and are working toward and hoping that it will communicate back with you, and that you are ready and willing to hear what it has to tell you.

When your Body-Mind accepts that you are open to listening and resolving your unresolved conflicts, it will begin to help you. This process may be slow and tenuous at first. If you stick with it, it will ultimately provide you information about your unresolved conflicts and how to resolve them. Even better, your Body-Mind can tell you what you need to do to accomplish your goals. It does this through dreams, feelings, emotions, physical, mental, emotional, and spiritual symptoms and signs. If you are journaling, it gives you crucial information to write in your journal.

We have all heard the expression, *"The pen is mightier than the sword."* Many people are more willing to accept what is written in a newspaper or magazine than what they see with their own eyes or hear from others. This is because the Body-Mind ultimately believes that the written word is truth. For many people, journaling is an excellent way to discover exactly what their truths and beliefs are. Your Body-Mind will be telling you what to write so that you will know what is going on within it. Your Body-Mind does this so that you can believe it and see what it believes is the truth. Because you can refer back to it again and again as you work, you will find important clues and previously unknown truths which your Body-Mind believes you will need to know in order to determine how to resolve your current problems and illness.

2. WE MUST ACCEPT RESPONSIBILITY FOR OUR PROBLEMS AND DECIDE TO RESOLVE THEM

To better understand this process, here is another example. Jed H., a 41-year-old male, had a history of recurrent sore throats for more than 30 years. Jed had his tonsils removed as a child because of recurrent episodes of tonsillitis. Jed initially came to us after many episodes of sore throats when his doctors could find nothing wrong with his throat. Ultimately, one doctor told him that there was nothing physically wrong him, and that his sore throats were "all in his head." For more than six months, Jed used a number of techniques we taught him. He learned that he suppressed his emotions, and that he usually took no action until his body communicated through some form of illness, usually a sore throat. He realized that he most frequently had a sore throat when he was not saying something he really wanted or needed to say.

At one visit, he told me that a few days earlier, upon arising and readying himself for work, he found that he had a "scratchy throat." In the past, he would generally have a full-fledged, painful sore throat by early morning or late in the afternoon.

Apparently, once his throat really hurt him, in the past, he would go to see his doctor to get a prescription for an antibiotic in order to "cure" it. However, that day he did something different. He sat at the edge of his bed, closed his eyes, and asked himself silently what he should be saying and to whom. In a flash, the answer came to him. His boss had told him the previous night that he wanted him to start a new project. He wanted to tell his boss that he had not yet completed the project he had been working on for the past week, and that he couldn't possibly start a new project.

"If I start a new project," he thought, "I would have to leave what I have been working on unfinished, or I will have to work overtime, working on two entirely different projects for the next several weeks in order to get them both done." He then related what he did. "Later that day when I arrived at work, I went directly to see my boss. I came right out with it. "Mr. Johnston, how important is this new project? I have not completed the work on the Henderson account. Should I put it aside and get on with the new project or should I finish up on the Henderson account?"

His boss, Mr. Johnston, sat for a minute or two not saying a word, appearing to be deep in thought. Then he asked Jed, "How much work do you have left on what the Henderson account?" Jed explained that the art department had been held up for a week on another project and that he needed at least another week to complete it.

"Henderson is just as important as the new project," his boss finally told him. "Finish your work on the Henderson account and as soon as you're done with it, let me know. If everything is good, then you can get to work on the new project."

Jed then told us that as soon as he turned to leave his boss called him back. "Jed, thank you for letting me know that you still have more work to do on the Henderson account, but why didn't you tell me yesterday?" Jed told us that he had felt flustered, and at first did not know what to say. Then he told his boss, "When you asked yesterday, I did not want to disappoint you. Therefore, I thought that I might be able to try to do both accounts at the same time. I guess I thought I could do it. But last night, I realized I could not do them both as well as I might if I finished one before I started the other." His boss then asked him again, "But why didn't you tell me that yesterday?" Jed answered, "I needed the time to think about it and decide if I could do both of them as well. I decided that I would have to tell you the truth and let you decide which project was more important."

Jed's boss looked up at him and shook his head, and said, "Thank you. I am glad you kept me up on it. You know both accounts are important to me, and I want them done right. Thanks."

As Jed left the boss' office, he suddenly realized that he no longer had any discomfort in his throat.

Before solving any problem, you must take responsibility for it. If you blame others or the problem itself, it is unlikely that you will do what is necessary to heal yourself. In fact, when we make others responsible or blame them and we know that this is not true, we will likely end up sabotaging ourselves because of these lies.

Jed had originally made his boss out to be an ogre, and it soon became clear that Jed was afraid of him. Jed had been unwilling to take the chance of being wrong or looking bad. He paid for this with sore throat after sore throat. He had been afraid to speak his mind for many years and his Body-Mind communicated this conflict by producing sore throats to let him know he had a problem that needed resolution. This had been his pattern since childhood.

With the first two steps, identifying problems and conflicts and taking responsibility for them, we start the process of resolution and healing into motion. However, before beginning the actual healing process, it is of value to take full responsibility for the creation of the problems and forgive yourself for this and for any hurt or problems you have created for yourself or others.

Do Everything You Must Do To Get Well

Taking responsibility is also the first step toward deciding whether you not only want to get well, but whether you are willing to do everything you need to do to solve your problems. Remember that whatever you do, you should not intentionally cause hurt to yourself or to any others. If you do, you will worsen the situation.

It has been our experience that many people say that they want to get well, but often they are not always willing to do everything necessary to make this happen. Jed recognized what was wrong and took the risk of confronting his boss and it worked out for him. Some people are just not able to do this or they simply may not be ready to solve their most complex, painful problems. They may not be ready to take full responsibility, or to say, do, or change what is needed to attain optimal results. Many people not only refuse to take medication, but they believe they can't change and clean up their lifestyles. Some may require necessary surgery; a special diet; or break their addiction to smoking, alcohol, or drugs. Some people are not willing or able to stop lying to themselves or to others. Therefore, their lies continue and they continue to undermine themselves. Under these circumstances, they may not be ready or able to find their problems and conflicts and then resolve them. The unknown is scary. When this happens, healing may happen very slowly or not occur at all. Even if and when some healing does occur, it may not be complete nor permanent.

In order to understand this better, let's look at another example. Terri W. was a 37-year-old female who had recurring upset stomach, abdominal pains, and sporadic episodes of diarrhea. She had seen her family doctor many times for these complaints. He repeatedly treated her with a barrage of different prescription medications. Early on, she seemed to respond well to these medications, but gradually each medication simply stopped working. As Terri stopped responding to the medications, her doctor repeatedly performed numerous laboratory and diagnostic tests. All the tests taken were found to be entirely normal. Her doctor ultimately referred her to a specialist in gastrointestinal diseases. The specialist repeated many of the previous tests, and then gave Terri an entirely new set of medications.

After weeks of suffering and several more visits to the specialist and changes of her medications, Terri became convinced that none of these new medications was helping her any more than those given to her by her family doctor. A friend of hers whom we had helped several months earlier referred Terri to us. Since her family doctor and the specialist found nothing, it was obvious to us that Terri's problems were not strictly medical in nature but probably a Stress-Related Disorder.

The first question we asked Terri was, "What is going on in your life?" Her immediate response was, "I think my husband has been having an affair."

"What makes you think that?"

Terri thought for a few seconds and responded, "Just little things, I guess, nothing I can really put my finger on. He is no longer as attentive to me as he used to be. He comes home late more often than in the past, and has been working through most weekends, telling me that he has 'business meetings.' He has done this ten or more times in the last six months."

"What if he was having an affair?" We asked.

"It would kill me."

"Would it really?"

"Well no, I didn't mean I would die, I meant, it would hurt me a great deal."

"How was your marriage prior to this?"

"Well, we had our problems, doesn't everybody?" She responded.

"What kinds of problems?"

She hardly hesitated. "Look, I just was having difficulty with his snoring, so I asked him to move into the spare bedroom. He couldn't hear himself snore and his snoring was keeping me up all night."

"How did he feel about it?"

"He was angry, but it's not my fault, I wasn't the one who was snoring."

"Did you ever suggest that he get medical help?"

"I told him to see a doctor, but he didn't consider it to be a problem."

After talking to Terri for an hour, it was clear, even to her, that she was no longer happy with her husband when, "He did nothing to control his snoring." She did realize that she had contributed to distancing her husband from her. They no longer had a relationship of any kind. She agreed to talk to her husband and take full responsibility for her behavior. It was not about who was right or wrong, but rather about making the relationship good for both of them.

During the course of our meetings, we talked about the same process we discussed above. About her taking responsibility for her role in this situation, about her willingness to do everything she needed to do to heal and about forgiving herself and her husband for what was happening to them. Terri listened to and understood everything we discussed.

Three weeks later, she returned a different person. She had finally talked with her husband. He went to his doctor, a new treatment was prescribed that decreased his snoring, and they were once again sleeping together.

"Was your husband having an affair?"

"You know, I never asked. I realized after we talked that I had driven him away. Whatever had happened was my fault. I forgave myself for doing it and I apologized to him. We dealt with a number of issues that I had not previously even known about. I decided that I had greatly contributed to what had happened, so I forgave myself and I forgave him. We have started all over again. We are seeing a marriage counselor and I believe we will be fine now."

3. IDENTIFY THE CAUSES AND CREATE AN INTENTION TO HEAL THEM

By now it should be evident that the illness or illnesses that have been plaguing you are Stress-Related Disorders. You may now also recognize that you must begin the process of taking responsibility for them, if you want to heal. What is the next step?

The next logical step must be discovering what conflicts or faulty belief systems triggered your Stress-Related Disorders. In order to do this, you must identify as many of these conflicts as possible. Once armed with this information, you can set the healing process into motion. Since you are reading our book, you have likely realized that this can be the most difficult part of the entire process. This is because, even though we are aware of our many unresolved conflicts, there may also be many unresolved conflicts that are hidden even from us. We may simply be unaware they exist. They are unknown to our Conscious Aware Self. Since we now understand SRDs and what causes them much better than in the past, we may now be able to see that many of our unresolved conflicts and the lies that have caused us to sabotage ourselves and others may be hidden from us either because we have been unable or have not wanted to acknowledge that they existed. They caused too many problems, too much fear, suffering, and pain, so we repressed them.

On the other hand, many people may feel "naked" without their problems. For many people, their problems are all they talk about. In many cases, their "problems" so occupy their awareness that their "problems" soon openly control their lives. In some cases because of fear and potential pain, their Body-Mind may not want to solve these "problems." Hence, the old adage, *"It may be better to live and accept with the devil you know, than open your door to the devil you don't know."*

Fully recognizing how conflicts can create a living presence within us can give you a much better understanding as to why these conflicts now activate your survival mechanism to protect themselves from being recognized, attacked, and possibly eliminated. Once created, they take on a life of their own. In a sense, they become living entities within us. They often do this by causing pain, anxiety, tension, fear, and a host of other negative, and occasionally positive, emotions that force us to move away from dealing with them and eliminating them.

This makes much more sense once you remember that these conflicts are ideas, thoughts, and memories located within cutoff parts of our inner self, for example inside your Child Within. This is especially true for unresolved conflicts contained within our subconscious mind. Some of those were created during childhood when we were three years old or possibly when we were fifteen year old selves. We were still children and unprepared to deal with or solve painful and traumatic conflicts that may have been forced upon us. It is as if these conflicts still live within us operating as they did back then, even though we are now adults and the trauma is only a memory from years long past. Since they are simply negative memories, their existence today is maintained by the power we give to all ideas and thoughts, positive or negative. Added to this is the power given to them by the fear, pain and anxiety they generate as we get too close to them, or when the Child Within fears they will be allowed to resurface. Consider how Cindy was affected by the negative ideas and thoughts her father placed into her Subconscious Aware Self when she was a child.

As discussed earlier, these problems and conflicts can and do take on lives of their own. When threatened, they fight to survive. Because they fear that we will eliminate or kill them, they often choose to fight with every bit of power they can drain from us. The Child Within feeling guilty or fearful may unwittingly become their ally and act to block or mask them from us as a child would try to protect their dog, cat, or doll from being destroyed. The Child Within may even fill our heads with reasons why they are not problems, or it may divert our attention by creating an illness that takes our minds off resolving the specific conflict it is trying to protect. Either way, without identifying the causes of our underlying conflicts, it will be very difficult to focus on them and resolve them amicably so all parts of us feel happy and healthy once these conflicts, faulty beliefs and lies have been resolved.

Healing does not occur by accident. While prayers can come true and miracles can happen, healing requires work, and the ability to develop solutions to the problems that underlie your illnesses. Healing happens best when we intentionally make it happen. Healing is more likely to take place in the exact way we want it to happen when we do everything possible to ensure that it will happen.

We have all heard the old saying, *"The road to hell is littered with the bones of good intentions."* The Conscious Aware Self usually wants us to heal and overcome our illness. However, remember that it also played a significant role in initiating our illnesses. Fully trusting the Conscious Aware Self to do everything needed to heal us can and may be foolhardy.

The same is true of the Subconscious Aware Self. It also played a role in our becoming ill. To heal ourselves, we must create a plan where we have both the capacity to heal ourselves and the ability to enlist the help of others who can help us heal ourselves. People who can and will support our healing process and help us monitor our return to wellness and optimal health and well-being. This is often the role of the "healer." Good intentions and desire to heal are not enough. We must create a workable plan. It must ensure that we easily move past simply having "good intentions" to exercising our utmost "desire" to heal ourselves and accept that we will need to be ready to do anything and everything we must do to make our journey into healing a full and complete reality.

The truth is that you can only start at the level of your Conscious Aware Self. It is important that you empower your Conscious Aware Self by letting it know that you are serious. To accomplish optimal healing, you will need to determine what your true intentions are toward healing yourself. If you are not able to do this on your own, then you may need to seeking out the best help possible to accomplish your goals.

Creating A Wellness Mentality

Once you decide that you truly want to heal, you must create a plan for healing and set specific goals to accomplish it. For example, if you are "always" catching colds or get the flu each winter, you must truly desire not to catch a cold or get the flu this year. You must first intend to remain well, in spite of the time of the year, weather, or germs. It should make no difference what is "going around" or not going around. This is called, "believing in wellness." The first step for creating a "wellness mentality" is to believe more in wellness than in illness and to understand and believe that wellness will always win out over illness. Finally, recognize that the only way illness can win over you is if you give it any amount of power over you. When you operate from a "wellness mentality," you take all of the power away from illness and you give it to your own continuing and ongoing, forever, wellness.

In order to maintain a healthy wellness mentality, you must first recognize that illness is a lie. Now that you know the real causes of illness, and you know that your body has layer upon layer of both Offensive and Defensive, Healing, Repair, and Maintenance Systems protecting you, you now can begin to think differently and to recognize that you have all the power you need on your side to create and maintain perfect health and wellness. It is your acceptance of illness and your welcoming illness into your life that will ultimately bring illness to you. When you expect it to happen, you are actually giving it power over you and at the same time instructing your Body-Mind to accept illness and its power over you. Any form of belief in illness undermines all later efforts for your body to work toward protecting you. Any belief in illness, no matter how small, can and will end up sabotaging you and all of your Offensive and Defensive, Healing, Repair and Maintenance Systems. Any belief in illness, again no matter how small, can and will, directly or indirectly, act to give permission to allow illness to enter and take hold of your body. To stop and reverse this process requires that you change your way of thinking from accepting illness to rejecting its very existence. This is the best and most productive way for you to protect yourself, and your overall health and well-being.

Simply pledging to yourself, "I will not get sick." or "I will not give any power to illness," is not enough. You must live wellness. Remember once again that most illnesses, especially Stress-Related Disorders, are Intelligent communications from your Body-Mind to you requesting that you make necessary changes in your beliefs, actions, diet, environment, or lifestyle that your Body-Mind believes are necessary to solve one or more unresolved conflicts. If you listen to what your Body-Mind and your body have to tell you, and acknowledge that the signs and symptoms you are experiencing are Intelligent communications to you, then you can start reading your body and finding out what you have to do to finally heal yourself. Again, always remember that your most natural state of being, in life, is to be fully and completely well. Illness is an unnatural state of being and not the norm. Wellness is our most normal state of being.

Do not give even a moment's thought to future or potential illnesses, except only by doing what is needed to prevent them from occurring. If you think about illnesses, you empower them. When you do, you give some or all of your healing power away, and when you do this, you will in turn be repaid with illness, pain, suffering, and possibly substantial risk to your life and overall well-being.

Always see yourself being perfectly healthy and being your highest, healthiest, and best Self. Always be willing to learn, grow, and evolve.

4. Create And Act On a Personal Plan For Health And Wellness

In this section, we discuss creating a personal plan for health and wellness. You will also learn how you can use this plan to solve problems, think positive thoughts, work on self-love, and find and become your highest, healthiest, and best Self.

Once you complete your wellness plan, you must put it into action. You will learn how to begin your wellness process through solving problems, resolving conflicts, and correcting lies. Taking action on your plan is easy if you believe in it and your ultimate success will be using it and creating healing. By giving wellness your complete attention, you clear out all past lies and conflicts that are sabotaging you. By using this plan, you will also work toward creating a positive, healthy self-image and generate a positive attitude toward wellness.

As we have repeatedly stated above, wellness and good health are natural states of being. To maintain this process here are six tips you can use when you need them:

1. Always believe that wellness is your natural right.
2. Always live a healthy and productive life.
3. Never unnecessarily expend more energy than you need to create

and support your good health.

4. Always live in harmony with your Body-Mind, your body and your Higher Self.
5. Always resolve conflicts which block you and do not ensure that you can live a happy, healthy and productive life.
6. Always listen to your body and your Body-Mind when they talks to you.

We repeat these constructs over and over again because they are crucial for you to keep in mind on a daily basis. Bad habits (such as believing that illness might exist) often die hard. In the early stages of your healing process, you will need to be ever vigilant not to fall back into old bad habits or sabotage yourself through hidden blocks and obstructions from your past.

There are three steps needed to start your Personal Wellness Plan. These three steps ensure that your Personal Wellness Plan is most effective for you.

Step 1: Create a clear picture of your signs and symptoms (illness) so you can better understand what they have been trying to communicate to you.

In order to help you establish a clear picture of your illness, the following exercise may help:

1. Write out a history of your illness process.
2. List all of the physical, mental, emotional and spiritual signs and symptoms you are experiencing in the order they initially occurred, if possible.
3. When did each sign or symptom start? (Chronology is important.)
4. How has each affected you? Describe all effects, sensations, or changes in your body that you felt or experienced.
5. Describe what was happening around you in your life when each of these signs or symptoms occurred. List them as you remember them: include the events, people, and places that were involved.
6. Next, list where in or on your body these signs or symptoms occurred. List which side of your body and how you were affected by them.
7. List all of the signs of the diagnosed illness you experienced.
8. List all of the physical, mental, emotional, and spiritual changes you felt or experienced, whether related or unrelated to the signs, symptoms, or illnesses you experienced during this same time period.
9. Repeat this process for as many past illnesses as you remember up to and including the current illness.
10. Seek competent medical attention if and when you need it.

What you just accomplished above is writing out your detailed medical history, as well as a list of your present and past illnesses. This can help you better understand not only what is happening but how to approach healing yourself and solving your unresolved conflicts.

Why It Is Necessary To Seek Medical Attention

The reason you want to seek competent physicians or alternative medical attention available to you at this point is that you want a physician to define your specific illness(es), make an accurate diagnosis, and provide you with the best medical support team, if you should need medical help, to solve your problems and treat your illness. The physician's role should be that of an advisor to you for all things medical. Your goal is to use all of your advisors to learn as much as is possible about your condition, so that they can assist you in managing your education, find the right diagnosis, treatment options, and surgery if necessary.

Remember that your goal is healing yourself. However, you may need medical help to do this. Not looking for and finding the best-qualified, competent physician possible, before you need them, leaves you vulnerable to having to take a less-qualified physician when and if your illness should become life-threatening. Remember, as you begin your healing process, your unresolved conflicts will do anything they can to survive, even try to kill you. Finding optimal help before it reaches this point is in your absolute best interest.

In addition, remember that while you are within the Dis-Stress to Dis-Ease Stages, finding knowledgeable and competent physicians who are not invested with an illness mentality may be difficult. Therefore, finding the right physician for your needs when you are still reasonably well can be to your greatest advantage.

If you show no physical signs or symptoms consistent with a defined disease pattern or illness syndrome and if all laboratory and diagnostic tests are normal, this is a good sign that you have not yet reached the Disease Stage. In this case, your life and well-being are probably not in any immediate risk and it is likely that what is happening to you can be 100 percent reversed.

If your diagnosis indicates that you do have a defined disease process, then generally we recommend following your doctor's instructions and prescribed medications or other treatments. Whether surgery is needed depends entirely on whether or not your physician feels you are in immediate danger. Simply believing that it is the only treatment available is not necessarily a good reason to have surgery unless your life is threatened. If your life is not immediately threatened, ask your doctor why surgery is needed, and whether or not you will have time to consider alternative treatments. If the answer is "yes," read on. If the answer is "No," ask "why not

Research Your Illness And Conflict

After completing the steps described above, you should now have competent medical support and a medical history that allows you to better understand what is happening to you. This next step moves you closer to doing what you need to heal yourself, as well as recognizing and resolving unresolved conflicts that are driving your Stress-Related Disorder.

1. Do whatever research you may feel is necessary to best understand your unresolved conflicts, the signs and symptoms or illnesses or disease processes you are experiencing. Initially, your interest should be general and directed at developing information about what is going on and how to heal it. This book will be an excellent resource for initiating your healing process.
2. Be diligent and know as much as is possible about what you are dealing with so that you fully understand what is happening and can best support your healing process.
3. Use books, the Internet, physicians, and other healers to obtain all the information you need to heal yourself.
4. Remember that you must always base your Personal Wellness Plan on facts. When appropriate, use intuition and instinct that are supported by the facts you know about yourself, your medical history, and the diagnosed conditions. You must never base your ability to heal on untested or unclear emotions, fear, wild or untested guesses, or misunderstandings. Listen to others, as well as your own inner knowing, but trust only that which makes sense from what you know about yourself, and your signs and symptoms. In the end, your final Personal Wellness Plan must be designed to accomplish your healing needs. It should not be based on making anyone happy except yourself, or to avoid any medical treatment that is in your best interest.
5. Become a lay expert. Understand as much as possible about the commonly assigned causes for your diagnosed condition. Learn how this condition or disease normally acts in time, its symptoms, signs, complications, and various treatments. Discover what can or will happen when it is not treated or treated correctly. Be aware of and understand the most appropriate treatments, their risks and benefits, and your treatment and non-treatment options.

Become An Expert In Yourself

1. Look carefully at yourself and begin improving your lifestyle. This should begin immediately, but will continue on a daily basis during the entire period you are healing yourself. It should continue afterwards as well to maintain the healing

and ensure optimal health and positive well-being.

2. Improve your diet. Eat only healthy foods, well-cooked meats, and whole grains. Avoid empty calories, such as are found in junk foods and candy. You can have sweets on occasion, but it should not be a regular part of your diet. Avoid sugary or diet soft drinks on a regular basis. Reduce coffee and highly caffeinated teas or drinks, to a minimum. Drink more water.

3. Stop smoking, chewing, or using tobacco products.

4. Reduce or eliminate alcohol. An occasional beer or a glass of wine is okay, provided you are not an alcoholic.

5. Use seat belts in your car, and use a competently designed crash helmet if you ride a motor cycle.

6. Improve home safety. Make your home safe for yourself, your children, family, and friends. Check fire alarms regularly. If you are at risk for carbon monoxide poisonings, make sure you have a qualified carbon dioxide sensor and alarm system.

7. Look at your job, relationships, and family.

8. Determine whether there are unresolved conflicts, small or large, that might exist between yourself and others; if so, who, why, and what might be required for their resolution? Determine whether there are unresolved conflicts, small or large, that might exist between yourself and others; if so, who, why, and what might be required for their resolution?

9. Ask and determine if you are giving your best to those you love and those who love you and require your support. If not, why not?

10. Are you receiving and accepting all of the love and support offered to you by friends, family and loved ones?

11. Do your main relationships enliven you? Do they promote your best interest? Do they promote and support your health and well-being?

12. Look at your connection with the Intelligent Universe:
    a) Are you involved in your chosen religion? Is your involvement appropriate, excessive, or too little?
    b) If you have no chosen religion, then you may want to do one of two things:
        i) Open yourself to finding a religious or spiritual view in which you can believe and be comfortable.
        ii) If you do not belong to an already existing religion or have a strong spiritual viewpoint, can create your own. What you ultimately believe requires only two important qualities to protect and increase your overall health and well-being:

c) It should not cause, lead to, or profess harm to any human or animal, and It should not cause, lead to, or profess harm to any human or animal, and

    i) It must ultimately promote your personal well-being, as well as the well-being of all humans and life on Earth and elsewhere in the Universe. To create a spiritual view that professes or causes hurt or harm to any other living being ultimately undermines all support for your well-being and health, and sabo tages your ability find and evolve yourself to your highest, healthiest, and best Self.

    ii) Another important point that is often overlooked and frequently hard to accomplish is to think only positive thoughts and say only positive words.

    iii) Lastly, forgive yourself and anyone who has or will harm you. Forgive them fully, even before they can cause you or your family any harm. Holding hurt, vengeance, or anger is one of the most potent conflicts. It is therefore one of the most common causes of illness and disease.

13. Create healthy reasons for living.

a) Set up a series of life goals and the steps needed to reach these goals. Set up goals for tomorrow, next week, next month, next year, and so on. These goals should be clearly defined and stated, yet flexible enough so that they allow for the constant changes for which our Universe is so famous. Base these goals on opportunity, not rigidity. As with your spiritual viewpoint, design them to cause no harm to you or to any others.

b) Find a career, hobby, or both that excites and stimulates you. This allows you to get up every day of your life, looking forward to the day and the rest of your life. While this is not always easy, it is possible to attain if you work on this goal on a steady daily basis.

c) Get involved in giving to others. This can be through your work, charity, or your personal way of living. We suggest, "Perform random acts of kindness on a daily basis." Giving stimulates wellness and physical, mental, emotional, and spiritual well-being.

d) Make your life worth living as best as you can, as often as you can.

Step 2: More on preparing yourself to create the best possible personal wellness plan.

Once your fact-finding is complete, you are ready to start creating your Personal Wellness Plan. However, before you go any further, make sure that you understand the rules that normally operate to ensure healing. Following these common sense rules can help ensure that your Personal Wellness Plan has been created considering everything necessary so that there are as few loopholes and blocks as possible to undermine or sabotage you.

Use the following rules to help you build and support your personal wellness plan:

1. You must insure that whatever you do, or are going to do, will not create injury, or harm to you or anyone else.
2, Your Personal Wellness Plan should prevent future problems by not creating any new problems now.
3. Your plan must work toward solving all, or at least as many problems as is possible, as well as create an openness into looking for problems you might not yet recognize, whether hidden or not.
4. Your plan must allow you to evaluate your results as you proceed. If along the way, any problem or conflict is not completely resolved, your plan must allow you to re-evaluate of your Personal Wellness Plan at that point. It must also allow for change when you need changes to accomplish some or all, of your goal. It must allow you to make new and even completely different effective changes so that you can do what needs to be done in order to fully and completely heal yourself.
5. You must be ready to move forward, invoke, and update your Personal Wellness Plan repeatedly until all problems are resolved.
6. Your Personal Wellness Plan should allow you to use one or more of the following to support your efforts and help implement and use your Personal Wellness Plan.

    1) **Introspection**: You should be able to look at your symptoms, their time of onset, pattern, timing, areas of involvement, the organs involved, and how and why they might be trying to communicate to you regarding unresolved problems or conflicts. Follow how these symptoms and signs respond to your plan and the changes you make. Do your symptoms and signs get better or worse, as they change and how is their message changing?

    2) **Communication**: Work with a good therapist on known problems or unresolved conflicts to both understand and resolve them. Determine how they had originally occurred and whether they were caused by your illness. Learn how to communicate with others. The better you communicate with

others, the more effective your communications with yourself, your Body-Mind and your Higher Self will also be.

OR

1) **Take Positive Action**: Work with a healer or physician who can help you solve problems and clear up your lifestyle issues. Inaction, procrastination, hesitancy, and suppressing feelings can play a significant role in creating your illness and slowing down or even blocking your healing process. Taking positive actions will help you greatly to accomplish your healing.

2) **Use Prayer or Meditation**: Using meditation and prayer can help you make contact with your unresolved conflicts and your Higher Self. Your Body-Mind will only "speak" with you when it believes that you are open and actually listening to what it has to say. It will communicate with your Higher Self, and your Higher Self will communicate with you when you meditate and when you are relaxed and open. Your Higher Self and your Body-Mind can be extremely helpful in identifying and resolving conflicts and problems.

3) **Practice Deep Relaxation, Breathing Exercises, & Hobbies**: Your Body-Mind and your Higher Self are more likely to communicate with you when you are relaxed, open, positive and enjoying yourself. These conditions are more likely to occur when you have reduced all stress and released all tension from your body. Doing things you enjoy, such as hobbies, can open the pathways between your Body-Mind and your Higher Self so that they can communicate to you what you need to know and in doing so help facilitate your healing process, reverse illnesses and also prevent potential future illnesses.

7. Get in touch with life and living.
   1) It is important for your ability to heal yourself that you make a clear and decisive decision to live, to live life to its fullest, and create a life worth living. This means creating positive health habits and goals that help you live a positive and healthful life style. Practice this every day.
   2) It is important to actually live fully and to enjoy life. Do this through your daily actions, but supplement it through other means.
      a) Getting in touch with your true nature and your inner Self.
      b) Make lists of everything good in your life, everything that makes your life worth living.
         (i) Create plans and To Do lists of what you can do for yourself with or without others on a daily basis that

will make your life better and more worth living.

ii) There are a number of ways to do this: introspection, journaling, meditation, and prayer are four of the more common ways.

c) In our role of working with many "sick" people through the years, we learned that there are two things that are very important. The first is coming to a place of peace within yourself. The second is coming to peace with the idea of death, your death, and the death of those you love and care about. Everyone dies. Birth is an absolute contract to die. This is an immutable law of the Universe. While it is right to fight to stay alive, it is also right to recognize that death is not the enemy. We all die; hence fighting it will only create stress and stress creates illness. It is important to prepare for your own death by accomplishing everything you need to accomplish in life and also to get everything in your life in order. Also of importance is being ready for and accepting the deaths of parents, siblings, and other loved ones. Frequently, this is not done. When a loved one dies, many people look at the death as if God has betrayed them. The death can and often does cause deep, painful wounds and conflicts. We may feel as if we were sabotaged or intentionally targeted. These conflicts can lead to depression and side track us away from our wellness path, onto a path toward illness or disease and even premature death.

   (i) Some of the more common problems related to unexpected death of a loved one are: guilt, anger, hostility (once again, often directed at God, but also frequently at anyone the individual perceives might have played a role in the death. For example, the spouse of the deceased person may blame the doctor, boss, or others). These negative emotions may even be directed at the deceased because of things he or she did or didn't do, such as not taking medication, drinking too much, etc., even if these factors were not associated with the cause of death. Once again, these negative emotions and conflicts can sabotage everyone involved. The problems they create are often the basis of illness in the mourner.

   (ii) Fear of death along with fear of pain or fear of illness can create a fertile ground for causing even more illness. These negative emotions and the conflicts they create negatively affect the individual's Repair and Healing Systems, hence allowing the creation of new illnesses or the worsening of existing illnesses.

(iii) Whenever we work with someone suffering from a life-threatening or near life-threatening illness, we work with them only when they are willing to give up their claim on life, thus allowing and even accepting death as an inevitable part of life. Once an individual fully accepts that he or she is going to die, then we can begin the work of choosing life and good health over death.

TINA R. A CASE EXAMPLE OF SOLVING PROBLEMS:

In order to fully understand what your Personal Wellness Plan is and how you can use it, let's look at another example. One morning, 62-year-old Tina R. noticed a spot of blood on her sleeping gown. The blood was at the level of her left nipple. Her first instinct was to panic, but she fought it off. At first she was too afraid to call her doctor, so she spent the next few days thinking and talking with various people whom she believed were knowledgeable about breast problems and breast cancer. She learned that blood from a nipple could be a sign of breast cancer. She also learned that it could be from other causes.

Upon seeing her family doctor, a smear was taken from her left nipple. When the smear returned, it was negative for cancer. Her doctor told her that this was a good sign, and suggested that she wait and see if bleeding recurred. Tina was concerned and did not want to wait, so she made an appointment with a surgeon for a second opinion. The surgeon first did a detailed examination of breasts, heart, lungs, and lymph glands. He then ordered a series of tests including a mammography and a breast CT scan. A suspicious area was noted on the CT scans, but no clear diagnosis could be made.

At her next visit to the surgeon, he suggested a biopsy. Tina agreed. The biopsy was performed the next day. Two small cancerous areas were found. The surgeon wanted to admit her to the hospital immediately and perform a mastectomy.

Tina, while scared, wanted to know what her options were. She refused immediate surgery and set up an appointment with an oncologist to discuss what type of cancer she might have and how it might act. She learned from the oncologist that she had a very slow-growing type of breast cancer. She also found that the type cancer she had was rarely discovered at such an early stage. She then learned that one of the lesions was extremely close to the biopsy sample's margin.

The oncologist informed her that she now had three choices. One, undergo another wider biopsy, essentially a lumpectomy. Two, do nothing right now and wait to see what happens. Three, have a mastectomy. Tina thought long and hard about her options. She talked with her husband and several friends and finally decided to have a mastectomy.

When we asked her why, she explained, "I knew immediately I didn't want to wait any longer, but I was not sure whether I wanted to just do another wider biopsy or go for a complete mastectomy. After a while, I realized that I was going to have to be deal with the cancer, one way or another." She continued, "Most likely surgery was going to have to be done either way. What if I had another biopsy and it was positive? I might still have to have a mastectomy, but if I had the mastectomy right now, it would all be over, and done. I elected to have the mastectomy because I wanted to get on with my life. The more I thought about it, the more I realized that my breast was much less important to me then having a long and healthy life."

Use Everything In Your Power To Heal

It is common for people suffering from Stress-Related Disorders to want immediate relief. Unfortunately, by not recognizing the causes of their symptoms, they are not always willing or able to do everything that is necessary to regain their health and well-being. They may try at least to give the appearance of diligently solving problems, clearing up old lies and guilt, or resolving conflicts that need to be completed, but they may consciously or unconsciously have drawn the line at doing some things, hence limiting what they can and should do to recreate their wellness and optimal health.

They may be unwilling to change their diet, create, and maintain a regular exercise program. They may not make important changes to further improve their life, find professional, skilled help, or choose a career that enlivens them. They may resist finding or creating a hobby that supports them. They may resist getting a new job or leaving an unhealthy relationship. By resisting or being unable or unwilling to solve important problems or making important life changes, they may block their full and complete healing, ultimately preventing them from reaching for and finding their highest, healthiest, and best Self. Subconscious fears, such as fear of being successful or fear of what life would look like if they were to fully heal themselves, can and often do hold them back and undermine them.

One of the most common reasons people fail to heal themselves is because they do not truly believe they have the power to do so. They often surrender their power to a medical doctor or to an alternative practitioner, making the doctor or alternative practitioner responsible for them and for healing them. Since these individuals don't believe that they can heal themselves, they may not do everything they can to bring about their healing. They may actually create significant limitations, blocks, and obstacles that may ultimately impair their ability to heal and return to their natural state of wellness.

The most important ally we have for creating healing and wellness is our

Body-Mind. It is well within our ability to program and reprogram our Body-Mind through what we believe, and the instructions we give it, so that it can lead us back toward the path of health and wellness. It is vitally important to us that we enlist its help and power in assisting us to do everything we need and must do to create optimal wellness. We must create a clear and precise image of what our life will look like as a healthy person. To do this, we must believe in this process and in ourselves (all three Selves), and our ability to heal. If you don't already have a clear picture or believe that you can't develop a clear picture, it may be helpful to work with a healer who can help you solve problems and teach you how to create a clear picture of your future healthy life. This healer may be a physician or non-physician healer, but they must believe, as we do, that wellness is your natural state of being. They must believe and help you understand that you can return to your natural state of wellness simply by guiding you to resolve all of your unresolved conflicts that have undermined you in the past.

Never allow anyone to sabotage you. Do not work with anyone who is not clearly part of your healing process. Do not work with anyone who gives power to illness or acts to take your power away from you. This includes medical doctors, alternative healers or any other health care professionals who only believe in treatment, do not believe in cures, or do not believe in their ability to help you or in your ability to heal yourself. Do not work with anyone who does not believe in your ability to return to full and complete wellness.

Many medical doctors believe only in treatment with drugs and surgery. This does not necessarily make them bad people. They may believe that all that is available to them, and hence to you, are drugs and surgical treatments. They may not be aware that there is more available to both of you.

Many doctors are unwilling to help their patients other than with drugs and surgery. Many do not recognize that healing can occur, or that their patients can heal themselves.

These doctors are not healers; they are simply technicians. While they may be good or even excellent technicians, they will most likely not be supportive of your needs and abilities to heal yourself. On the other hand, if you need surgery or interventive medical treatment and you cannot find a skilled healer to help you, these physicians may be excellent choices to perform the technical work of treatment or surgery that you may need right now in this moment to save or protect your life and well-being.

Whether a physician is a good technician, or even a good physician, whether or not they can best treat your symptoms or remove body parts that are diseased – if you are presently working with such a medical doctor, you do not necessarily have to leave their care. You may want to find a more caring, loving, and sup-portive healer who can help you find the causes of your problems and return you to your natural state of wellness. Your Western interventive physician adds whatever skills or experience they may have to assist you and help you by

providing those services that you might need to help you and your healing process progress.

A Personal Example – One of Our Own:

Several years ago, Lisa, began having increased cramping, irregular bleeding and spotting between her menstrual periods. I suggested she see a local
obstetrician-gynecologist for a pap smear and a pelvic examination. A small
fibroid tumor was found during the examination. The doctor I had referred her to
was quite competent, but he did not believe in healing. After his examination and
a pelvic ultrasound verified the presence the fibroid tumor, he told Lisa that she
had five choices: 1) she could have a Dilatation and Curettage (D&C) to control
the bleeding; 2) he could give her medication to "try" to shrink the fibroid tumor,
but warned her that this medication could cause depression; 3) she could have
the fibroid removed or have a hysterectomy removing her uterus, or 4) she could
get pregnant and the fibroid tumors might "go away during the pregnancy." 5) Or
she could wait another month and see if the bleeding stops.

Because of my background as an OB-GYN physician, I knew that what he
told her was both reasonable and appropriate from the standard medical point
of view. However, knowing Lisa and Body Symptom Language™, I also knew that
there was something else going on, and so did Lisa.

Instead of choosing any of the standard OB-GYN choices, we decided to do
something different. We decided to perform a technique that we often use with
our patients, Body Dialogging™. We will speak more about this concept and what
happened to Lisa in the next chapter.

Accept Responsibility For Your New Health And
Correct All Associated Areas To Support It

In order to maintain good health, we must be willing to accept responsibility for our past problems, and take full responsibility for our present and
future well-being. This means not only allowing healing to take place, but also
maintaining it and making it a life-long process. This is best accomplished by
constantly making good, healthy choices and by making wellness a priority.
It is essential to keep a constant vigil against all the forces that would try to take
wellness away from you. Telling the truth to yourself and others is essential, for
as soon as we start lying, we start creating conflict, and this conflict impairs or
even blocks our healing process.

I, Allen, created such a problem for myself. While I wanted to enjoy good
health and protect myself from illnesses, I was not willing to always eat a
healthy diet, exercise regularly, or work at what I knew was best for me.
Fortunately, I was able to start letting go, working at, and eliminating many of
the faulty belief systems that held me back. I eventually recognized that healing
is a life process. It is not always easy for us to give up all our fears and faulty
belief systems instantly.

Once I recognized this, I began working on those fears that , in the past, I had allowed to have power over me. Those which I was not able to release I accepted and stopped fighting. There is a fine line between allowing growth to happen and trying hard to force it. I found that when my intentions came from a natural desire to heal myself, it was much easier to resolve conflicts than when I tried to force myself to deal with my conflicts. We must always allow the healthy part of us to keep some pressure on us to grow, improve, and enlighten our lives. We should never try to force it, especially, when we are not yet ready.

We have stated that to acquire and "own" complete health and well-being, each of us must do everything in our power to make it happen and support it. This means if we have lost our good health, we must find out what we need to know and work to re-acquire what was lost. We must find the right path to reduce our stresses, see the beauty in our life, educate ourselves, and work diligently to return to good health and support ourselves in maintaining it once we have re-acquired it. If we only work on the obvious and most problematic parts of our life, we may ignore other important needs without realizing it. We may then find that we have created gaps and problems which most likely will have to be dealt with sometime in the future.

Develop A System Of Intuition And Insight.

Along with taking responsibility and improving all areas of our current lives, we must also prevent future problems. It is easy to fall victim to people and situations that can take our well-being away. It is also very easy to subvert our well-being on our own. We do this in ways that are often so subtle that we might not even realize that it is happening. It can start innocently with small, meaningless lies. For example, not eating healthy foods or giving away power or decision making ability over yourself, to your family or to others. This may slowly grow in time until we are entangled in a web of lies, deceits and faulty belief systems that can push or pull us into harm's way.

To prevent this, we must learn to come from our enlightened and healed Selves. We must also create tools and develop our intuition and insight in order to protect us. In order to help ourselves, we must learn how to recognize when we have created problems and how to identify them as early as possible. One time or another in our life, each of us has experienced at the "feeling" that we shouldn't be doing something or that someone we are dealing with is not trustworthy. When we act appropriately, we must learn from what we shouldn't have done and how not to do it again. These are what we mean by intuition and insight. We may not always have paid attention to these insights and intuitions in the past. We must learn to tune into ourselves and into our primary defense mechanism to learn how to protect ourselves all the time. By acting on signals from our protective senses, we can then protect ourselves and carefully guard what we know is right for us.

Develop Your Spiritual Self And Become Aware
Of The Intelligence Of The Universe

A natural extension of the healing and growth processes is enlightenment. The word "enlightenment" has two meanings. One definition is entering into the "light" or truth that is, shedding "light" on who we are and our own existence, even in the process of life itself. It also has a second meaning, to "lighten up," to take things much easier, to not be so hard on ourselves, others, and life itself. When we become enlightened, we grow more knowledgeable about ourselves and the world around us. Light is shed on what we need to know and how to use it. By doing this, we become less stressed and less conflicted. We then "lighten up." This process allows us to function better and to increase our ability to survive on the physical, mental, emotional and spiritual levels.

As we gain spiritual enlightenment, we accept more of the truth of our lives. We recognize that we are the embodiment of the Intelligence of the Universe and that our growth and evolution is what is most important to us and even to the world around us. We better recognize our limitations and faults, we better understand how our actions affect us and others around us. We better understand ourselves as being human and at the same time unique and part of the Intelligence of the Universe.

Many people believe that God controls our destiny. We believe that God (or the Intelligence of the Universe) gave us free choice to evolve in any way we choose. However, certain choices take us closer to the Intelligence of the Universe (God) and to who we really are while others take us farther away from one or the other or both. The choices we make either guide us toward our highest, healthiest, and best Self or away from it.

To move toward God and our highest, healthiest, and best Self, the choices we make must never cause intentional hurt or injury, either to ourselves or to others. If we do cause intentional hurt or harm, we are sabotaging our own healing process. When we make healthy decisions, we are guided and chosen. When we reach for our highest, healthiest, and best Self, we not only evolve ourselves, but also further evolve the Universe in a direction that heals and strengthens it. This enlightens it and all beings within it.

Upon joining with the Intelligence of the Universe, we begin seeing life as part of an ending and undying process, one that continues in an endless chain of life, death, and rebirth. Each generation passes its wisdom on to the next. This may happen slowly over hundreds or thousands of years or it can occur in leaps and bounds within generations. We all affect this process by what we think and do, and who we are. When we change, we change not only ourselves, but also everyone and everything around us. We change our spouses, children, friends, co-workers, and we may even change all of the generations yet to come. Who and what we are, our positive and negative ideas, beliefs, thoughts, and actions, all have an effect on everyone and everything. The sum total of these effects has brought mankind, planet Earth, and all living creatures to where we are today.

It is so easy to believe that each of us or any one person means nothing and that what a single individual does may have little or no real meaning. However, this is not true. Because of the limited ways our sensory and nervous systems work, we are often caught up in faulty belief systems, thinking that we are separate and alone. The truth is that everything we do is important because we decide the ultimate fate of humanity itself. We are all connected. We are all part of the Intelligence of the Universe. This Universe is infinite. It has always been and always will be. It is in no hurry to get anywhere. Time is merely a human perception. For us, just as for the Universe, life is an evolutionary process. We

> **The truth is that everything we do**
> **is important because we decide**
> **the ultimate fate of humanity itself.**
> **We are all connected.**
> **We are all part of**
> **the Intelligence of the Universe.**
> **This Universe is infinite.**

grow, learn, and evolve every day of our lives. As we evolve ourselves, we evolve our species, all life, the planet, and the Universe we live in. When we evolve and become healthier, we become one with our own Intelligence and with the Intelligence of the Universe.

Continually Strive To Find And Become
Your Highest, Healthiest, And Best Self

We can choose to accept the challenge and move toward our highest, healthiest, and best Self. We can choose to cower in fear, or we can do nothing at all and let opportunities pass us. We can evolve or merely become a lesson to others about what not to do. You do not have to go out of your way to evolve. Neither do you have to be a Thomas Jefferson, Thomas Edison, nor an Albert Einstein. You just need to be your highest, healthiest, and best Self. You need only enjoy the things you do and do the things you enjoy. Put your heart and soul into whatever you do. Allow your creativity to emerge. Be true to yourself, and do what gives you the most joy. What could be easier?

It is important to remember that what you are today may not be the true you, especially if who you are today makes you sick. What you do for a living may have been chosen from what was available or necessary at some other time. What you do tomorrow is what is important. If you like what you do, that's great. If you hate what you do, continuing to do it is being dishonest to yourself. To find your highest, healthiest, and best Self, you may need to extend and expand yourself. Find what you love to do with your time and energy. Being your highest, healthiest, and best Self does not entirely have to be related to your job, as long as your job doesn't diminish you. It can be your hobby, your volunteer work, an art form, an area of study and interest, or how you relate to people. The list is endless. What is important is that you find what allows you to be the best person you can be. Your talents and abilities are yours alone, but they become higher and greater when you share them with others.

While many people spend their entire lifetime searching for their "right" place in life, others find it even during childhood. Our highest, healthiest, and best Self is always that part of us that loves what it is doing. It is that part of us that grows from what it does, and so makes the world and the Universe we live in a much better place for all.

Truth

If illness is based on the lies and faulty belief systems we integrated into the Body-Mind, and if healing is based on our creating solutions to our problems and unresolved conflicts, where does truth enter into the formula?

The recognition of a lie or problem alone is not enough to attain healing. To create healing, you must go one step further and transform those lies in a way that both undoes them and resolves the problems they created. If you simply substitute one lie or set of problems for another, resolution will not occur.

You must find solutions that create truth. Truth is that solution that most fulfills the person's authentic needs. Truth gives you what you really need, not what you or others think you need and not simply what society or others tell you that you need. Truth produces positive reality and healing, which lead to our highest, healthiest, and best Self. Finding our own individual truths is the single most important action we can take to make our lives whole and healthy.

In the example regarding Cindy W., she was able to free herself, not simply because she recognized that she accepted her father's faulty belief system about "a woman's place," but that she recognized that this was a lie.

Even better for Cindy, she was then able to release the empowerment of her father's faulty belief systems and replace them with her own, newer and truer for her, set of beliefs. These newer and healthier beliefs, *"I can do anything I want to do. All I have to do is set my mind to it and do it,"* changed her life. She acknowledged that she had accepted and unwittingly adopted her father's faulty belief systems without checking what she herself really believed. She recognized and did something about reversing the power she gave to these faulty (for her) belief systems to work against her. She realized that she had operated from them without thinking about what was really right for her. She recognized that, not only did they not work for her, but that in doing what she did, she had made herself ill. This was now a clear indication that what she had been doing was wrong for her. Now, in order to heal, she replaced these faulty belief systems with newer, healthier, and truthful (once again for her) belief systems.

This allowed her to solve some of the most important problems blocking her ability to live her life in the healthiest way possible. Her new, more realistic belief systems represented her personal truths. Using her new life views enabled Cindy to create a higher state of health and well-being.

THE STORY OF NORMAN L.
ANOTHER ILLUSTRATION OF HOW ILLNESS IS CREATED:

Norman started film school while in his late thirties. During his early twenties, he spent two years in college, but then quit because he didn't like studying and hated being told what to do. For the next ten years, he worked from job to job. He rarely stayed at any job for more than a year, and sometimes for only a few months. His passion was movies. No matter what job he did, the moment he finished working, he would be off to the movies. As time passed, he began thinking about creating movies. He soon believed that if he tried, he could create great movies. His only problem was his poor track record at everything he did.

Norman's parents constantly chided him for his lack of drive and inability to hold a job. They criticized him for "living in a fantasy world." They believed that going to the movies so frequently was his way of hiding from the real world. They could not understand his fascination with movies and repeatedly told him that it was childish to always be thinking and talking about movies. They scolded and also repeatedly told that he should, "Get a stable job, find a nice woman, settle down, and have children."

One weekend just before his thirty-fourth birthday, he made a decision to go to film school. He signed up at a local state college and took a communications course. He did extremely well. As soon as he had all the prerequisites, he applied to one of the best film schools on the West Coast and was accepted.

Norman turned his passion into opportunity. His fears about "his failures in the work world" were soon turned into life experiences upon which he could draw in making his movies. His eagerness to talk and live in the world of movies created many new friends and contacts. One of these contacts was later instrumental in getting him his first directing job.

During the next ten years, Norman made eight movies and became a multi-millionaire. He became a very successful director. He found his true calling in life and all because he had taken the opportunity to become his highest, healthiest, and best Self. When it presented itself, he evolved and became highly creative. He also married a wonderful woman, settled down, and had three happy, healthy children. His parents were finally happy. So was Norman.

The ultimate mastery of healing depends on our ability to identify the lies we empowered in the past, and make the decision that we can no longer live by them. We each need to discover our own personal truths. We must remove all negative power from the lies which block us from being who we are meant to be. We must give this power to those healthy truths which move us toward our highest, healthiest, and best Self. While most of the lies we live with are extremely elusive and exist deep within us, many are superficial and easy to see and eliminate. Often, many of the most damaging lies are not thought of as lies, but rather as "facts of life" or "the way things are." They often come from our childhood or inaccurate conclusions we made through the years. They are judgmental and frequently the reason for our separation from others ourselves, and who we really are.

The significant people in our lives may see these faulty belief systems; we ourselves often cannot see them in operation. On the other hand, sometimes we are actually aware of the faulty belief systems of our friends and family members, including our spouses. These faulty belief systems are constantly with us. They act as filters through which we see our world. They are often the things that we think about for a good portion of the day and maybe even what we dream about at night. They are our fears, blocks, limitations, and our prejudices. They are the beliefs that siphon the vitality out of our life. When we talk about them to others, they are often preceded by statements such as, "You can't," "I won't," "I can't," "Aren't you afraid of," or "Anyone who." They are generally limiting and restrict of our capacity to reach for and find our highest, healthiest, and best Self.

These lies invade our lives and take the joy from us. They can also be condescending or pejorative, sexist, racist, or ego-centered. When we listen to people parading their lies in front of us, we usually feel uncomfortable. On occasion, these lies may seem to have an air of truth. Because of the nature of these lies, the people who rely on them may feel the need to hold onto them or to create new lies to preserve their egos' needs. They may even couch them as benefits or goals to achieve.

Consider the white supremacist who entices others to join his cause. He believes his lies, and he couches them in such a way as to make them sound believable and even enticing to others. No matter how colorful and attractive they are created to sound, they are still lies, and just about everyone else in the world knows that they are lies. Alcoholism, smoking, gambling, having affairs, over-spending, getting into debt, spousal abuse, child and sexual abuse, not taking care of health problems, and feeling superior or inferior are just a few of the more conspicuous lies and unhealthy actions people use to cover up their lies.

Some lies are much less obvious than others. For example: fear of success, anxiety about past events, fear of someone telling the truth about something, fear of solving problems, or fear of taking the risks necessary to succeed in life, unwillingness to complete relationships, not having the job we want, or even not being able to consider or decide what we want to do with our lives. The lies that result in illness are also the same belief systems and behaviors that diminish us or keep us from reaching our highest, healthiest, and best Self.

Belief in illness, getting ill to avoid certain situations, not taking care of yourself, and using illegal drugs, often may not be seen as problems but instead circumstances that "just happen," "rebellion," or simply "circumstances beyond our control."

Fear itself can be a lie. If what we fear is not a real threat to our lives or overall well-being, then being afraid is not meaningful–it is a lie. If our fears are not real threats and ultimately lead to illness and disease, they are definitely lies. Fear is only real and meaningful when our lives or overall well-being is threatened. Everything else is illusion. Fear initiates the Stress Mechanism that must eventually have resolution to turn it off. If fear is continuous, the stress reaction becomes continuous and the Stress-Illness Mechanism is triggered. While being fearful in a certain situation may be appropriate, at least until verified, holding onto it and not verifying its reality and not doing what needs doing to eliminate it leads us toward danger and hence constitutes lies.

Truth makes life much easier. It promotes health and supports us in being our authentic and real selves. It is important for you to learn to recognize your lies and correct them. Apologize to those to whom you have lied. Forgive those who lied to you. Build your life around truth, and you will build a strong, meaningful, and healthy life.

In the next section, we will look at blocks and complexes, how they form, how they undermine us and how they ultimately lead to conflict, illness, and finally, disease.

*Stress
should be
a powerful
driving force,
not an obstacle.*

~Bill Phillips

Chapter Sixteen

STRESS — BLOCKS AND COMPLEXES

BLOCKS AND COMPLEXES

Throughout our lives, each of us lives with, experiences, integrates, and rejects many positive and negative experiences. Some hardly affect us at all, while others may traumatize or nearly destroy us. In order to remain sane, rational, and healthy, we must handle these situations in such a way as to minimize their negative effects, and encourage and expand their positive effects.

Healthy people realize that life is filled with threats and dangers of all types, but they also recognize that it is filled with great beauty and love. Healthy people take danger and negativity in stride. They are aware of what they can or cannot handle. The healthy individual creates a series of positive support systems, which he is able to use to support himself. He also takes advantage of all available resources, and his support systems are always ready to go into action as protection for himself and his loved ones (at its most basic level, this is what Fight or Flight is about).

The unhealthy person often reacts differently. He is generally less able to integrate past life experiences. He often neither fully deals with nor learns what he needs to know from his life experiences. He is often less likely to be prepared for the challenges he meets along the way. He is often unrealistic about his goals and circumstances. He is frequently obstructed and limited by these experiences. Because of all this, these unhealthy individuals are usually less prepared to face the rigors of life. For many unhealthy people, life becomes a living nightmare.

Because they do not fully deal with life experiences, they are often filled with fear of further insult or injury. They worry about physical, mental, emotional, or spiritual injury, and about their ability to protect themselves from future negative experiences. All of this worry and stress turns on the Stress Mechanism. Because they are not problem solving, this entire process now leaves them unable to fully use their internal and external resources. They become less capable of counting on the support of others around them. They may be afraid to ask for help. They may not know how to ask for help, or whom they can really trust. Because they have created many faulty belief systems, they learned that when they do not have to face or deal with most of the important issues at hand, they feel better and may be even safer, at least in the short run, avoiding conflict. While this all may be true in the short run, it is a very poor strategy for growing, evolving, and solving problems.

When faced with positive or negative life experiences the Body-mind must experience these events. The Body-Mind must then decide whether what is happening in any moment is meaningful and appropriate for the Conscious Aware Self to know. If what is happening is negative, threatening, or traumatic, the Body-Mind may limit what the Conscious Aware Self is allowed to become aware of and know. This process of information selection is essential, for if it does not happen, the Conscious Aware Self can quickly become bogged down in minutia and over stimulation with which it may not be able to deal, hence reducing its ability to make decisions and survive.

RECOGNITION

The process by which the Body-Mind deals with each event is called "recognition." It must recognize and then incorporate the substance of the event into the life picture. The life pictures are created by the Conscious Aware Self. All new events must fit into both the personal and overall world view.

These processes, our personal view and world view, exist to protect us from surprises and unexpected threats. At the same time, we gain a more meaningful sense of what is around us and the reality in which we live. These are created by the Conscious Aware Self and instruct the Body-Mind what to expect in both the short and long term. An example might be if you see a person coming toward you, your Body-Mind must recognize whether this person is a friend or enemy. If the Body-Mind believes that the person is a friend, it instantly looks at and tries to make meaning of the person's body posture, speed, facial expression, whether they have a weapon in their hand, and whether they appears hostile or friendly. It then uses its deductive logic and it compares what it knows about this person with its current experience and decides whether they present an immediate threat or not.

In this example, the events are happening in the present but all decisions must be made quickly based on information from the past. If certain clues, such as a threatening posture, a weapon, or some kind of threatening movements occur, this might suggest a hostile intention. The Stress Mechanism is immediately activated, even before any further thought or consideration occur (Fight or Flight).

This process works in the same way with events that have occurred in the past or are expected to occur in the future. For instance, a person is involved in an auto collision during which they were injured. In the same accident, their friend, who was a passenger in the car, is killed. Upon awakening, he calls for his friend but is told that the friend was killed in the accident. He may not want to believe this, and the pain of his friend's loss may cause him to totally block events related to the accident. He may experience amnesia in regard to the events surrounding the accident and his friend's death. It may take him weeks or even months before memories return. He may experience guilt about the accident, even if he had absolutely nothing to do with his friend's death. Eventually, he may rationalize what happened. His memory may return and the guilt he experienced may subside, as he is finally able to accept that there is no legitimate reason to blame himself.

When experiences are too traumatic or when they cannot be immediately rationalized, the Body-Mind may suppress the experience altogether. In such cases, the Conscious Aware Self may not have any memory of what happened from just before the accident until sometime after the event. This is not done intentionally by the Conscious Aware Self, but rather by the Body-Mind to protect the Conscious Aware Self. When the Body-Mind believes that the Conscious Aware Self is unable to face issues that are too painful, it often suppresses them.

The Body-Mind may initially do this only to protect the Conscious Aware Self at that the time these events occur. It may also need time to process the experience and fit what happened into the individual's personal life picture, which is held in the Body-Mind for the Conscious Aware Self. It may need time to heal. Since life continually moves on, the Body-Mind may lose track or soon become occupied with other momentary or important experiences. As time goes by, the memories of these events move further and further away from the present and become less important to the Conscious Aware Self. While they are never completely expunged, they may become "past" experiences (memories).

Positive experiences often become "good" memories, while negative experiences usually become "bad" memories. The degree of "good" or "bad" attributed to these memories is decided upon by the Body-Mind based on how threatening these events feel, whether or not the Body-Mind perceives them as positive or negative, whether it judges that they need resolution, and how strongly the Body-Mind desires resolution. When an experience is judged as negative and the Body-Mind believes it requires resolution, this is called a conflicted situation or simply a conflict.

It may be clear that the Body-Mind knows that these suppressed conflicts still exist and that it also knows that they must eventually be resolved and rationalized but it may not in the "now-moment" be ready or willing to take either of these on. It may want to complete the rationalization process. It may want to forget it and make believe it never had happened. Most negative experiences are eventually rationalized, even if it takes many years to do this.

Meanwhile, some part of the Body-Mind, which never forgets anything, still wants resolution. This means that on and off, these unrationalized, negative, "conflicted" memories push up and out into the Conscious Aware Self. This may happen in the form of dreams, nightmares, flashbacks, or emotional outbursts that sneak out before the Body-Mind can suppress them.

The Body-Mind actually does want completion. To accomplish this, the Body-Mind may allow memories of these events to leak out into the Conscious Aware Self to stimulate action. In the best of all worlds, this might work well, but in many people, it represents years of pain dealing with traumatic experiences that are old history.

RATIONALIZATION

The Conscious Aware Self uses a slightly different process to protect itself. This process is referred to as "rationalization." To make sense of the world around us, the Conscious Aware Self must fit events into what it believes life is about, its personal life picture, and its overall world view. For example, if we want to believe that someone is our friend, we consciously look for clues proving their friendship. We may also consciously or subconsciously ignore or avoid suspect information, so that the total of the evidence we accept fits our picture. Hence, if a person whom we believe is our friend says something negative to us or about us, we may rationalize it away. We may tell ourself that he really didn't mean it or that what he said was only meant jokingly.

We do the same thing when we work at a job we hate. We may choose to ignore our feelings. When we do something wrong, we may rationalize it or lie to cover it up so that others will not be angry or dislike us. The difference between what happens in the Body-Mind and Conscious Aware Self is that when it comes from the Body-Mind, we are unaware of the truth. When the Conscious Aware Self rationalizes something as good or bad, we know exactly what we are doing, even if we ignore or disregard the truth. Rationalization is used for both good and bad events. We may not want to believe someone does not like us, so we may consciously interpret everything they do to "prove" that they do like us. We may also decide that someone does not like us, and no matter what that person does, we rationalize that the person really had an ulterior motive and what they are doing in the "now-moment", in the past and in the future proves that they truly dislike us.

If a person is experiencing negative emotions and internal conflicts, it soon becomes important to work toward bringing all of these experiences up into the light and recognizing how we may have rationalized them. We do this so that they can be appropriately rationalized and integrated into our personal life picture and our overall world view. Only by doing this can we release the Stress Mechanism, which in turn releases us from its negative effect so we can live wholly and realistically.

As an example, consider a young girl who has been molested. Fear for her life, or guilt created by the molester, blocks the memory of the actual events. For many years, she may have flashbacks or nightmares. They may be distinct or fragmented, but since she has suppressed the painful events and has no conscious memory of them, they may be misunderstood or seen simply as "some traumatic event." The Body-Mind suppressed them for her protection. As her previously unconscious memories now rise into her conscious awareness, she may at first feel that she needs to deny them, and subsequently rationalize them away in order to prevent feeling the pain that these memories bring back.

Only through working on what actually happened, bringing her traumatic experiences into the open, openly experiencing the pain and rationalizing it appropriately, recognizing that she was not responsible, that she was and is blameless, can she finally be set free. If these experiences are not dealt with or are inappropriately rationalized, this unresolved conflict eventually triggers the Stress Mechanism. Once triggered, the Stress Mechanism must ultimately be shut off. If not, this may eventually lead to physical, mental, emotional, or spiritual illness.

It is important to learn the lessons from these experiences, and gain and grow from them. We must, for health's sake, learn to accept reality, even if or when we do not like it. Then, and only then, can we let go and be free to be our real and true self.

All of these mechanisms are part of the strongest and most important mandate of life – the Survival Mechanism. When negative situations are not resolved, they can begin to act as blocks to our future growth and to realizing the joy of the gift of life. They block us from getting what we want out of life. They lead to illness. When we have one or more blocks linked together, no matter their causes, we call them "complexes."

MORE ABOUT BLOCKS AND COMPLEXES

To best understand the concept of blocks and complexes, we must give you more information. When the Body-Mind, Conscious Aware Self, and the body are well integrated and working together, the result is wellness and good health.

When these three work together to resolve conflicts, you have the best possible situation and the most likelihood of attaining a good solution. However, when these three entities do not work together to resolve conflicts, many problems can be created. Generally, these entities are more likely to create problems when blocks and complexes exist, a situation which undermines their healthy interaction.

Blocks and complexes often arise from faulty interaction between the Conscious Aware Self and Body-Mind. Blocks and complexes are simply devices the person (the combined Conscious Aware Self and Body-Mind) uses for protection when overwhelmed with fear, threat, or conflict.

At first glance, one might believe that these protective devices are always working against us. This is not true. They work for us most of the time. If you touch a hot pot and burn yourself, the memory of this event associated with the pain that was created will work to keep you from making the same mistake again.

Blocks are simply memories that, under normal situations, help us to not repeat the same mistakes. In certain situations, when an individual is in an altered state of consciousness – during sleep, when ill, drugged, under anesthesia, has a head injury, during a traumatic event – the trauma that occurs is confused with the cause and the effect. Rather than being helpful, blocks created by these situations may become a source of anxiety and negative behavior.

Blocks and complexes can also result from positive interactions between the Conscious Aware Self and Body-Mind or others. Take for example a two or three year old poised on the edge of the curb ready to run out into the street to retrieve a ball when his mother yells, "No! Johnny, No! Johnny, stop! Don't you run into the street, or I will spank you!" The child, who may have been spanked before, does not want to be spanked again. Possibly because of his fear of being spanked or possibly because of the urgency, demanding or pleading tone of his mother's voice, Johnny stops and does not run out into street and into on-coming traffic. Clearly, Johnny does not really understand the risk of running out into traffic or into the path of an on-coming car, nor the intricate consequences of being struck by a car; but his mother does. However, the child may well understand the consequences of being spanked. When the mother takes his hand and says, *"Now, Johnny, before you can go into the street to get a ball, you must first look both ways to make sure no cars are coming. Take my hand; let's look both ways. Okay, no cars are coming, now we can get the ball."* Through this series of events, Johnny begins to learn that running into the street without looking both ways and making sure there are no cars coming is unacceptable to his mother and that it should also be unacceptable to him. A positive protective block is created, In the future when the ball goes into the street, he will think twice about just running out after it. This simple action, stopping and looking both ways, might well someday save his life.

WHAT DO BLOCKS AND COMPLEXES REALLY MEAN TO US?

We can easily say that blocks and complexes are simply subconscious belief systems that interpose themselves between the requests and commands of the Conscious Aware Self and the actions of the Body-Mind. While they may be positive or negative, the ones that cause the most problems for us are the negative blocks and complexes. For simplicity's sake, we will refer to these negative blocks and complexes as "faulty belief systems."

They are faulty belief systems because they often end up sabotaging us. They limit our abilities and potentials. They are fears and unresolved conflicts, remembrances of negative experiences, and old hurts. They operate through the Stress Mechanism. While they were created with a very specific intelligent reason for protecting us –and many do operate to protect us – negative blocks and complexes may also act to undermine us and even cause more conflict, pain and suffering.

Blocks and complexes, both positive and negative, often start emerging as soon as the nervous system develops, even while in the womb. They initially occur as external and internal data inputs into the nervous system regarding real or imagined threats. Rather than reading them simply as an "input of information", the Body-Mind may give them power to affect some or all of our future responses to life events.

In a sense, they act as filters. They screen the information we receive over the course of our life. They persist until they are no longer necessary and are either eliminated or replaced. Since the blocks and complexes we are primarily discussing here are negative, they often act to block or interfere with positive information and actions. They can cause us to see the world differently from the way it really is. This can even force us to see the world in a negative or distorted way.

One example of how negative blocks and complexes can distort the world around us is bigotry. Bigotry changes us and how we see the world. In the case of bigotry, the individual may only be capable of seeing though a very limited and distorted belief system regarding other people. It forces the individual to focus on only certain attributes, such as religion, race, or ethnicity. Rather than the bigoted individual seeing others as unique individuals, his bigotry blocks and complexes filter thoughts, beliefs, ideals, and how he reacts to others through his faulty belief systems. The bigot often holds a point of view that all people of a certain color, gender, sexual orientation, race, religion, or age are somehow inferior, bad, dangerous, threatening, stupid, or worthless (to name only a very few ways bigotry may cause people to think or believe). The intelligent person knows that this viewpoint is not true, but the bigot sees nothing else. The bigot's view of the world and others is not just limited, but is controlled and directed by faulty belief systems, bigotry, and the blocks and complexes that have created them.

While the person who is the victim of the bigotry certainly suffers, it is also true that the bigot suffers because he is living in a complex of lies. Because of this, the bigot is often unable to see and experience the real world. This limitation distorts not only his world view but also his self-view. When the faulty belief system is bigotry, we usually don't feel sorry for the bigot. We may instead see the bigot as angry, narrow-minded, evil, or simply as a "bad person."

However, when faulty belief systems lead the bigot to a sense of lowered self-esteem, failure, or fear, the bigot is just a hop, skip, or a jump away from illness. At that point, we may begin to change our point of view and see the bigot as a casualty of life. This may not help the bigot's victims, but it can put his action into perspective regarding the ultimate cost of bigotry and the cost of blocks and complexes that distort and undermine them.

In the end, all blocks and complexes, and the fears and restrictions they create, are simply faulty belief systems accepted at some time or another during our lives, either consciously or unconsciously. Like any other belief system, they can be discarded or replaced at anytime. We see this happening every day of our lives. Someone might say that he hates a particular food until he tries it and decides he likes it. A woman thinks a particular style is awful until she tries it on and finds she loves it. Faulty belief systems exist whenever we hate something, when we are afraid of something, or when we feel threatened by something. Our true view of the world is biased by false information, negativity, or faulty decisions from the past.

Faulty beliefs exist because at some point in our lives, we believed that they presented a threat to us or had some other important meaning that negatively affected us. When they are based on something that threatened us, or when we feel that having it taken away from us renews a prior threat and will cause harm, they automatically trigger the Stress Mechanism, and the situation is given negative power. Whenever power is given to any possible threat, real or imagined, or to any idea, belief, or situation which activates fear or a threat to our existence, a block or complex is created. During this process, we may make decisions or create opinions about these beliefs.

Because we feel threatened and these beliefs may suddenly appear as a way out, we may not only want to believe these faulty belief systems, but may even fight to retain them. We may fear giving them up or losing them because if they are taken away, this might lead to some sort of injury or harm. In order to protect ourself, the Body-Mind may act to give power to these faulty decisions and opinions.

These beliefs continue to be powerful because we continue to give them power. We may even repeatedly re-enforce this power. This usually requires finding or even creating some kind of evidence that "proves" that this belief system is right (or everything else is wrong) and continues deserving the power given it.

The same is often true of emotions. Emotions are simply belief systems that became associated with physical feelings and sensations. The body sets specific chemical reactions and pathways for stimulation when certain types of events occur.

When emotions are triggered, a series of very specific neurochemicals are released. When emotions are triggered, it is because these pathways and the release of specific neurochemicals were triggered. Often the physical response, what we think of as emotion, is immediate. Yet, in the end, emotions are merely blocks and complexes, either positive or negative, depending on the circumstances.

Our job in life is to find as many of these negative blocks and complexes as we can, then rationalize and eliminate them. Then, and only then, can we be safe, sane, whole, and healthy.

BLOCKS AND COMPLEXES AND ELIMINATING STRESS

Whenever we eliminate stress – especially when we also eliminate faulty belief systems, lies, blocks, complexes, guilt, and resentment associated with them – we return our body to its normal state of operations. Since most stressors are not life threatening, one of the best ways available for reducing or eliminating stress is changing faulty belief systems into reality-based pictures that positively support us. This helps us create a realistic positive self-image. When we operate from a realistic picture of who and what we are, we also form more realistic pictures of the world around us. This creates a reality-based world view, and this removes many or all negative influences that trigger stress and lead to illness.

Doing these things can help us set our life up so that it works for us with little or no lies, faulty belief systems, or faulty or unrealistic illusions. Instead of illness and confusion, we can now return to moving forward and finding our highest, healthiest, and best self.

In the next chapter, we look at how to you can find harmony and balance in your life, and how you can restore any lost balance.

*Maturity
is achieved
when a person
accepts life
as full of tension.*

~Joshua L. Liebman

Chapter Seventeen

CREATING WELLNESS
THROUGH HARMONY & BALANCE

WELLNESS IS A STATE OF HARMONY AND BALANCE

In order to understand the concepts of disease and wellness, we must first do away with the myth that disease and good health are enemies of each other. Disease is the condition that occurs when we are "out of ease," out of harmony and balance with our true selves. It is during these times when our Immune, Repair, and Healing Systems, which normally protect us, are most likely to fail. Good health is the state when we are in balance with ourselves and in harmony with the world and Universe. What we call "good health" is really a state of harmony and balance between all of the major aspects in our life.

There are at least six major aspects that make up each of our lives: the physical, personal or self, mental, family, work, and spiritual aspects (See Figure: 17-1).

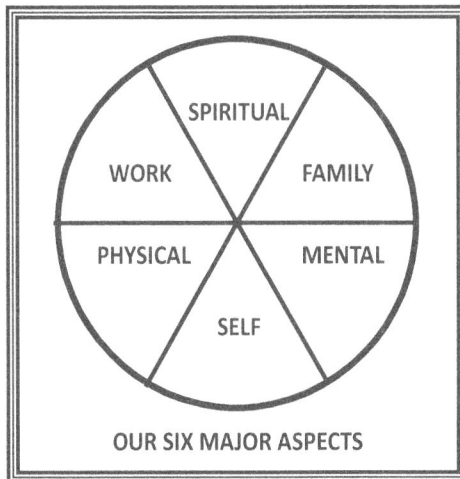

OUR SIX MAJOR ASPECTS

Figure: 17-1

Each of these aspects may involve one or more subcategories, and each touches on and interacts with each of the other aspects in a multiplicity of different ways.

The Physical aspect is composed of how we see and deal with our physical body and its needs–grooming, physical fitness, physical activities, body image, touching and being touched, and so forth. It often overlaps with how we feel about ourselves in relations to others, our work, and even spiritual beliefs.

The Self aspect is a compilation of how we see ourselves in our lives and with the world around us. It includes our self-image, politics, need and ability to self-nurture, all the factors that affect, increase, or decrease our self-esteem, and ability to create self-love. It also includes how we relate to the world around us, our hobbies, how and with whom we play, our skills and interests, how we utilize our work, and how and what we contribute to the world around us.

The Mental aspect relates to what we think, our intellect, what stimulates us, and even our levels of education. Examples are what we think about our self, what we think about the world around us, and how we see others and ourselves in life. It can also interrelate with our emotions, which are a combination of our mental attitudes, physical feelings, and attitudes. We can also have mental pictures and belief systems about most things that affect us, whether real or imagined, positive or negative, during the course of our lives. Mental aspects also overlap with family, work, emotions, self-image, physical states of being, and spiritual aspects. We are who we are because of them.

The Work aspect represents both the jobs we do and the careers into which we enter. When work is a job, it suggests a vocation, something we do to make a living. A career, on the other hand, is a path, a calling in life, not just simply a job, but something that fulfills inner need. Work is also an integral part of becoming your highest, healthiest, and best Self. A career can be all encompassing. It can be the center of our lives, defining who we are; or it can simply be something that we do, or something we use to fulfill an inner physical, mental, emotional, even spiritual aspect of ourselves. It can replace family, as the people at work can become a surrogate family. The same is true of organizations, such as unions, employee, employer, and professional groups.

The Family aspect. Family has many different meanings. It can be related not only to our immediate family and relatives, but also to friends, co-workers, people with whom we play, or whom we need. While our own families may be supportive, our spouses may be soul mates or simply friends. Children are the product of the pro-creative needs of a husband or wife; or their pride and joy, identity, or a vehicle of immortality. Once brought into the world, children can become the focus of the family. It may either bind it together or be perceived as a negative force. Alternatively, the many problems associated with being a parent can split a family apart, leaving one or both partners conflicted on multiple levels. The problems of a single child or of one of the parents can end positively or negatively directing the lives of everyone in the family. A family may work together, or the actions of one or more members can create problems that tear the family apart and dominate all future decisions. The family can also be the basis of a deep, **spiritual** root that steadies and balances its members, as they reach out into the world around them.

Work, career, family, and child rearing are intimately intertwined. To be healthy, one must master these aspects and their many subtleties. When the major aspects of our lives are in balance and harmony with whom and what we are, we generally have good health. However, when one or more of these aspects are out of balance, we have the potential for creating problems, conflicts, and then illness. While initially the stimulation of a conflict may increase the body's defensive response, if left undiscovered, unchecked, or unresolved, imbalances will occur. These imbalances can then operate through the Stress Mechanism causing a reduction in the body's ability to defend, repair, and heal itself, hence leading to illness, specifically Stress-Related Disorders.

WHAT BALANCE LOOKS LIKE

Harmony exists when life is in balance. Balance exists when life is in harmony. Any aspect can change, as long as it is balanced by a corresponding change in another area. While any balance is always precarious, the balanced life in a healthy person has flexibility that allows for periodic upset and disturbance. Unless such disruption is extreme, the balanced person usually finds a new balance point and returns to normal (see Figure: 17-2)

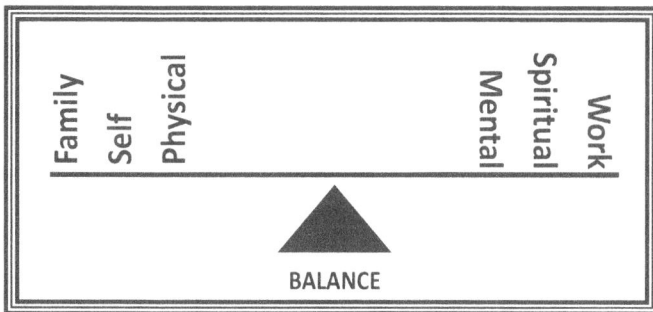

Figure: 17-2

WHAT IMBALANCE LOOKS LIKE

An imbalance occurs when one or more of these major aspects become either excessively or persistently disturbed and the Body-Mind is unable to re-establish a state of normalcy. Lies and faulty belief systems most commonly create imbalances. However, they can also be created by injury, natural disaster, other disease states, or any significant physical, emotional, mental, or spiritual trauma or stress. When an imbalance becomes significant enough to impair the body's ability to cope with outside invaders, then we have, by definition, entered into the Illness-Disease Mechanism. In order for a disease to take hold, not only must the body's Defense, Immune, Repair or Healing Systems be undermined or have failed to some degree, but there must also be some diminished capacity for directing and controlling the healing and repair process. Without a completely competent Defense-Immune-Repair-Healing System, invaders can take hold, grow, and flourish. Disease occurs when the body falls out of balance and is unable to protect itself.

Figure 17-3, below, demonstrates a state of imbalance. In this case, since everything else is unchanged we would interpret this as a temporary imbalance due to the Work aspect of this person's life being excessive. Even though this person has lost balance, all other functions remain stable. When this conflict within the person's work situation is finally resolved, all is likely to return to normal.

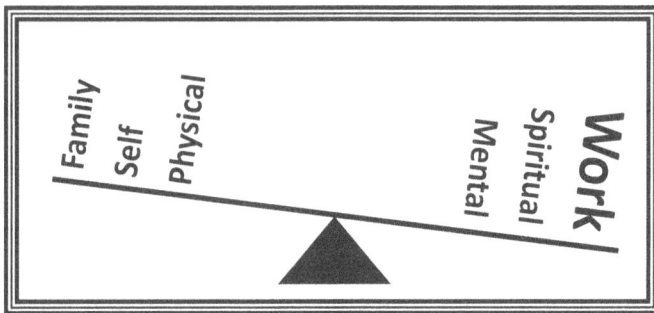

Figure: 17-3

WHAT DISEASE LOOKS LIKE

Figure 17-4 demonstrates what happens when the imbalance in the work situation persists or grows large enough to create a significant negative effect on the Body-Mind.

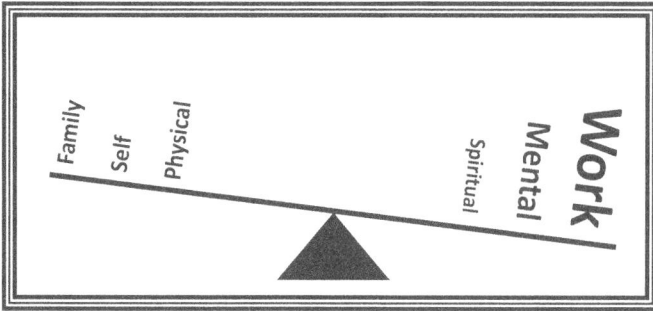

Figure: 17-4

Here, the time and energy expended at work take a significant toll on the person, drawing time and energy from Family, Self, and the individual taking care of their health and body. As the imbalance persists, time and energy are also drawn from the Spiritual aspect. Only the Mental aspect appears to stay in perspective with the Work aspect being greater than what is healthy. This person needs their mental faculties to ensure they function optimally at work. This misalignment of the six major aspects may cause the other aspects to either work harder or lose the time, energy and balance they need. In time, this can eventually lead to further imbalances and even breakdowns within the body, the organ systems, mental issues, emotional outbreaks, a breakdown in time and energy associated with the family, self, physical and spiritual aspects. These imbalances often open us up to illness.

The imbalance we see here may be due to excessive time and energy this person is putting into Work. He may eventually find himself becoming distressed, fatigued, and his resistance to illness might diminish. The Body-Mind is stressed, and this puts a strain on his Physical body. Ultimately, he becomes sick. This might occur in the form of frequent colds or flu, headaches, asthma, allergies, or even bleeding ulcers that may require surgery such as with Peter in one of our earlier case histories.

While we have used an imbalance in an person's Work aspect to demonstrate the results of life imbalances in this example, we could have used any other aspect or combination of aspects since they all act in much the same way as the person's life becomes unbalanced. When one major aspect is pushed or forced out of balance, this imbalance eventually affects one, some, or all of the others aspects. We are all familiar with people who have conflicts with family members, or conflicts about relationships. These conflicts are blamed on "work," or "drinking too much," "working out too much," or some other conflict or imbalance within their life. All that is needed here is for one or more parts or aspects of a person's life to fall or be pushed out of balance and illness is just around the corner.

We all know or have seen people who work too hard, avoid working, stop taking care of themselves, work out too much, smoke or drink too much, hate themselves, are too introverted or antisocial, people who lie or cheat, overspend, or who have become mentally or emotionally unbalanced, or spiritually conflicted. We are aware of women who become bulimic or anorexic, men who eat too much, people who abuse their bodies in one way or another. These are all examples of people who fell out of balance in one or more aspects of their lives.

It should now be apparent that imbalances can and do lead to physical, mental, emotional, and even spiritual stress. We also recognize that all too often, these same individuals eventually end up suffering from physical, mental, emotional or spiritual illness, or disease if they do not deal with their problems and unresolved conflicts.

In summary, to be healthy, we must create a sense of harmony and balance in our lives. If illness exists, it is likely that an imbalance already exists somewhere within one or more of the six major aspects. It should now be obvious that these individuals must resolve these imbalances as part of their process of healing in order to create full and complete wellness and well-being.

THE PROCESS OF HEALING

Healing occurs in many ways. Sometimes, it occurs with the use of traditional or alternative medical treatments, such as medication, surgery, acupuncture, hypnosis, massage, chiropractic treatment, herbal, or nutritional therapies. These treatments are only temporary or secondary methods.

They are given to us without our having to do anything other than take the medication, submit to surgery, or show up for treatments. While the sick person may choose to take advantage of them, they do not actively involve life changes or problem solving. These treatments do not directly change or resolve the conflicts that caused the person's problems or illness. The treatments and procedures may indirectly affect our conflicts.

This is good, especially if it somehow eliminates the conflict or allows our Body-Mind to resolve the conflicts on its own. We often see this happening in medicine, where it is commonly referred to as the Placebo Effect. Too often, the original conflict is merely sidetracked and unchanged. The negative energy persists. With time, the person may move closer toward the stages of Disease, Chronic Disease, and even Death. Our primary healing mechanisms are always ready and available within us. They are built into us for healing any injury or illness to which we are subjected. Medication and surgery can help it, but do not do the exact same job of curing the problem's root cause.

Our healing and repair mechanisms are Intelligent; they "know" what they are supposed to do. We do not have to tell them what needs doing. They learn from their experiences. These healing mechanisms are based on cooperative interaction of their component parts; our Defensive and Offensive Systems, our Maintenance, Repair and Healing Mechanisms; our brain and nervous system and their many neurochemicals and neurohormones; our Endocrine System; our Stress Mechanism and the many other protective and healing systems that have been designed to not only help us get well, but also to keep us well.

They all operate through an Intelligent strategy called "Feedback." This occurs when information regarding bodily responses are relayed back to the source of the each of these healing systems and mechanisms hence controlling the status of the healing process. It lets each system know when to turn on or off, the level of neurochemicals, neurohormones, and hormones as well as a host of other chemicals to release, slow down or speed up.

When this feedback system is allowed to work, it acts much like a conductor managing a symphony, telling each component when to act and when to turn on and off, how much to give and when to reduce or increase its function. In the end, this feedback system ensures that neither too little nor too much of anything is done, but only the right amount to get the right result.

Within our bodies, we have many survival-healing feedback systems. When we are presented with a threat, our bodies initially invoke the Stress Cascade. Once activated, the many feedback mechanisms turn on and off to manage it.

If we are injured, special chemicals are released at the injury site. These chemicals and hormones feed information back to the healing mechanism describing where the injury is and how serious it is, in other words, the extent of injury or injuries. This tells the brain and the Body-Mind the exact location, nature, and pattern of the injury. This information allows the Body-Mind to orchestrate the necessary adjustments in the amounts and types of hormones and chemicals needed to defend and repair all injured areas. Other hormones and chemicals signal the Body-Mind that healing is progressing. When healing is complete, another group of neurochemical messengers notify the Body-Mind that healing is complete so it can shut down all further healing and repair efforts. Once the crisis is over and healing is complete, the Body-Mind returns us to a state of a harmony and balance.

When an imbalance occurs within the Defense-Repair-Healing Systems, this feedback mechanism may function inappropriately. The delivery of proper hormones, chemicals, and neurohormonal substances may become disturbed, timing may suffer, and feedback may be interfered with as well. This can impair the healing process and even create faulty signals, which could provide false information to the Body-Mind. At some point, the Stress Mechanism may be triggered again by this "new" threat.

If these problems are not quickly resolved, the Stress Mechanism may remain in a state of continuous activation, which once again can lead to a state of Chronic Stress, Dis-Ease, Disease, Chronic Disease, and eventually Death.

In the end, as it is with most problems in life, the best treatment is always solving the original triggering problem. The sooner a solution is reached, the less likely any long-term or highly problematic imbalance will be created. For example, if someone works too hard and subsequently loses their resistance, they may get a sore throat. While penicillin might be prescribed, it is not likely to solve the triggering problem that originally created the imbalance. If the problem persists, the imbalance also persists. As time passes, the Defense and Healing Mechanisms may be undermined and even damaged. The person may then suffer a series of sore throats and possibly other illnesses. They may repeatedly return for medical treatment, each time resolving the acute illness but never solving the underlying conflict. While some relief from symptoms may be accomplished, this is usually short-lived, and the old symptoms return or a new illness appears. Again, treating the symptoms, an antibiotic will likely be prescribed. While there may be acute resolution, there may be no permanent results.

When this happens, many physicians and patients blame the antibiotic. Sometimes, the physician blames the patient. Sometimes, it is decided that the wrong organism was treated. However, the real problem is missed again and again. The underlying unresolved conflict that has triggered this series of illnesses and possibly impaired the patient's immune system, has not been resolved and the individual is not cured.

The same thing might happen with stress problems. For example, you become sick and your physician tells you that you're working too hard. Your doctor suggests that if you reduce your hours you will decrease your stress. However, if you believe that you need to work hard to succeed or pay bills you may not be able to take time off from work. Hence, the doctor's advice instead of reducing stress may only trigger new fear of financial insecurity and potential disaster. If you then try to follow your physician's instructions, it will not help for very long. It may even increase your overall stress levels, hence worsening the process. Once again, if the original conflict is not resolved, the imbalance will likely persist and the affect may be more problems, an inability to maintain balance and harmony and ultimately a worsening of the illness process.

For those with frequent recurrent sore throats, colds, sinus infections, bladder infections, bronchitis, allergies, accidents, or recurrent injuries or other problems, be aware that these problems might actually be Stress-Related Disorders. If medical treatment does not resolve your problems, consider that you have a Stress-Related Disorder. If you want to return to excellent health, look for and find your underlying problems and conflicts, the problems your Body-Mind wants you to resolve.

Remember, if these conflicts are not resolved, your Defense and Immune Systems may eventually lose their ability to protect you. This could lead to more serious illnesses or even disorders such as autoimmune diseases, cancer, or to a Chronic Disease State where your overall ability to function becomes severely impaired. Remember the severity of the ultimate disease process will likely be directly related to the following three variables:

1) How important it is to your Body-Mind that you find an appropriate resolution,
2) How much you resist or ignore finding the right solution or solutions,
3) How long the underlying imbalances are allowed to persist before a solution is found and implemented.

Generally, the development of most diseases will take many years. The original conflict may have long been forgotten by the time the disease process is recognized and a diagnosis is established. Generally, by the time identifiable symptoms are recognized, the individual is no longer able to associate cause and effect with any specific prior conflict.

CASE HISTORY: MARY JANE F.

Mary Jane F. offered a clear example of this situation. We first saw Mary Jane F. when she was thirty-five years of age. She had a long history of recurrent vaginal infections. Mary Jane had seen ten to twelve medical doctors and gynecologists during the previous ten years. In the course of her most recent episode of vaginal infections, she was also found to have a Class III Pap Smear suggestive of moderate-to-advanced cervical dysplasia. There was already sufficient inflammation to cause her cervical cells to demonstrate a pre-malignant condition.

Mary Jane was an interesting young woman. When we first met her, she was very blunt, "I'm tired of doctors. They never solved my problems. They just use me as a guinea pig. They obviously don't know what they are doing, since none of them have cured me!"

We immediately recognized at least four clues in what she had just said. One clue was the way she said it. She was angry, even though we had never met each other. Second, she was hostile toward doctors, as if the doctors (all male) had something to do with causing her problems. Three, she had apparently been making her doctors responsible for her problems. And finally, no one had solved her ongoing problem, not even her.

Usually, treating vaginal infections is not a complicated or difficult problem. It immediately became clear to us that her problem was not just that she hadn't been cured, but that her vaginal infections kept recurring. Each time, she would end up blaming someone beside herself for the re-occurrence. This is a childlike response. This suggested to us that we would be treating a conflict that had its roots deep in her childhood. One more clue: she was unaware that she had a conflict at the base of her problem. While taking her medical history, she gave us several other pieces of information that led us to some additional conclusions.

Mary Jane was brought up as a strict Roman Catholic. However, she had been married and divorced three times. She described all of her former husband's as "jerks." Her current "live-in relationship" was with a man she described as "a creep." "He's so unsympathetic," she told me, "he just doesn't care that I always have vaginal infections."

Putting this all together, it became clear that the result of her recurrent vaginal infections were that they kept her from having sex, even though she said she "loved sex." This, along with her anger at men and her inability to get any long-term relief, led us to ask two more questions. First, "How old were you when you had your first vaginal infection?" She told me that she was fifteen years old at the time of her first sexual encounter. However, when she told me this she looked away, dropped her voice level and then stared off into a space for a minute or two. She had lied. Our second question was much bolder but seemed to us to be the next logical piece in the puzzle, "Who sexually molested you?"

Mary Jane looked up, her eyes dilated widely and she quickly laughed. In fact, she laughed much too quickly. Almost predictably, she denied that she had ever been sexually molested. Then, almost out of nowhere, tears flooded into her eyes and she cried. We patiently waited. After awhile, she looked up and asked, "How did you know? I've never told a living soul."

She then related the story of how her brother had sexually molested her on several occasions between the age of eleven and thirteen. She then admitted that she had felt so ashamed that she never told anyone, that is, until now. After regaining her composure, she admitted that by the time she turned fifteen, boys had already started "hitting" on her. She thought that they must have known that she was no longer a virgin, she felt ashamed and humiliated. It was about this time, she related, that she began to have her first vaginal infections. She told us that when any boys approached her she felt "dirty and unclean." She believed that she was impure and that no one would ever truly love her "if they knew." After this, she subconsciously chose boys who were rowdy and intellectually beneath her. She believed that no decent boy would ever love or respect her.

We referred Mary Jane to an excellent rape crisis counselor. Mary Jane returned a few times afterward to talk about the dynamics of her situation. At the time of her initial visit, we treated her current vaginal infection. With time and follow-up treatments, we resolved her abnormal Pap smear. Within a short period, she got rid of her "creepy, live-in" boyfriend. She stopped dating and started working on loving herself. We saw her several times during the next three years, and she has not had a single vaginal infection since her initial treatment. The last time we saw her, she was engaged to a man she described as "her most understanding soul mate."

Mary Jane's situation was not at all unusual. Many women have problems with recurrent vaginal infections, abnormal Pap smears, pelvic pain, and other gynecologic problems because of conflicts regarding sexuality, relationships, and even nurturing. While her particular story was about incest and sexual molestation, which is more dramatic than most, each story is a unique situation. They range from rape to bad marriages, fears about masturbation, or anger at a prior partner, inability to trust men and inability to trust themselves. We have seen many women whose specific issues were much less dramatic than Mary Jane's but a lot more dangerous to them.

As with Mary Jane, when the Defense-Immune System begins to fail, there is usually a number of signs of disharmony and imbalance occurring, often for many years before we seek or find help. While the issues are different, the same types of unresolved conflicts occur in men with erectile dysfunction, chronic prostatitis, nonspecific urethritis, and a host of other nonsexual illnesses or medical problems. For example, men and women often develop problems and conflicts regarding work, financial matters, family, conflicts with partners or children, deteriorating self-images, episodes of fatigue and depression, and of course, general unhappiness.

Relationship problems often spill over to affect the children or relationships with other family members, neighbors, co-workers, and bosses. Sometimes, children may suddenly develop ear infections, recurrent colds, flu, sore throats, allergies, asthma, and other stress-related illnesses when their parents are having problems.

Children acting out may well be secondary to the imbalance and disharmony created by their parents' problems, or those of other siblings. While we may blame children for tantrums, behavioral problems in school or other types of acting out, their behavior may simply be their attempts to communicate their unresolved conflict over their parents or classmates' behaviors or school problems. "You're never around," "You don't love me," "You don't care anymore," or even "Something is wrong with you, and we don't know why and we're scared," or "my teacher hates me."

When Stress-Related Disorders exist, they indicate that there may be problems in the family and that the family may be in the process of eventually breaking down. Divorce, the irreversible breakdown of the "marital body," may occur because of the inability to resolve unresolved conflict. Unfortunately, the unresolved conflicts of the parents may be passed on to their children and become the unresolved conflicts of their children. This can ultimately lead the children to Stress-Related Disorders, illness and even Chronic Disease and premature death.

Situations like these are often mistakenly considered, "just a normal part of life." They are not recognized as signs of a destructive imbalance. When medical problems arise, they may only occasionally be associated with the patients' events and conflicts. Only the most perceptive physicians tend to make any effort to identify the original unresolved conflict and then treat the conflicts rather than merely their later signs and symptoms.

Today, most medical doctors miss the true nature of Stress-Related Disorders. When patients present symptoms related to Stress-Related Disorders, they are commonly treated with medications. Often the root cause of the problem is never identified and the problem itself is never resolved. Hence, these patients are treated with medications and not with problem-solving. This happens because most doctors are not trained to see their patients as whole beings. We human beings are not just our body. We are the totality of our existence. Only through maintaining harmony and balance, integrating mind, body, and spirit, can we stay whole, healthy, and happy.

WITHOUT RISK-TAKING, HEALING MAY NOT BE POSSIBLE

In order to get well, it is essential, possibly even mandatory that we take risks. In the traditional sense, seeing your doctor is taking a risk. You might not like what he finds. You may have to remove your clothes. It may cost a lot of money. You might be told you need an operation. You may experience pain during the examination. Taking medicine is risky. You may have side effects or an adverse reaction to the medication.

Dealing with unresolved conflicts also creates risks. You may re-experience old pains, old turmoil, and events you would much rather forget. If you are still in pain about your conflicts and can't face your problems, they remain unre-solved. The pain involved may be too great for you to face. It is often easier to take medications and hope that you will get well than it is to experience the pain these conflicts have in the past created within you. Many people would rather risk death, as way out of the pain, than revisit old pains, anger, or humiliation.

The problem is that unless you find and confront these conflicts, your Body-Mind may activate the Wellness-Illness Mechanism to force you to face them. It often requires that you re-experience them so that they can be resolved. If you have symptoms or disease, your Body-Mind is already crying for you to resolve these conflicts. In the end, both alternatives are unpleasant. However, one leads to health and wellness, while the other leads to illness, more pain and suffering, chronic health problems, and possibly premature death.

Risk-taking can be positive or negative. Positive risks are those that help us grow. Their results are constructive and enliven us. They usually take the form of challenges to master and opportunities to learn. Positive risk-taking leads to physical, mental, and emotional growth and sometimes even spiritual enlightenment.

Negative risks are dangerous adventures where we can lose something or everything, feel pain, and get hurt. Some examples are driving too fast, having an extramarital affair, or staying at a job where you are underpaid or unappreciated.

Mary Jane dated and married the same types of destructive men. She was afraid of taking any risks by dating "decent men" who might reject her and cause her even greater pain. Negative risks generally end up producing negative results.

Whether we perceive a risk as positive or negative has much to do with our desired goals and how the situation finally turns out. If good health is our goal, then everything we do to accomplish this goal is a positive risk with a positive outcome. Negative risk-taking is more likely to lead to illness, disease, or distortion of our lives since it is always a lie and not in our best interest.

In general, positive risk-taking – accepting healthy challenges – leads to healing because it supports the truth of our being. It is also positive because it leads to a positive result.

Every day, we are exposed to examples of illness and healing. It is helpful to recognize these positive and negative models. Negative risks are our teachers. They demonstrate what happens when we allow illness to take root. Recognizing this can help determine what is really happening and what is really in your best interest. It can give you the direction and power to undo the illness process and work towards reversing your illnesses and returning your Body-Mind to optimal health and well-being.

If used correctly, this knowledge can help you find the problems underlying your own conflicts and gives you the courage to resolve them. By using what you learn from others, you can compare the benefits of wellness to the risks, and the limitations and negativity of illness and disease. You will soon recognize that illness is never preferable to wellness. Illness is an unproductive state, even when you learn and grow from it.

The most demanding risk-taking is when you face the truths of your life. However painful this is, illness is worse. Healing requires telling the truth. This is often difficult. You have to be ready to be well when you can face your problems and admit to the lies and faulty beliefs you have created in your life.

The Body-Mind always wants to heal. It continually works toward this goal. If properly directed, it gets you there sooner and with less pain and struggle. Unwillingness to take risks suggests that a lie exists somewhere within. Lies also demonstrate their existence when we are only willing to take less-productive risks instead of solving problems. Another way of recognizing that lies exist is when we substitute one risk for another rather than solving the problem at hand.

Mary Jane so feared rejection that she chose partners who were not right for her and left her feeling unloved and unlovable. Somewhere inside herself, she believed that she took less personal risk if they later rejected her. Yet, she still felt emotional pain even when these partners rejected her and left. Positive risk-taking would have meant for her to only choose partners who were kind, supportive, stimulating, loving, and emotionally healthy. Her feelings of unworthiness tripped her up. It wasn't until she was able to see how much her fears had cost her that she finally became willing to take positive risks to resolve her hidden conflicts.

Mary Jane's story represents a perfect example of how healing can be subverted. In her case, there were a series of distortions and lies sustained by her fear of exposing her molestation. For some people, the fear of acknowledging and exposing old conflicts or traumas is so threatening that they will do almost anything not to have to face their problems. Some people run away or even attempt suicide, believing that this is the only way they can be free of their pain.

Chronic illnesses, such as infections, autoimmune diseases, and cancer, are often the result of resistance to resolving conflicts. They become a form of suicide in that these individuals would rather die than resolve their problems. This feeds and generates their illnesses. Unfortunately, many people die from illness which could have been cured, simply because they were unaware of the relationship between the unresolved conflicts and the Stress-Wellness-Disease Mechanism.

To understand the power of negative risk-taking and the conflicts that originally caused them, look at how often death seems unnecessary. If you believe that the universe is an unreasonable, stupid, thoughtless, random, and cruel place, it is easy to think of death as just another example of the tragic things that happen to people. However, if you believe in an Intelligent Universe, then death must have some purpose or meaning. Not immediately seeing the specific reasons, purposes, or meanings does not mean they don't exist. The underlying reasons, purposes, and meanings are often so deeply hidden within us or are so old that they are not recognizable. However, the underlying cause for the problem is often apparent to others. We all have heard people say, "It's such a shame Harold drank himself to death. He must have felt so alone since his wife died," or "It's a pity June just couldn't make her life work, but she would never listen to advice so she just destroyed herself," or "After Ralph retired, he made no plans and had nothing to do. I guess he just died of boredom." These same reasons are often missed by the person who either can't or doesn't want to see them.

One of the best ways of eliminating stress and converting negative risks into positive risk taking is by transforming conflicts into challenges and opportunities. When we do this, we can eliminate their negative aspects. Then it is easier to recognize that these conflicts are our teachers and that we have things to learn from them. As we master our challenges, we gain opportunity to grow and empower ourselves in many positive ways.

Let's take a moment to see how we can do this. Suppose you're afraid of the water. The fear of drowning terrifies you. To transform your fear into a challenge, you must learn as much as you can about swimming. You could use visualization techniques to imagine yourself swimming successfully without even entering the water. You could take swimming lessons. You could practice your swimming ability so that you could swim in all types of water. This would be an example of transforming a negative fear into a positive skill through creating a challenge that helps you resolve and master this previously unresolved conflict.

We see this happening around us all the time. People who fear flying learn to fly. People who are afraid to drive learn to drive. People who are afraid of success learn to be successful. In all cases, what appeared at first glance to be a negative situation can became a positive opportunity. This can only happen when you accept your conflicts and transform them into challenges and opportunities. We must do whatever is necessary to meet the challenges of life so that we can ultimately take advantage of the opportunities that are all around us.

LIFE WITHOUT ILLNESS

A life without illness can occur only when we are always telling the truth and only when we clear our life of all lies, conflicts, and unresolved problems. If we are able to recognize that the symptoms of Stress-Related Disorders are not really a sickness but an Intelligent communication from our Body-Mind to us that one or more unresolved problems and conflicts exist, then we can begin healing ourselves.

The truths and lies of our lives are always holistic since they have mind, body, and spiritual components as well as social, physical, and cultural components. They encompass the totality of our lives and they ultimately become our lives. We define ourselves by our truths, lies, and belief systems. We may see ourselves as a Northerner or Southerner, smart or stupid, handsome or ugly, healthy or sickly. We do this rather than see ourselves as a person with many attributes, both positive and negative, who may need help in order to resolve our negative attributes. These self-imposed descriptions are simply decisions we made about ourselves or that others made for us about how we decided to live our lives. These descriptions tell others and us what we believe about ourselves.

These definitions are the key to what the Conscious Aware Self is telling the Body-Mind. When they are truthful, what the Body-Mind knows to be true and what the Conscious Aware Self knows to be true are the same, and this allows harmony and balance exist. When our self imposed definitions are lies or are controlled by faulty or distorted belief systems, they end up producing imbalance and disharmony. Inevitably, our Body-Mind becomes aware of all of our truth and lies. It wants to set matters right. It is then when the Stress-Wellness-Illness Mechanism initiates. Healing requires that you see yourself as a whole, healthy human being, already healed in all levels of your life. That which blocks healing is a lie. That which encourages healing is truth. Since nothing exists without mind and belief systems, we must recognize that what we believe about ourselves is what decides what is a lie and what is truth.

*A sad soul
can kill you
quicker
than a germ.*

~John Steinbeck

Chapter Eighteen

HEALING OURSELVES
— HEALING THE WORLD —

REVERSING ILLNESS

You can begin healing yourself once you understand how and why your Stress-Related illnesses were caused by those unresolved conflicts. Most of your unresolved conflicts have at their core, faulty belief systems. Start by recognizing that your signs, symptoms, and illnesses are actually clues that can help you determine their underlying causes. As you learn how to recognize these clues, you will heal yourself more fully and faster. Your Body-Mind chose these specific signs, symptoms, and illnesses to provide you with all the information it can give you to help you resolve your unresolved conflicts. To accomplish healing, use these signs, symptoms, and illnesses to direct you to uncover and resolve these conflicts. They will help you find the conflicts that are causing you health problems so that you can finally eliminate them.

As we stated earlier, most Stress-Related Disorders can be stopped anywhere along the Wellness-to-Illness process by solving the underlying conflicts causing them. However, even when these conflicts are fully resolved, the Illness-Disease Mechanism may not immediately reverse. Once allowed to reach the Disease Stage, this process often takes on a life of its own. If illness is not resolved early, it may advance to a point where complete reversal is impossible without medical or surgical intervention and treatment. At the point where the condition reaches the Chronic Disease Stage, irreparable damage may have already occurred making complete resolution less likely.

If significant damage has been done, the illness or illnesses already created may not be completely reversible, since part of the body's integrity may have already been lost. An example would be breast cancer where surgery and possibly radiation or chemotherapy were required. The cancer may be gone, but so is part of the woman's breast. Radiation or chemotherapy may irreversibly damage both the remaining breast and surrounding tissues. In such situations, the woman is left with both emotional and physical scars.

Even if the original conflict has been found, reversed, and eliminated, the physical and emotional scars remain. Once removed, the breast that was can never be replaced.

People often have an illusion that healing is "a return to the way I was before. ..." This is not always possible, since we can never go backward. At best, we can stop the negative illness process and get back onto a positive, healthy path. There is a parable on healing from the New Testament in which Jesus comes upon a cripple who begs to be healed. Jesus says to the man, "Are you willing to forgive yourself your sins?" The word "sins" is a code word for the lies we create in our lives. "If so, pick up your bed and walk." In this parable, the bed represents his lies and their consequences.

The symbolism here suggests that by picking up his bed, he is finally taking responsibility for his prior actions. Putting it on his back suggests that he will now accept the consequences and responsibility of his past actions and lies. Walking is moving forward and onward in life. It is our lies, "our sins," which ultimately cripple us and cause our illnesses. Since not all the harm we've created can be undone, we must carry these consequences figuratively on our back. People who've been impaired by disease must live with what is done and bear its burden until they truly forgive themselves and create sufficient truth and love in their life to overcome the consequences of their past. Only then will they be fully healed. However, they may not necessarily return to their former "perfect state" or physical condition. In fact, they might not want to go back to what they were. Their new selves are often considerably better than were their old selves. People who have had an extremity amputated cannot expect it to grow back, but they can learn to accept their loss and maximize their existing capabilities. When they do this, their amputation is no longer a disability – only a fact of life.

All illness represents opportunities to learn, grow, and evolve. The lesson learned may be the real purpose of the illness. It may even define the purpose of our life. We believe the purpose of life is to grow and evolve. Therefore, the lessons learned from illness are part of our growth and evolution as persons and individuals. People who transcend their illnesses or use them to better themselves or others are often considered heroes.

Yet, usually their intention was simply to get better. In their process of getting well, they reached for and created their highest, healthiest, and best Self. This frequently can inspire others.

The Illness-Disease Process can stop on its own anywhere along its path. The exact time and place this might happen depends on how much power you gave to the originating conflicts or lies. Conflicts can burn themselves out, and they can be outgrown. They can even spontaneously resolve themselves like a child who one day just lets go of his favorite teddy bear or blanket without a word or threat from anyone else.

However, significant, unresolved lies or conflicts may evolve and lead to chronic degenerative diseases, surgery, destructive medical treatments, or even death. If the process of finding the underlying problems and conflicts is started and taken seriously before the disease becomes chronic, healing may spontaneously occur. Once the ability to reverse these lies, create truth, and problem solving is learned, it is never forgotten. This skill must, as with any other skill, be constantly practiced if we are to remain healthy for the rest of our life.

Thomas Jefferson said, "The price of freedom is eternal vigilance." Perhaps we could paraphrase this to say, "The price of wellness is constant vigilance." This vigilance ultimately must take the form of self-knowledge and self-discipline concerning what we say, what we think, and do.

> # The Price of Wellness is Constant Vigilance

BIRTH, DEATH, AND REBIRTH

We are constantly healing and deteriorating. The processes of birth, death, and rebirth are the nature of life. The forces of destruction are always working, tearing down the old to make room for and even create the new. Cells and tissues begin dying from the moment of their birth. They are born, live, are injured and repaired, regenerate, die, and are replaced. This is the cycle of all life. Our Healing and Repair Systems facilitate this process. Our ability to regenerate maintains it. Since our bodies are constantly breaking down and rebuilding (supposedly, every seven years we entirely regenerate ourselves), the choice of direction toward illness or health is ours. We each have the power to control our lives, even when we are unwilling to admit this or do not feel good enough about ourselves to make it work for us.

THE PHYSICIAN AS A HEALER

A healer can be just about anyone. In our society, the person we most think of as a healer is the physician. To be a healer, a physician must fill three roles.

The first is to evaluate, diagnose, and treat illness with necessary medical procedures. Most physicians do this well.

The second is assisting the patient in finding underlying conflicts, the causes, and then help them resolve these conflicts. The average physician does not rate very high in performing this role.

The third and most important role for the physician is helping his patients prevent illness from occurring in the first place. He does this first by helping his patients solve problems as soon as they are recognized, then also through teaching them how not to have unresolved conflicts in the first place. This is generally not done at all by the majority of medical doctors.

To be an excellent healer, the physician must also be an educator. He must educate his patients about the causes and effects of illness, describe anatomy and physiology when necessary, and clearly explain any abnormality and what can be done about them. Education should help to allay the patients' fears and facilitate healing whenever possible. The excellent physician advises his patients about medical and surgical treatments, alternative treatments, possible complications, side effects, or adverse reactions. Using this information, the physician helps patients make the healthiest and best decisions regarding their safest and best processes for treatment and healing. The healer-physician can withhold medical treatment if the causative problems can be eliminated without it. Medical or surgical intervention should be a last resort.

The healer-physician's most important role is believing in healing and inspiring their patients regarding their own ability to heal themselves. He should work diligently to teach each patient how to do this. The healer-physician should always see their patient as healthy and on a voyage of exploration to learn, grow, and evolve. His ability to facilitate doing this makes all the difference in the world whether he is a healer or simply a technician, and whether his patients are ultimately healed or allowed to progress negatively to illness, disease, chronic disease, or even premature death.

Once the patient is on a healing path, the healer-physician can then monitor meaningful information, changes their patient is making, watch for side effects, and help the patient avoid complications and adverse reactions from medications and other medical treatments. When problems are found, the healer-physician guides the patient out of harm's way. Through the entire treatment process, the physician-healer should educate, inform, and advise but never undermine the patient's progress. The healer-physician acts as a guardian of his patients' safety and well-being. He must always remember that all healing is accomplished by the patient's will, not by medical treatments alone. If the patient's desire wanes or if the patient is not achieving good results, the healer-physician can help by working with the patient, investigating, and looking for new problems and better solutions. If the healer-physician is not capable of helping his patient, he must refer the patient to someone who can give the most correct and the highest level of care available. Most of all, the healer-physician must always acts as a caring friend, working toward complete cure and resolution of all illness, as well as all inciting problems and unresolved conflicts.

The healer-physician always does his best to help all of his patients to prevent illness even before it can occur. Unfortunately, few medical doctors today assist their patients in self-healing. Even fewer are involved in problem solving or prevention. Most medical doctors do not have the training or much interest in finding their patients' underlying conflicts or in preventing illnesses before they happen. Most medical doctors are too busy making a living, trying to keep up with insurance company requirements, or are too burned out to extend this level of care.

Another problem lies in the fact that even if medical doctors were trained as healers, medical insurance companies work against healing. They even frequently work against their client-patients getting the needed quality of care. The best insurance companies believe in prevention and psychological care. Unfortunately, many insurance companies today deny their policyholder's payment for services that are preventive, or where the insurance company believes it is unjustified because it is "not considered usual and customary care." Since they are based in the standard, interventive medical model of treatment, anything that does not fit their specific criteria may be considered to not be normal care, to be experimental, or belonging to nontraditional medicine, hocus-pocus, or simply, "not covered."

Many patients come to their physician uneducated, angry, and scared. Because of this, they are unwilling to do everything necessary to get well. Many even come with such blatant death wishes that the physician may quickly lose interest in working with them. Sometimes, the physician has to accept that the best that can be done is to treat their patients' symptoms and hope this makes them happy. However, in the best of circumstances, this should not be the only thing done – and certainly not the first step.

The sad truth is today, most physicians would rather treat with medications or surgeries because it's more expedient than help a patient discover the underlying conflicts that caused their illness, even if this means that the patient is going to be left with only temporary results and without a real cure. In the future, physicians must be better trained in techniques of healing.

THERE ARE MANY OTHER HEALERS

The healer does not have to be a medical doctor. A healer can be an osteopath, chiropractor, podiatrist, massage therapist, nutritionist, body-work therapist, physical therapist, acupuncturist, dentist, psychologist, marriage and family counselor, clergy, spiritualist, astrologer, or tarot reader. A healer can be from any field that ministers to individuals who are physically or emotionally sick or out of balance. A healer could also be someone not normally thought of as being part of the healing profession, such as a parent, relative, friend, neighbor, attorney, teacher, accountant, insurance professional, banker, or financial counselor. In fact, a healer can be any person who helps others solve problems, look for and find problems, or resolve conflicts that have created any physical, emotional, mental, or spiritual problems. Healing is often a team process requiring more than one healer and lots of support.

A serious problem in today's society is that many people, including physicians and other health professionals, are afraid to get involved. Many professionals are afraid to give love and personal one-on-one care. Unfortunately, many non-medical professionals, even those who are most willing to make a difference in helping others solve their day-to-day problems, are either not trained or are not able to help those people with the most serious health problems, such as diagnosed illnesses or life-threatening problems. This may be because they are afraid of being sued or are unwilling to take on problems they do not feel qualified to treat. This may be a smart choice for them, but it leaves many sick people with few or no meaningful resources since the medical profession is also unwilling to provide any other form of treatment other than standard Western medical treatments.

Another major factor is that medical doctors often refuse to work with non-medical professionals. This once again denies their patients the skills and services they themselves do not possess. Medical doctors may also demean the non-medical healer's approach to problem solving, which they themselves cannot provide. Too often, medical doctors consider anyone who doesn't fit the Western medical treatment model, as being an incompetent outsider, a charlatan, or con artist. They may refer to individuals practicing alternative healing techniques as "quacks" or "frauds," and so undermine any good these other people could provide. While there are indeed unscrupulous people who prey on the sick, it is inappropriate for physicians to condemn healing practices they haven't looked into or cannot provide themselves.

To be able to provide the highest quality healing care may require that the physician goes beyond their medical training, keeping an open mind to healing patients, and not just treating them. Unfortunately, for many physicians this only occurs when they themselves become ill and discover that their colleagues are not able to heal them. The door to healing was opened this way for both Lisa and me.

HEALING YOURSELF

The body's ability to defend, repair, and heal itself is truly miraculous. It is a process that can create and return people to optimal health and wellness. This same type of process, problem solving, fixing things that have been broken, checks and balances, creation of harmony and balance, prevention and constant vigilance, works the same way in the world around us as it works within our bodies. We work this way ourselves every day.

The same general concepts involved in healing are used in setting up and running businesses, governments, or other organizations. We use it every time we start or manage a project of any kind. Most people become confused about this process, since they do not always see it in action. They take it for granted and only think about it when it is not working.

Only when our lives are in turmoil do we begin thinking about how to find and undo problems and to create preventive solutions.

Those who do not yet understand that their problems are both clues and keys to needed solutions often consider themselves failures. Many people are still caught in this kind of insanity and miss the wheat for the chaff. Many people think of failure as being bigger than real life, but this isn't true. Failure is only an illusion of the moment. Real life is about living fully, enjoying life, problem solving, fixing things that are broken, managing, learning, growing, evolving, and becoming our highest, healthiest, and best Selves. To do this, we must try new approaches and take risks. When we do this, we might fail from time to time, but if we do nothing, we will surely fail. The old adage, "nothing ventured, nothing gained," tells us exactly how important it is to be ready to fail.

It is this book's principal goal to help you understand the illness-healing-repair process so that you can completely heal yourself and live your life fully and joyfully. Another goal of this work is to help you become so proficient in creating wellness for yourself that you can help others.

Before beginning the healing process, it is important to understand the basics of the process we are about to discuss. If you are not committed to getting well, this process is doomed from the start. Once you are willing and able to do whatever is necessary to heal yourself, you are ready to go on to the first step of this six-step process.

STEPS TO HEALING

1. Admit That You Have a Stress-Related Disorder.

2. Accept Responsibility for Healing.

3. Find the Conflicts That Caused Your Illness.

4. Solve Problems and Correct Faulty Belief Systems.

5. Transform Negative Beliefs Into Positive Growth.

6. Thank Yourself.

Table: 18-1

SIX STEPS FOR CREATING HEALING AND WELLNESS

1. **Admit That You Have Become Ill from a Stress-Related Disorder**

    The first step requires admitting that you are ill and are suffering from a Stress-Related Disorder. You must be willing to acknowledge or accept its possibility. Once this is accomplished, you must next be willing to take full responsibility for your illness. *"I am sick and I caused my own illness (injury)."* This is never done to create blame or establish guilt, but rather to empower us to heal ourselves.

2. **Accept Responsibility for Healing**

    Once you take responsibility for causing your illness, you must next take responsibility for healing yourself. *"I am the only one who can heal me. I am completely responsible for my own healing."* If you deny that you are sick, believe it is someone else's fault, or the fault of a bacteria or virus, you are not taking full responsibility for the cause of your problems or for the illness itself.

    This does not mean assuming guilt or shame. Guilt and shame are destructive and will block your healing process. Holding onto any negative thoughts or behaviors will only make healing more difficult, since this would be a lie and faulty belief system which would act more to maintain the problem, than to resolve or heal it. This would eventually sabotage your healing process.

    Only through taking responsibility for your symptoms and illnesses, with the intent of accepting that they exist and are real, can you now use them to help you find and remove all of the blocks and obstacles which are causing them. If you use your symptoms and illnesses in this way, you will better be able to help yourself and ultimately create full and complete healing for yourself.

3. **Find the Conflicts That Caused Your Illness**

    Next, look for the causes and triggers of your illnesses or injuries. This process requires that you search out all underlying lies, faulty beliefs, and unresolved conflicts. If there are belief systems or other conditions triggering your Stress-Illness Process and they are clearly apparent, acknowledge them and forgive them for causing your stress and your illnesses or injuries. They were only tools your Body-Mind used to get your attention and direct you toward solving them. They are not against you and you should consider them on your side. They are merely providing information and lessons you need to learn and resolve.

    Next, forgive yourself for not recognizing this information and lessons earlier and for having allowed or even forced your Body-

Mind to create illness for you to finally experience what is happening.

Look for, find, and write down all negative thoughts, feelings, beliefs, ideas, or habits you recognize, now and in the future. Each time you will find a new unresolved conflict, negative or positive, write it down as well. With time, you find that patterns will unfold and that these patterns provide new clues to help you heal yourself. Everything you learn along the way will help you better understand what is actually causing your illness, subverting your energy and feeding the progression of your illness.

All negative conflicts are clues and should be seen and recognized as your teachers. Life is not about negatives. Life is about transforming negatives into positives. Life is about learning, growing, and evolving. Everything we think of as being a negative is illusion, a block or unresolved conflict that is testing us and forcing us to learn, grow, and evolve. Truthfully, many people may argue with this way of thinking, but the reasons they argue is because they are unhappy and do not have better answers. Many of these people are simply blocked by their own unresolved conflicts and have not yet found their way toward healing their own issues.

As time passes, the picture of what is causing your illness will unfold. When you finally recognize what your Body-Mind is telling you, you will be able to not only stop your illness process, but also reverse, eliminate, and cure these illnesses.

4. **Solve Problems and Correct Faulty Belief Systems**

Once you have identified your problems, do whatever you need to do to correct them. You can use whatever problem-solving techniques you have available, or you can learn new ones. Recognize what each problem was trying to teach you. Learn from it, grow, and evolve. It's okay if you're not immediately able to recognize the lessons or the answers. The answers will come to you along the way, often when you least expect them. The problem-solving process is more important than the problem itself. Learning to prevent illness and solving problems helps you grow and reduces the occurrence of problems in the future.

You can use the techniques outlined in this book to identify the problems. However, be aware that the blocks and complexes you created through the years will work to undermine your efforts. Also, be aware that you will recognize your blocks and complexes and will have to deal with them to obtain optimal results. This is all part of the process. When you decide you want to paint a wall in your home, it requires choosing a color, buying and mixing the paint, spending whatever time is required applying the paint to the wall, cleaning up the ground and surroundings, cleaning your brushes and containers, and finally cleaning yourself as well. If you chose to do less, you may get not get the entire job done to your satisfaction. It also helps if you enjoy what you are doing and have fun doing the work. Each step listed above is a necessary part of the process.

Think of the work you have to do to heal yourself in the same way, everything you will have to do will be a necessary part of the process. When negative thoughts, feelings, ideas, or beliefs enter into your life, they are merely blocks and complexes. You may want to recognize and respect them, but not let them take you away from your work. Once you are able do this you will also be able to solve your unresolved conflicts faster and more effectively. You will be more effective at reaching your goals, healing yourself, and creating a new and healthier life.

5. **Transform Negative Beliefs into Positive Growth**

Once the lies and conflicts are recognized, the next step is transforming all lies into truths, resolving all conflicts, and solving all problems. When this is done, you can return to a truthful place within yourself. Discovering and eliminating all death wishes is also important. These simply negative belief systems can be transformed into positive learning and growing situations.

At first reading, this may seem to be a complex and daunting task. Remember that these are your blocks and complexes talking, not reality. We always use the construct of the *"glass half-empty and the glass half-full."* When you find a negative belief, ask yourself what is its polar opposite.

In the case history of Mary Jane, she recognized that her greatest fear was of rejection. The polar opposite of rejection is being loved. She wanted to be loved. She not only recognized this, she also recognized that once she had forgiven her brother for molesting her and accepted herself as she was, she had finally opened herself up to accepting and being loved. When she did that, love found her.

This is the way healing works. This is why it is about learning, growing, and evolving. Find the conflict, learn from it, let it give you the information you need, transform it from a negative to a positive so that you can then grow and evolve. To do this, use and do everything you can to become your highest, healthiest, and best Self. Do this, and what you most desire will come to you.

List all of your conflicts to the best of your ability. Then list their polar opposites or what you know to be true. Remember, this is an ongoing process; this is an exercise you will start but you will never completely finish it. Like peeling an onion, as you resolve one issue another will surface. The process is lifelong. This is okay, since it ensures that you spend your life as you should — learning, growing, and evolving.

6. **Thank Yourself**

As wellness returns, thank yourself for your efforts and the lessons learned. Always appreciate yourself for your accomplishments. With this success, your self-value increases and you begin experiencing more self-love and respect for yourself and others. Remember, the Universe is Intelligent. See yourself and your body as part of the Universal Intelligence.

This is the way healing works.

Find the conflict,
learn from it,
let it give you
the information you need,
transform it
from a negative
to a positive
so that you can then
grow and evolve.

Do this,
and what you most desire
will come to you.

WHAT ELSE CAN I DO?

There are many stress reduction techniques and programs that you can use to reduce stress while stopping, eliminating, and curing your illnesses. Some of these techniques and programs include relaxation exercises, breathing exercises, massage, acupuncture, acupressure, healthy diet, and regular exercise. There are many good books on reducing stress even on healing stress.

Our next book, When Your Body Talks, Heal It!, will outline some of our most productive and favorite methods of reducing and healing stress. Until it is released, use what is available.

MAINTAINING YOUR GOOD HEALTH

In order to maintain your good health, remember to always tell yourself and others the truth and problem-solve to the best of your ability. When you tell a lie, apologize to yourself and anyone else affected. Then forgive yourself for any lies in which you ever believed. Forgive yourself and all others who participated in these lies.

When a problem presents itself, solve it. When you discover an unresolved problem, solve it. When you are exposed to trauma, deal with it. Be aware that unresolved complexes may exist. Work on finding them later when you are once again stable and ready to problem-solve. Forgive yourself for all problems left unresolved and complexes you have yet to find. Continue working on them. Ask your Body-Mind to give you clues and information without making you sick. Pay attention to your thoughts, dreams, fears, fantasies, and lies you find. These are all clues. Write them down, journal, use the Polar Opposite Exercise, do everything you can, always making sure that you live by the One Sin Rule: hurt no one else, and certainly not yourself, in this process.

Do nice things for yourself. Live your life in harmony and balance as much as possible. Surround yourself with people who love you. Work at a job that not only supports you, but also facilitates your reaching for and obtaining your highest, healthiest, and best Self. Create hobbies and goals that allow you to expand yourself and keep challenged. Eat well and do nothing to harm yourself or your body. Live within your means. Develop friendships and spend time with friends and family. Consider yourself part of the Intelligence of the Universe. Pray and believe in God. Consider everyone around you as a part of this Intelligence, no matter their religion, ethnicity, race, color, or their personal beliefs. Remember the biblical injunction, *"Do onto others as you would have them do onto you."* Learn from your mistakes and do not criticize yourself or others. If you do, apologize to them and to yourself. Value yourself and your life. Love yourself and love life.

If you are not able to recognize or solve your problems or if you feel too intimidated or fearful of them, seek help. If you are not able to solve your problems, don't worry. It is not possible to solve every problem. Simply recognizing that they exist, and coming to peace with them may be enough. We must work on resolving those issues that are causing pain and suffering. We must even work harder on those issues that cause problems which might lead to or cause serious or life-threatening illness. Those conflicts that simply cause discomfort or minor problems can wait until you have resolved any serious or life threatening illness.

If you have completely assumed responsibility for causing and healing your illness, you will soon realize that you will only need to use medical doctors or other healers as tools to accomplish your goal of healing. Use their advice, skills, support, and abilities to perform medical treatments in helping your process of healing. For this reason, it is important to never work with anyone who does not believe completely in your getting well, that is UNLESS they perform a task you know is needed to get you well again. If you must work with someone who is not invested in your being fully healed, be careful and allow them to be involved no more than necessary. If you can, work only with healers you feel are on your side and can help you heal yourself.

Remember that treating is not healing. Be sure that your healer-practitioner possesses the skills you require to heal yourself. If you aren't being healed, move on and find another person who can provide you what you need.

Remember to always appreciate and to thank those people you use in your healing process. Acknowledge their value and help.

These actions give your Body-Mind a clear message that you are respectful, worthy, and that you recognize and believe that you have value. It tells your Body-Mind that you are willing and able to do whatever is necessary to protect yourself from anything that could possibly harm you. It says that you believe you are valuable enough to maintain the highest level of protection against future illness.

Tell your Body-Mind frequently that you love it. Tell your body that you love it. Tell you Conscious Aware Self that you also love it. Show your Body-Mind and Conscious Aware Self through your actions and choices that you mean this and you believe in yourself and in being healed. Tell yourself over and over again that you are willing to do everything you can to protect yourself, to re-establish optimal health, and are willing to do everything needed to do to keep yourself healthy. Then, do everything you can to make this happen.

Create a picture in your mind of what your life can look like when you are completely healthy and full of vitality and creativity. Create a picture of how long you want to live. Tell your Body-Mind to "make all of this so" and expect it.

Lastly and of great importance, live your life as if everything you have asked for is your birthright. Create as few lies and conflicts as possible. Listen to your body to recognize and solve any new problems. Learn to trust your body. Know that you and your Conscious Aware Self are the Body-Mind's supervisor. If you both treat it well, it will be your friend and partner.

This common-sense approach is the ideal process for creating and maintaining good health and well-being.

While at first, this all might sound difficult or even impossible; it is not. It is done every day, all over the world by healthy people. You already create ongoing pictures of what you want your life to be like every time you make a decision, think of an idea, or perform an activity. The only problem is that this picture may not be exactly what you want. It may not be clear, and it may not even be positive. Start today to create clear, concise, positive pictures of what you want your life to be like. Work by using the healing steps presented in this book. If you do this, your life will turn out exactly the way you want it. All you really have to do is know what you want and tell yourself and your Body-Mind what to create.

We have all felt the pain of lying to ourselves and the joy of knowing we told the truth. We know the price we pay for dishonesty, and we know how good we feel about ourselves when we do things right. We know that things generally

> ### If You Avoid Making Decisions, Life Will Make Them For You.

turn out as we want when we plan carefully and keep to the plan. We know that the less we like ourselves, the more we are unhappy. We have all seen people fail because they didn't believe in themselves, and we have seen others succeed and become happy because they did.

You know what it feels like when you are well, and you have experienced the misery of being sick. It is entirely up to you and what you are willing to settle for in your life. As with everything else, it is simply another set of decisions.

This concept can only be experienced by living it. To change your life, have a desire to do it for yourself. Our role as healers is to provide the information you need to empower you to create a healthy and joyful life. You must ultimately find or create the needed skills to help yourself become your highest, healthiest, and best Self. We offer help to anyone who needs it because we believe that every person we help also helps us to heal ourselves.

Once you enter the process of healing, you begin seeing who you really are and how you want to spend your time. When I, Allen, started into my own healing process, I soon realized that healing myself meant healing others. We cannot be our highest, healthiest, and best Self without healing others by sharing what life has taught us.

IS THERE A CONFLICT BETWEEN THE ROLE OF THE MEDICAL DOCTOR AND OTHER HEALERS?

No! While most medical doctors are primarily involved in the practice of interventive medicine, treating illness with medications, medical procedures and surgical treatments, they have the same goals as the non-interventive healer: helping sick people get well. As I stated earlier, interventive medicine practitioners generally believe that the cause of illness is due to infectious organisms or parasites, chemical imbalances, or imperfect tissues, factors that are external to the individual.

Healers know that illness most often comes from within and is caused by internal forces such as faulty belief systems, lies, fear, and faulty beliefs, sins, blocks, and complexes, as well as unresolved conflicts. While the interventive medical practitioner believes that healing is in his hands, the non-interventive healer will more likely believe that wellness is primarily in the hands of the patient himself.

To most interventive physicians, the underlying causes of illness are considered secondary to the treatment of the acute or chronic condition. Medical doctors may treat a patient for many years without ever relating the patient's condition to conflicts in the conscious or subconscious minds. These doctors are less interested in the causes of the illness than in relieving or eliminating the symptoms. If the patient doesn't get well, interventive medical doctors refer the patient to a specialist. Medical doctors may accuse their patients of not cooperating, or they may tell their patients, "your problems are all in your head." In any event, most medical doctors soon lose interest in the problems they cannot solve.

Non-interventive healers are aware that the individual with a Stress-Related Disorder may go to a medical doctor for help but often ends up being mistreated. They also do realize that their client/patient's symptoms and acute illnesses may require medical treatment to relieve acute pain, cure secondary infections, and protect their client/patient's life. However, they may also know that unless the causative process is discovered, treatment will be incomplete and healing may only be temporary.

Individuals who are ill should first be evaluated and treated through the process of interventive medicine. Treatment may be necessary to clear up acute life-threatening illness. Once stable, physicians should either switch their approach and work as a healer or refer the patient to someone who can help him resolve any underlying conflicts.

Patients don't want to hear that the underlying problem is, "in their mind." They want their problems solved and illnesses cured. Because of the influence of Western medicine, many people are not aware that Stress-Related Disorders exist. They not only believe in illness, they believe that once sick the best they can hope for is to receive medical treatment. Many people are willing to spend good portions of their lives and their income being treated with no hope of ever being cured. **These people confuse treatment with cure.** They assume that the medical profession is doing their best for them. They have little thought of cure, and when they do, their doctors often tell them that is only a wishful fantasy.

Medical practitioners have a responsibility to educate and inform their patients that a Stress-Related Disorder underlies their illness. Medical doctors who simply prescribe medications, procedures, or surgery and ignore the stress-related component are acting irresponsibly and mistreating their patients.

If a patient constantly returns with recurrent or new illnesses, the causative problem has not been solved. Individuals suffering from Stress-Related Disorders need more than just medication. This is especially true if they don't respond to medical care. The same is true with individuals who manifest anxiety, panic disorders, chronic fatigue syndrome, or other symptoms.

While it would be ideal for every physician to learn to recognize Stress-Related Disorders and to treat them as outlined here, we realize that this is not likely to happen in the near future. At present, the best that we can hope for is that physicians will recognize that Stress-Related Disorders exist. When they have ruled out acute, life-threatening medical processes it is our hope that they will then refer these patients to a medical specialist, psychologist, or other non-interventive healer for counseling and help.

ATTRIBUTES OF THE HEALER

Unless the physician acts as a complete healer, the healer's role is different from that of the physician. While the physician defines and treats specific medical problems, the healer helps patients transform their life situations from illness to wellness, health, inner harmony, and balance. This means teaching problem-solving techniques, helping patients develop their spiritual Self, or find an appropriate career or lifestyle. It may mean helping them solve relationship problems, finding inner peace, and reducing other causes of stress. The healer helps clients love and value themselves. Once these qualities are clarified and integrated into the true self, their highest, healthiest, and best Self, they let go of their illnesses and become healed.

Healers know that we can only change ourselves by changing what we choose to believe about our lives and ourselves. They know that only we can know what is true for us. How we live our lives is the only true measure of who we are. Healers are not magicians or con artists. They are not directors or dictators. Healers are simply guides and teachers who work with patients to help them find their own true Self.

The true healer never tries to take the decision-making power away from the client. Instead, they help their client identify choices, and then help their client learn techniques of decision making, problem solving, and sorting alternatives. The individual does all the work of healing. Healers help their clients recognize their own power. They help their clients learn to use this power wisely and directly for creating health and well-being. For healers to use their influence differently would mean not healing but controlling, and controlling destroys healing.

Healers should not have a stake in their clients' success. Healers should not feel a personal need for a client to heal, although they can root for their client to heal. The healers' main concern should be that they are being their own highest, healthiest, and best Selves whenever they work with any client.

This takes the ego aspect out of the healer's role and allows the client to count only on the healer's healing skills and heart.

It is also important that the healer envisions their clients as already being well. The next chapter looks further into the problems and benefits of the interventive practitioner becoming an integrated healer or working with other healers. It is important for both the physician and the nontraditional healer to remember that the health and well-being of the soon-to-be-fully-healed person is more important than their personal desires, egos, or biases.

Working together, the patient has a much better chance of being cured. Working together, we have a much better chance to heal our communities.

*Diseases
of the soul
are more dangerous
and more numerous
than those of the body.*

~Cicero

Chapter Nineteen

WORKING TOGETHER TO PROMOTE HEALING

HEALING AND INTERVENTIVE MEDICINE WORKING TOGETHER

While the overall intention of medical treatment should be to cure, this is not happening at present. Medical treatment is currently directed toward treating symptoms with drugs, not toward problem solving.

However, healing is not about treating. It is about curing and the elimination of the illness process. Both interventive medical doctors and healers agree that in treating an individual with high blood pressure, for example, the goal is to return the blood pressure to normal. The physician does this by prescribing medications. The healer accomplishes the same goal using diet, exercise, meditation and non-medication processes. Healing is also about finding the physical mental, emotional, or spiritual issues that are causing anger and unrest. It is most important to help the client find the issues that cause them to "boil" and hence raise their blood pressure. Today, more and more physicians are using diet, exercise, and techniques such as meditation, visualization, and self-help training to accomplish the goal of lowering blood pressure. This is great. However, once a medical doctor normalizes his patient's blood pressure, he is likely to consider his job done except for follow-up visits. The true healer knows this is where the real work begins.

The process of working with the patient to create a cure is done in steps. The first step is lowering the blood pressure and getting it under control so that the patient is not endangered. This is often most efficiently accomplished through medical treatment.

Once the patient's blood pressure is controlled and stable, the healing physician must begin the next step of guiding the patient through the healing process in order to help them heal their illness. The patient should lose weight; next reduce salt in the patient's diet if these are causative factors. The patient should then be instructed on how to eat an appropriate diet to maintain normal blood pressure. These steps are taken with some patients but they are not always done and may be missed in many patients who really need this help.

The patient is now stable, blood pressure is normal, and the work must change to finding and healing any related unresolved conflicts such as concealed anger, guilt, or shame that may have triggered and sustained the patient's high blood pressure. Techniques such as meditation are also effective and should be recommended and taught by the practitioner or referred to someone who can teach this to the patient. Biofeedback, acupuncture, herbs, and chiropractic therapy can also have beneficial effects in certain situations.

The physician should know when and how to use them, or at least support the patient in finding a competent teacher or practitioner who does. These non-traditional treatments can be used alone or in combination with medication to relieve non life-threatening hypertension. Eventually, as the factors that have caused the high blood pressure are resolved, blood pressure not only naturally returns to normal, but its cause is resolved and it will no longer be a problem in the future. Once the patient is stable and on an appropriate diet, performing a regular exercise program, and finally starts to solve the problem that needed to be solved, the patient might now slowly be weaned off all medications that were temporarily used to help control their blood pressure.

While the healing process takes time, the goals are simple. First, prevent acute injury from the high blood pressure by using medications to temporarily bring the blood pressure to a safe and manageable level. Second, solve any related unresolved conflicts that can be found and resolved. Third, as blood pressure returns to normal and the patient is stable and has created a new and healthier lifestyle, steadily withdraw all medication so that the patient is finally controlling their blood pressure naturally, either without need for any medication or at least the lowest possible dosage of medication necessary to maintain a normal blood pressure.

Always consider the patient's lifestyle as a contributing factor and as a part of their problem, at least until it is clear that these factors are not involved. At the beginning of any well-constructed healing program, the patient and the healer must look at all lifestyle factors that are commonly considered to affect or cause their health problem.

The healer must educate their patients as to their own roles in creating and healing their present conditions. He should produce a list of appropriate lifestyle changes which address solving the underlying causes of the health problems, as well as those factors making these problems worse or feeding them. This may include changes in diet and initiation of stress-reduction measures. They may go beyond these basic changes to include a directed exercise program, marital or other counseling, working with a wellness or life coach, or consulting an accountant. Whatever must be done must be done. These actions help convince the Body-Mind that you really mean business and truly desire to get well.

Teaching patients how to communicate with their Body-Mind is also key. The first thing they need to learn is to recognize imbalances and unresolved conflicts their Body-Mind has been trying to communicate through the symptoms they experience. As these conflicts are identified, they should be written down. In time order, create the list with the most problematic conflicts at the top.

This list may take years to complete. However, the Body-Mind will likely give you a few of the most and least important issues to see what you do with them. As you recognize the more important unresolved conflicts, you will want to reorder the list and move the least important and easiest to resolve conflicts to the top of the list. To do this you will have to rewrite the list moving the lowest priority issue to the top and the most difficult to resolve issues to the bottom. This now provides a hierarchy with the easiest and simplest issues to resolve at the top and the most difficult to resolve issues at the bottom. If you have any issues that require immediate attention or are potentially life-threatening, put these on a separate list for immediate action. If there are no significant immediate or life-threatening problems on your list, start with the simplest and easiest conflicts to resolve, and start resolving each item on your list as rapidly and effectively as you can. Keep all three lists. Compare them periodically to see that no important issue is missed, as well to judge your progress. Also, check your lists periodically to see whether you were right regarding which issues would be the easiest to resolve and which are more difficult to resolve. Creating these lists and acting on them accomplishes several important goals.

1) They allow you to become aware of which of your conflicts are easily resolved and hence completed.
2) They allow you to get them out of the way, reducing the total number of issue while reducing a significant amount of negative pressure that is likely affecting you.
3) This allows you to subconsciously work on the unresolved, more difficult issues without having to directly take them on and spend time working on them. This can help reduce future work and conflict.
4) Since the issues at top of your To Do List are simple and easy-to-solve conflicts, they can be used as a learning experience, as you gain valuable problem-solving practice. They help you better understand the problem-solving process and teach you how to resolve conflicts.
5) The simple process of resolving these unresolved conflicts brings you closer to balance and harmony in your life.
6) Solving these conflicts demonstrates to your Body-Mind that you not only care, but are working on many of the most problematic issues which it has been trying to inform you exist. It tells the Body-Mind you are listening to it and taking it seriously.
7) Each of these conflicts can only be resolved through solving problems and forming healthier belief systems to replace less-workable or illness-producing belief systems.

As you resolve each issue you will move forward and gain confidence in your ability to heal yourself and use problem-solving techniques that can be used again and again throughout the remainder of your life.

Clearly, this is not going to be an easy task. It is also unlikely that merely solving one or two problems will allow everything in your life to return to perfectly normal. Rather, this will be an ongoing process that you will use repeatedly. You can reclaim your health and well-being, organize your affairs, and create new or re-establish old healthy lifestyle habits that can steadily bring you back to optimal health and wellness. This process takes time, work, and a great deal of energy. Your goal is a complete return to optimal health and wellness. While you can stop anywhere along the way, you will be working on this process for the rest of your life if you choose total health and wellness.

As you recognize and resolve your previously unresolved conflicts, you will steadily move forward toward optimal health and wellness. Eventually, your Body-Mind begins to believe and trust that you really want to heal yourself. It then allows some illnesses to fall away and some medications are no longer necessary.

As you work on resolving your underlying causes and problems, your physician can work with you to create a safe and effective process for withdrawing the now-unnecessary medications. The reduction in dosage or use of prescription medications should always be done under the close supervision of an involved physician. As the dosages and use of medications are reduced, the goal of your physician and any healers working with you is to accomplish this reduction as safely and successfully as possible. This requires careful monitoring and conservative decision making. Eventually when all is done right and you are healed, there should be no further need for medications. Whether or not you reach this point is not the main issue; solving your unresolved conflicts and problems is the primary goal. Reducing the dosage of your medications is merely a secondary benefit. **Remember, once any medication has been prescribed and started, only your prescribing physician should stop or reduce the dosage. Medication prescribed by a physician should never be altered or changed by non-physician healers or the patient**.

The idea of interventive medical doctors, healers, and patients all working together as a team is rare in Western medicine. However, this process can work for any condition that meets the criteria of a Stress-Related Disorder or any illness that has a stress component to it. By adopting this concept, the medical profession would be elevated from its present role of treating symptoms to its optimal role of healing. As medical schools begin teaching more about the relationship between stress and illness, we will hopefully see a significant reduction in illness in our society. Only then will physicians become full-fledged healers.

MEDICINE AND HEALING WORKING TOGETHER

In a society such as ours where the population believes so strongly in illness, medical care is extremely important. Physicians are seen as the gatekeepers of health. They not only perform physical examinations, but also care for and protect patients and their families–often for entire lifetimes. Most people give complete control of their bodies to their medical profession for safeguarding.

The established norm is going to one's family doctor whenever we don't feel well. Our doctor is the first line of defense against illness. However, **you** are the first-line protector and guardian for illness prevention.

As we have repeatedly suggested, the individual who sees his physician with vague symptoms, whose physical examination shows nothing abnormal, and whose laboratory tests are negative is most likely exhibiting a Stress-Related Disorder.

Physicians have two paths at this point. They may treat patients with medications, or they may recognize the symptoms of Stress-Related Disorders. Medicating patients may only lead to a limited result, the incomplete relief of symptoms, and the later return of symptoms.

If the symptoms are completely resolved, but the patient is back within a short period with the same symptom or an entirely new problem, the physician may have to re-evaluate whether this is a primary illness or a Stress-Related Disorder. If the physician recognizes his patient's condition as a Stress-Related Disorder, he must decide whether he has the capacity, skill, and interest to treat his patient's underlying problems. If he is able, he can perform the role of the healer by educating, counseling, and guiding the patient to wellness. If he is not capable of doing this, he should immediately refer his patient to a healer who is trained and able accomplish this. A good physician seeks to heal, not merely treat. A physician who only treats symptoms is merely a technician. A great physician is one who can help his patient heal himself and recognizes that there are other healers who can do a better job and refers his patient to them.

The natural history of the process of illness, the Wellness-Stress-Illness Mechanism (see Table: 19-1, below) requires an enlightened physician to head the team.

It is in the patient's best interest to be attended to by a physician who is capable of managing and directing the evaluation and treatment of the illness portion of this complex. The healer must always work with a physician. The job of healing an individual is a team process. If all team members know what they are doing, the patient gets the very best. The patient's needs must always come first in the healing process.

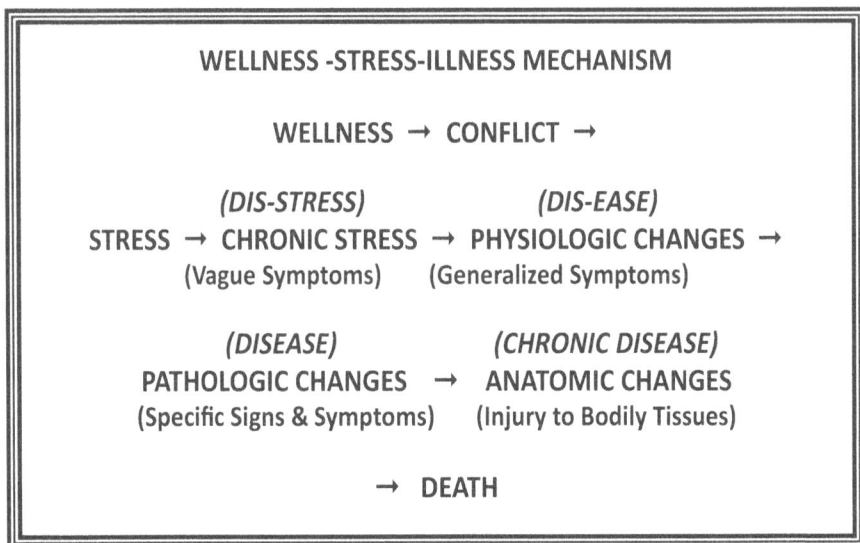

```
WELLNESS -STRESS-ILLNESS MECHANISM

WELLNESS → CONFLICT →

        (DIS-STRESS)              (DIS-EASE)
STRESS → CHRONIC STRESS → PHYSIOLOGIC CHANGES →
        (Vague Symptoms)    (Generalized Symptoms)


        (DISEASE)              (CHRONIC DISEASE)
PATHOLOGIC CHANGES  →   ANATOMIC CHANGES
(Specific Signs & Symptoms)  (Injury to Bodily Tissues)


            →  DEATH
```

Table: 19-1

The public and law at present see the physician as the most responsible caretaker, but this is changing. More people are choosing non-medical alternative care in the form of nutritionists, chiropractors, body workers, herbalists, acupuncturists, even tarot readers, and spiritualists. Some see this as a sign of the medical profession's inability to provide for the community's many needs. Others recognize, as we do, that there are many ways of helping a person regain harmony and balance. The likelihood of success is much greater when all parties work together.

What the medical profession will have to ultimately recognize is that physicians, unless trained as holistic healers, will most likely have to work with alternative healers for the patient's benefit. Both must remember that in the healing situation, which is very different from the present interventive medical system, the individual is always fully responsible for his own healing.

True healers are always working toward putting themselves out of a job, since they are always working to help their clients/patients cure themselves. A true healer is also dedicated to a healed world.

**The Healer Must Always
Work With A Physician.**

Some medical doctors may fear that if every one of their patients were healed, they would not only be out of a job but would have no value. This could never happen, at least not in our lifetime. Some medical doctors are too invested in their belief in illness and disease that they have no clear understanding of true healing. Some cannot envision a world free of illness, pain, or suffering, a world where sickness and illness don't exist. Some may not believe it possible that they themselves could reach for and find their highest, healthiest, and best Self through becoming a healer and healing their patients.

This concept has not been part of their training, and they do not know it as individuals. It is up to each physician to make an independent choice whether to simply treat signs and symptoms of illness, or work at healing the whole person. It is also up to each person seeking wellness to decide what is best for them—a technician dedicated to keeping them sick, or a physician-healer dedicated to helping them cure, repair and heal. It is also up to the medical establishment to choose between maintaining the old system, which clearly doesn't work, or joining other healers to forge a new covenant with their community, healing instead of treating.

Most doctors today are dedicated to getting people well through what they believe is modern and scientific treatment. In this sense, they are probably not significantly different from their physician counterparts some 150 years ago who bled and leached their patients as the most accepted form of medical practice at that time. Just as those treatments were built on faulty beliefs, so is treating only with drugs and surgery without finding a cause or creating a plan for a cure.

For centuries, well-meaning doctors have done their best to treat what they couldn't see or understand. In other words, they fought enemies they did not know or understand how to fight. Believing that the dogmas of the time were scientific truths, they drew blood, leached, flogged, purged, and starved patients all in the name of wellness and a desire to cure. We may think we are considerably more sophisticated today, but we still do much the same thing. We wait until the person is ill before we intervene. We treat symptoms instead of cure illness. We put off resolution and healing by simply treating, thereby risking side effects, adverse reactions, chronic irreversible diseases, dependency, addictions, and a great deal of suffering all while telling ourselves we are trying to heal. We do this even when we see and often know that we are neither healing nor curing our patients.

It is time that we move to the next level—curing and healing. It is time that the medical profession put emphasis on prevention and transforming illness into wellness. It is also time that the public take responsibility for its own well-being. We cannot entirely blame the medical profession for the current state of affairs. They came to their present situation because of decisions made by previous generations of medical doctors. Their predecessors believed in illness and gave it power, as one pays homage to a superstition. Most of the general population also believes that illness is inevitable and that taking medication and undergoing surgery is best.

We frequently have patients telling us, "Just give me something to get rid of the problem. I'm too busy for anything else," or, "I'm not here to talk. I'm here to get medication." Few patients are willing to change their diets, exercise, or create new habits or lifestyles. Yet when we sit down with these same people, we quickly see the layers upon layers of lies, faulty belief systems, confusion, and lack of self-love and self-caring they created for themselves through the years. There can be no productive changes for patients or our society unless the medical profession is willing to be educated and work at changing public opinion.

Possibly no single story demonstrates these issues better than that of a patient we saw a number of years ago. We shall never forget her. Her story demonstrates just about all of the principles we have been discussing.

THE STORY OF MARGARET N., A WOMAN IN HER 70'S:

Margaret N. demonstrates how illness is created and the consequences of giving power to belief in illness. Margaret put herself in the hands of her doctor, unaware that her doctor was much too busy to be fully aware or even care about what was happening in her life. While her doctor saw the events in her life unfolding right before his eyes, he was either unwilling or unable to stop and put together the pieces of the puzzle. He accepted no frame of reference for Margaret outside of his training. He treated her without understanding what was happening to her. Is this malpractice? No! Is this negligence? Maybe! He treated her for serious medical problems when she demonstrated symptoms and signs of Stress-Related Disorders.

What ultimately happened to Margaret N. happened not only because of her doctor's lack of knowledge or caring, but also because she had surrendered her power to him and to her fears. She also demonstrated neither interest nor desire to reach for her highest, healthiest, or best Self.

Margaret N. came to us with a long history of chest pain, weakness, dizzy spells, and occasional blackout episodes. We spent a good deal of time talking with Margaret trying to understand what was happening to her. We soon recognized that to understand what was currently happening to Margaret, we had to understand what her life had been about. We also knew that in order to really understand Margaret and her problems we also had to understand her relationship with her husband, and his problems as well.

The story unfolded as follows: Margaret first told us that she had been perfectly healthy and happy until her husband Tom died of a sudden heart attack. Later, Margaret admitted that she had been angry with Tom for several years before his death because he worked incessantly "for the good of the family" and never took any time off. Margaret and Tom often talked about traveling the world together after he retired. This never happened. Tom refused to watch his diet and never took care of himself. Through the years, he gained weight, became less active, and had episodes of fatigue.

Tom was a meat-and-potatoes man. He loved steaks and roasts, eggs and butter, cream in his coffee, and fried foods. He smoked two to three packs of cigarettes daily and drank heavily. When he wasn't working, he would be off with his friends gambling and drinking.

Margaret was a stay-at-home mother who took care of the house and children. She said nothing to Tom about his smoking, drinking, gambling, or incessant working. They occasionally argued about small things, but Margaret generally accepted her lot and allowed Tom to live his life as he wanted. Everything was generally okay until Margaret accidentally found out from Tom that the nurse at his work told him that his blood pressure was "higher than it should be." From that point, they argued a lot about Tom having high blood pressure and his refusal to see Dr. M., their family physician.

At one point, Margaret insisted so vehemently that he go to and see Dr. M. that Tom finally agreed, if for no other reason, according to Margaret, to "shut her up!" Tom had a complete physical examination. After the exam, Dr. M. told Tom that he indeed did have high blood pressure. During this visit, Dr. M. put him on medication for his blood pressure. The medication made Tom impotent. Margaret and Tom discussed his inability to get erections. While Margaret begged Tom to tell Dr. M., Tom refused to go back and get Dr. M. "involved." "All he'll do," Tom argued, "will be to put me on another medication that will do the same thing or worse." Tom told ultimately Margaret, "All I would be doing is just giving him my hard-earned money for nothing."

One Saturday afternoon shortly after Tom's fifty-eighth birthday, Tom complained to Margaret that he was feeling tired. Margaret suggested that he lie down and nap for a while. Tom agreed and started climbing the steps to their bedroom when he suddenly clutched his chest, fell over, and died.

After Tom's death, Margaret mourned for nearly three-and-a-half years. She wouldn't consider "dating," as her children suggested because this would be disrespectful to Tom's memory. Therefore, she remained lonely and unhappy. She lived alone and could not forgive Tom for dying. She couldn't let go of her anger at Tom for leaving her alone after all his promises and all of the plans they had discussed to be together into their "old age."

Four years after Tom's death, Margaret began having periodic chest pain. Her daughter took her to see Dr. M. While her electrocardiograms, chest x-ray, and blood tests were all normal, and she had no other signs of acute heart disease, Dr. M. told her that he believed that she was having episodes of angina. He prescribed nitroglycerin. Margaret returned monthly for a while as she continued having frequent episodes of chest pain. All further x-rays, electrocardiograms, and even a cardiac stress test were negative. Dr. M. changed her medications several times, each time adding new medications to the old ones. When Margaret asked Dr. M. why she continued to have chest pain in spite of the medications, he told her that she had "intractable angina."

At several of her regular visits, Margaret told Dr. M. that she was having trouble sleeping, was gaining weight, and was very unhappy about that. He gave her a prescription for sleeping pills and recommended she go to Weight Watchers to lose weight. She used the sleeping pills regularly but found after awhile that she could not sleep without them. She tried Weight Watchers but didn't lose weight.

During the next two to three years, her chest pain persisted—it was located directly over her heart. Subsequently a CT scan of the chest, a gall bladder series, an upper gastrointestinal x-ray series, and a small bowel series were all performed. All these test results were normal. They provided no explanation for her pain. Dr. M. changed her medications repeatedly. He added new and different medications a number of times during the next few years.

Eventually, Margaret began having the episodes of weakness, dizzy spells, and occasional blackouts that she soon called her "loss of awareness spells." She repeatedly told Dr. M. that they would leave her feeling weak, tired, and sad. Shortly after these episodes started, Dr. M. ordered a CT scan of the brain and carotid angiography. Both were normal. Dr. M. told Margaret that she was now suffering from "ischemic brain episodes," that her brain was not getting sufficient oxygen for her needs. Dr. M. told her that it was possible that she could have a stroke at any time. Several weeks later during a follow up visit, Margaret's blood pressure was quite low, and Dr. M. told her that she needed more exercise. Another new medication was prescribed to compensate for this new symptom.

During the next couple of years, Margaret's symptoms would come and go. Margaret told Dr. M. that she noticed that her chest pains always seemed to come when she thought about Tom and all she had lost because of his dying so young. However, Dr. M. didn't seem to think this meant anything, so Margaret disregarded it as having any meaning. Margaret never did start exercising, and Dr. M. never brought the subject up again. He also never asked her about her fears, dreams, thoughts, or frustrations, or even why she never got over being angry with Tom. He simply treated her symptoms and her acute medical problems.

During the next four to five years, her condition remained steady. She saw Dr. M. periodically, and he continued refilling her medications without ever examining her. By this time, she was taking eight different medications daily.

One morning, Margaret awoke and felt an unusual lump in her left breast while taking her morning shower. Her first thought was that it might be cancer. This so terrified her that she couldn't allow herself to think about it. For the next several days, she tried to ignore it and put it out of her mind. After ten days, she touched the area again and the lump was still there. Several more days passed before she told her daughter about it. Her daughter immediately called her own personal physician, Dr. S., and set up a quick appointment for Margaret later in that same day, and her daughter drove Margaret to his office for an examination.

Dr. S. examined Margaret, sent her for a mammography, and made an appointment for her with Dr. W., a general surgeon. The following day, Margaret saw Dr. W. He immediately scheduled her for a biopsy where the lump was removed and sent for pathology. Several days later, the surgeon's nurse called Margaret to tell her the tumor was benign (not cancer). Everyone was greatly relieved. A note of interest: Dr. M. had been Margaret's family doctor for nearly 20 years, had never done a routine breast examination on her, and had not done more than a cursory basic examination since the visit when she was having chest pain almost nine years earlier. Neither he nor she had discussed or thought about routine mammography.

Just after her sixty-seventh birthday, Margaret had an episode of vaginal bleeding. Once again, she called her daughter and again went to see Dr. S. He admitted her into the hospital and performed a D&C procedure. The tissue biopsy demonstrated a very early cancer of the uterus. No pap smear or pelvic exams had been done in more than twelve years. A hysterectomy was performed, after which radiation treatments were given. Shortly after her radiation treatments, Margaret began having episodes of diarrhea, sometimes with blood. A lower GI was performed and then a sigmoidoscopy, which is a tube placed in the lower bowel to check for cancer. The GI specialist later told Margaret that he believed that there had been some injury to the lower bowel caused by her radiation treatments.

Margaret was placed on a special diet and given more medications. During this period, she had fewer episodes of chest pain, but not only continued experiencing her "spells," but they were more frequent. While she later described that her "life had returned to normal," she also admitted that she continued experiencing intermittent chest pain and an increased frequency of her "spells." Margaret continued seeing Dr. M. who continued treating her for her chest pain and "spells."

We saw Margaret for the first time shortly after her seventieth birthday. Dr. M. recently died, and she came to an office where I was filling in for Dr. M. while his family was looking for someone to take over his practice. She and her daughter provided me most of the history I just related. I did also have Dr. M.'s chart and records to get his perspective as well as the results of the hundreds of test he had performed on her during the nearly twenty-five years he had treated her. That day I had time to talk with both Margaret and her daughter, so I did. Margaret's answers to my questions were very revealing.

Dr. Lawrence:	Do you still miss your husband?
Margaret:	Yes, I do! My heart is still breaking over his loss. I miss him so much. I feel empty without him.
Dr. Lawrence:	Are you still angry at him for dying?
Margaret:	No!

Dr. Lawrence: Never?

Margaret: Well, I was angry at him when he died.

Dr. Lawrence: Why?

Margaret: Well, because we had plans. I was counting on him. He hadn't taken care of himself at all. He had allowed himself to get terribly overweight. He wouldn't see a doctor for his high blood pressure. He wouldn't stop smoking and he drank too much.

Margaret paused at this point, took a deep breath and waited awhile.

Dr. Lawrence: What else?

Margaret: Well, he just wouldn't take care of himself. It was almost like he wanted to die.

Dr. Lawrence: How did you feel immediately after he died?

Margaret: I felt abandoned, I felt betrayed.

Dr. Lawrence: How do you feel now?

Margaret: I still feel abandoned and also lonely. For years I would wake up in the middle of the night crying and screaming at him for leaving me.

Dr. Lawrence: Is that when you would have your chest pains?

Margaret: Yes. They would start after I had cried for a while. First my chest would start hurting and then, when there were no more tears, all I would have was the chest pains.

Dr. Lawrence: Did you ever tell any of this to Dr. M.

Margaret: No!

Dr. Lawrence: Why not?

Margaret: He never asked and I wasn't sure that the two were connected.

Dr. Lawrence: What do you think now?

Margaret: I think that my heart was broken and I didn't know what to do about it.

Dr. Lawrence: What about all the medications Dr. M. put you on?

Margaret: Well, I trusted him. I assumed that he knew what he was doing. When he told me that I had an angina problem, who was I to disagree?

Dr. Lawrence: What about the dizzy spells and the blackouts that you had a couple of years later? What do you think they were about?

Margaret: I believed that they were due to the medications that I was taking. When I stopped the medication for a while the spells also stopped.

Dr. Lawrence: Did you ever tell this to doctor M.?

Margaret: Yes, once.

Dr. Lawrence:	What did he say?
Margaret:	He told me that it wasn't likely that the medications were causing it because he suspected that I was having Ischemic Brain Episodes. My brain wasn't getting enough oxygen.
Dr. Lawrence:	What did you do then?
Margaret:	I stayed on the medication, of course. After all, he's the doctor. He should know what he's doing.
Dr. Lawrence:	Are you still having these episodes now?
Margaret:	No!
Dr. Lawrence:	Why not?
Margaret:	He took me off the heart medicine that caused it because it wasn't helping to stop my chest pain. I don't have any more problems with dizziness.
Dr. Lawrence:	How did you feel when you found out that you were right?
Margaret:	Well, everyone is entitled to make a mistake. I don't think he did it intentionally. I've forgiven him.

Margaret and I talked on several more occasions. She remained angry with Tom. Then one day after talking for a while, she told me that it was time to let go of Tom and get on with her life. She started dating a man she met at a senior's dance. I had also referred her to an excellent cardiologist. He reviewed all past records and repeated some of the studies. He concluded that there was no definite evidence of angina, no heart problem, and no indication of problematic heart disease. Within two months, we had taken her off all of her medications. Her chest pain went away and she later moved in with her new boyfriend. When I last saw her, she thanked me and told me that if I hadn't started her thinking about what she had been doing and what she was missing, she would have continued living a dreary and empty life. Her last words to me as she left were, "I believe I have a new lease on life. I want to live and I want to enjoy myself. Nothing is going to keep me from doing that."

WHAT IS THE IDEAL SITUATION?

In the ideal situation, the physician should make the diagnosis, determine the extent of the illness-disease process, and help the patient design a wellness and healing plan. When the process is in its early stages and medications are either unnecessary or just to control discomfort, the patient should be referred to a healer, a specially trained physician, or counselor. This should be someone who can work with the patient to define their conflicts and help them reestablish balance in their life.

In the previous example, the family physician, Dr. M., apparently did not consider looking for a Stress-Related Disorder after Margaret presented herself with chest pain. Several clues were present suggesting a Stress-Related Disorder, her ECG, chest x-rays, blood and other tests were all normal, and she had no meaningful response to nitroglycerin. These clues, along with the relatively recent death of her husband, should have triggered some suspicion by Dr. M. Instead, he chose to label her with an unsubstantiated diagnosis.

As time passed, more illnesses occurred. Yet, she continued being treated with medications and then surgery. Margaret's emotions, conflicts, and fears were ignored. It is possible to support Dr. M. and his decisions. Yet, one must stop and think that had her family physician been more astute and considered a Stress-Related Disorder, how that might have changed the direction Margaret's life took. Possibly two surgeries, radiation therapy, years of taking medication, and considerable pain and discomfort, loneliness, depression, sadness, and anxiety could have been avoided.

It is too late to know if a different approach could have made a difference for Margaret. However, it is not too late for millions of other men and women who will see their physician for help this year and in the following years. It is essential that Stress-Related Disorders always be considered when the criteria for their existence are present.

WHAT ABOUT ADVANCED ILLNESSES?

When a patient goes to a physician with an advanced process, the physician must remain in close control of the patient. The healer should work directly with the patient and physician. The healer should ensure that the patient is regularly followed up and routinely examined. Medications should be monitored for side effects and adverse reactions until the physician can safely stop these medications. The goal of both physician and healer should be to help the patient cure and have resolution, not long-term treatment.

Healers should make sure that their clients have had a recent, complete physical examination and that the physician is aware of the patient's physical status and the level of Stress-Related Disorders. Healers should communicate with the physician and help create a plan of action. A Healing and Wellness Plan should be set up. When necessary, all prior medical records should be reviewed to determine the length and degree of the Stress-Related Disorders and associated problems. By doing this, the patient gets the best results possible.

In some cases, the client/patient may be unwilling to accept help or allow either medical or healing techniques to be used to solve their problems. They may not acknowledge that they have any underlying conflicts or any medical problems. In this situation, the cooperation of the entire team is necessary to support the patient while they sort through their fears and anxieties, unresolved conflicts and physical, mental, emotional, and spiritual symptoms. It may be a long time before some patients are ready to accept being involved with or starting into a healing process. The healer may have to accept that some individuals may choose to remain on medication for the rest of their lives.

The healer may have to accept that some patients will not want to be healed. Physicians may have to accept that some patients will refuse treatment even when the physician truly believes that certain medications are essential for protecting their patient's health, life, and well-being.

The medical profession will also have to accept that some patients will be unwilling to submit to medical evaluation and examination, and that only the healer may be trusted. It is up to the medical profession and the healers to put aside their differences, egos, and financial interests and join so that their patient feels confident that both are only interested in the his/her well-being.

Both must learn to identify Stress-Related Disorders and then learn to treat and heal them. Working together openly signals to everyone that wellness, health, and healing are the only enlightened goals. Awareness of Stress-Related Disorders and their symptoms should be made more available to the public, so that anyone can easily recognize the physical, mental, emotional, and spiritual symptoms that may indicate unresolved problems and conflicts. Only then will people be willing to do something about these conflicts and problems before they escalate into the Dis-Ease or the Disease Stages. Only then will we be able to positively affect the Stress-Illness Mechanism.

Imagine A World
Where Everyone Is Healed,
Where Everyone Is A Friend,
And Where Life Exists Without Illness.

Wouldn't That Be
A Wonderful World To Live In?

Only through widely based educational and public programs will the message get out. People educated in this process will be less fearful of both medical treatment and non-medical healing. The hope is that many more people will be more willing to heal themselves, and that the healing process will be easier and more productive. With community support, people will learn much more quickly how to solve their own problems and our entire society will change for the good. These changes can benefit everyone and our entire society will learn, grow, and evolve with it.

*If I'd known
I was going
to live so long,
I'd have taken
better care of myself.*

~Leon Eldred

Chapter Twenty

THE EPILOGUE

The concept of healing is certainly not new. It long predates modern Western medicine. The arrival of quantum physics initiated a new paradigm for medicine. The changes taking place now require support from all who believe, as we do, that it is possible to have a world without illness, a world of brotherly love and tolerance. This is because illness is nonproductive. It robs us of great talent and opportunities to evolve ourselves and our society.

While we will never be without stress, it is possible that we can become sufficiently knowledgeable about it that we can create systems that can both control and eliminate it before it causes harm. Life can be less stressful. We can also learn to harness stress in productive ways, turning negative stress into positive challenges. We can also learn to recognize it early and gear our physiological systems to more effectively assist in this transformative process. We can prepare people to deal with stress more effectively and easily.

We believe that knowledge about stress, health problems, and illness prevention is so important that it should be taught in our schools starting in kindergarten. Everyone should be taught self-help techniques. Physicians, nurses, medical educators, dentists, chiropractors, nutritionists, podiatrists, optometrists, exercise and fitness instructors, as well as all other health-related practitioners should be involved in defining a program that teaches children and their parents how to prevent illness and optimize their health and well-being.

It is unfortunate that in a time when communications are so easy, health professionals still have so little contact with each other. It is essential that health practitioners of all types get together and share knowledge as part of their training and daily routines. No sick person should be denied this kind of integrated approach. When we are finally capable of doing this, our society will have evolved from one interested in dollars to one interested in life, joy, and the well-being of all humanity. When we can do this for the whole planet, we will have evolved from being merely men and women to being gods (with a little 'g').

Our goal with this book has been to introduce stress, what it is and what causes it. In the course of this book, we have looked at the many processes which create stress and make stress meaningful to you. Through understanding stress, you should now know how it can and does affect your health, what causes it, what it is trying to tell you and finally, even more importantly, how you can heal it.

As we become more and more adept at recognizing the signs and symptoms of stress and Stress-Related Disorders, we can recognize stress earlier and we can learn to resolve the many underlying problems and unresolved conflicts which trigger and drive it. Once we can recognize and eliminate our stress we can, with little effort, return ourselves to complete wellness and total well-being.

It is most important to remember that **When Your Body Talks**, take time, and pay attention, **Listen!** to it and what it has to tell you.

The Beginning.

* PLEASE NOTE:

The lists of symptoms, signs, illnesses,
diseases & conditions
presented here in all of these tables & appendices
are by no means exhaustive nor complete.

The conditions suggested represent primarily
examples of manifestations & conditions
that are most commonly associated with stress.

You may be aware of other conditions
associated with stress. Please feel free
to add them to these lists.

While stress is not the only cause
for most of these conditions,
it should be noted that stress does play
an important & direct role
in the creation & causation
of some while leading to or causing
the triggering or worsening of others.

APPENDIX A

EXAMPLES OF PHYSICAL SYMPTOMS
CAUSED BY OR ASSOCIATED WITH STRESS*

GENERAL
Cold, clammy hands &/ or feet/
    increased sweating
Faintness/ dizziness/ numbness/
    paralysis
Frequent bouts with flu-like
    symptoms (possibly related to
    lowered immune system & body
    resistance)/ more colds than
    normal
Increased appetite & obesity/
    decreased appetite & being
    too skinny
Inability to work
Sudden bursts of energy
Rashes/ acneform rashes/ eczema /
    urticaria (hives)/ allergic reactions

IMMUNOLOGIC
Reduced resistance to infection
Tumor promotion

**EXTREMITIES-MUSCULOSKELETAL
SYSTEMS**
Arthritic-like joint pains
Muscle aches (especially neck, shoul-
ders,
    back or legs) cramping/ tightness
Neck pain/ backache & pains/
    sharp, momentary, shooting pains
Numbness/ paralysis of extremities
Unexplained fatigue/ recurrent or
    chronic fatigue/ muscle weakness/
    lethargy/ tired feelings

GASTROINTESTINAL SYSTEM
Nausea/ vomiting/ diarrhea/
    constipation/
bloating/ biliousness
Stomach or abdominal pain/
    acid-indigestion/ reflux of acid
    into esophagus

URINARY-REPRODUCTIVE SYSTEMS
 Frequent urination/ difficulty
    starting & stopping urination
Discomfort on urination/ impotence
Irregular Menstruation/ menstrual
    cramps/ worsening of premenstrual
    syndrome/ skipped menstrual
    periods/ stopped menstrual periods

HEAD-EYES-EARS-NOSE-THROAT
Dry mouth/ bad breath/
    difficulty swallowing
Eye strain
Facial tics & twitching
Frowning or frequent wrinkling
    of the forehead
Headaches/ migraines/ tension
    headaches/ sinus headaches
Jaw clenching/ jaw pain/ bruxism/
    tenomandibular joint syndrome
Ringing in the ears
Teeth gnashing & grinding

**RESPIRATORY-CARDIOVASCULAR
SYSTEMS**
Crackling, hacking, chronic cough
Chest pains/ shortness of breath/
    angina-like symptoms
Hyperventilation
Rapid heartbeat/ irregular
    heartbeat/ arrhythmia/
    palpitations

APPENDIX B
COMMON BEHAVIORAL AND OTHER MANIFESTATIONS
CAUSED BY OR ASSOCIATED WITH STRESS*

GENERAL
Frigidity/ Loss of sex drive increased or chain smoking increased or decreased appetite/ Insomnia/ Nightmares/ Frequent day-dreaming

EMOTIONAL
Altered moods/ feeling like there is a fog/ Cloudy/ Curtain separating you from your life/ Nagging
An awareness that while you are organized and working hard, you are not producing or accomplishing much
Crying episodes/ Laughing episodes with no apparent reason
Episodes of fear/ anxiety/ Feeling on edge/ feeling tense/ Nervousness/ Panic episodes
Feelings of frustration/ inability to define the reason for frustration
Feeling you must always have something to do/ can't sit still and enjoy life
Poor judgment/ Confusion

PHYSICAL
Persistent ache in the center of your being
Restlessness/ Unnecessary hand-waving/ Wild gestures
Stuttering
Unconscious foot or finger-tapping/ Nail biting/ Scratching/ Picking at body
Pacing

MEMORY AND THOUGHT PROCESS
Difficulty concentrating/ Must continually re-read material/ Inattentiveness/ Shortening
of memory or attention span
Foggy thinking/ Racing thoughts/ Impaired judgments Indecisiveness/ Feeling confused/ Fear of making decisions
Memory slips/ Loss/ Inability to remember familiar names and faces/ Reduced instant recall/ Reverie
The knowledge that the little problems you've been experiencing disappear completely when you are absorbed in a movie or something pleasurable to you but return immediately when the activity is over.
Stuttering
Waves of anger/ Feeling hurt/ disappointment/Depression/ Irritability/ bad temper
Traumatic and post traumatic stress syndromes

DIGESTIVE
Eating problems/ Anorexia
Abdominal pain
Obesity

APPENDIX C - 1
STRESS-RELATED DISORDERS *
COMMON MEDICAL PROBLEMS AFFECTED BY OR RELATED TO STRESS

GENERAL
Accidents/ Injuries
    (to all areas of the body)
Anorexia
Bad Dreams
Chronic fatigue syndrome
Edema
Excessive use of alcohol/ Alcoholism
Excessive smoking
Hair loss
Pain of various sorts
Poor eating habits
Premature aging
Sexual addictions

CARDIOVASCULAR
Arrhythmias
Coronary artery disease
Hardening of the arteries
Heart Attack
Heart diseases of various kinds
Hyperlipidemia
Hypertension
Hypercholesterolemia
Stroke

EAR-NOSE-THROAT
Allergic rhinitis
Ear infections/ Otitis
Flu syndrome
Post nasal drip
Sinusitis
Sore throats/ Pharyngitis
Upper respiratory infections/ Colds
Vertigo
Visual problems

ENDOCRINE-METABOLIC SYSTEMS
Age onset diabetes
Hypoglycemia
Menopause
Obesity
Premenstrual syndrome
Thyroid disease (hyperthyroidism &
    hypothyroidism, Hashimoto's
    Thyroiditis hypothyroidism)

IMMUNOLOGIC
Allergy
Autoimmune diseases
Cancer
Collagen diseases
Food allergies
Hay fever
Infections
Reduced resistance to infection
Tumor promotion

GASTROINTESTINAL
Colitis
Constipation
Diarrhea
Esophagitis
Flatulency (Excessive gas)
Gastritis
Gastroesophogeal reflux
Hemorrhoids
Hyperacidity
Indigestion
Irritable bowel syndrome
Pain of various sorts
Peptic ulcer disease
Polyps
Rectal itching

MUSCULOSKELETAL/VASCULAR SYSTEMS
Arthritis
Cervical pain, spasm, &
    stiffness/Torticollis
Claudication - blood vessel spasm
Joint pains & stiffness
Low back pain spasm & stiffness
Migraine headaches
Muscle aches & stiffness
Problems of the hands & feet
Sprains of ankles & knees
Tension headaches
Thoracic back pain, spasm, & stiffness

APPENDIX C - 2
STRESS-RELATED DISORDERS *
COMMON MEDICAL PROBLEMS AFFECTED BY OR RELATED TO STRESS

REPRODUCTIVE SYSTEMS
Breast cancer
Breast pain, lumps, tenderness, &
   tumors
Cervical & uterine pain,
   infection & cancers
Dysfunctional uterine bleeding
Failure to Menstruate
Hypermenorrhea (Excessive menstrual
   bleeding)
Impotence
Infertility (When no physical
   abnormality is found–male &
   female)
Oligomenorrhea (Missed menstrual
   periods)
Ovarian pain, infections, & tumors
Pelvic pain (when no other reasons
   are found)
Tubal infections, pain, & blockage
Vaginal & vulvar infections &
   symptoms

RESPIRATORY
Air Hunger
Asthma
Bronchitis
Cough
Difficulty breathing

PSYCHIATRIC
Addictions of various types
Anxiety
Bulimia
Depression
Emotional diseases/ Insecurity & fear
Neuroses
Panic attacks
Post-traumatic stress syndrome
Transient situational disturbances

SKIN
Acne
Dandruff/ Seborrhea dermatitis
Eczema/ Eczematoid dermatitis
Fungal dermatitis
Non-specific dermatitis
Pruritus
Skin Tumors
Urticaria (Hives), Non-specific
Warts

URINARY TRACT SYSTEMS
Bed wetting
Bladder infections/ Cystitis
Incontinence
Prostate Infection, enlargement &
   tumors, including prostate cancer
Stress incontinence
Urethritis

**NON-MEDICAL PROBLEMS
AFFECTED BY STRESS**
Business problems
Criminal behavior
Financial problems
Gambling addiction
Job problems
Lying
Marital problems & affairs
Misused life
Parental problems
Problems with children
Spiritual problems
Stuttering

0

APPENDIX D - 1
TYPES OF ILLNESSES*
BIRTH RELATED ILLNESSES AND INJURIES

BIRTH RELATED ILLNESSES & INJURIES
Intrauterine
Basic Prenatal Matrix I Conflicts
Genetic
Injury (Cord Around the Neck,
    Positional)
Intercurrent Illness of the Mother
    (Thyroid Disease, Heart Disease,
    Sepsis, etc.)
Infectious Disease (German Measles,
    Syphilis, Toxoplasmosis, etc.)
Nutritional
Toxic (Alcohol, Smoking, Exogenous
    Toxicity, Drugs [Prescription,
    Over-The-Counter or Illicit Drugs]
Environmental
Labor Related
Anesthesia
Basic Prenatal
    Matrices II - III Conflicts
Birth Process Trauma (Physical -
    Cord Around the Neck, Hypoxia,
    Anoxia, Breech)
Iatrogenic
    (Failure to Deliver During
    Emergency, Excessive Use
    of Oxytocin)
Maternal Illness (Hypertension,
    Metabolic Disease, Fever, Sepsis,
    etc.)
Preeclampsia, Eclampsia
Birth Injury
Basic Prenatal Matrix IV Conflicts
Iatrogenic
Maternal Illness, Herpes, Monilia,
Prolonged Labor
Thrombosis, Stroke,
Cardiovascular
Disease
Vaginal vs C-Section Delivery
Post Partum Conditions
Failure to Thrive
Infection
Nutritional

GENETIC
Disease Passed Through Genetics

METABOLIC ILLNESSES & DISEASE
Genetic
Nutritional
Organic (Thyroid Disease,
    Kidney Disease)
Toxic

IATROGENIC
Injuries caused by Physician,
    Hospital, Pharmacy, Nurse or
    Treatment Program

TOXIC
Energy (Heat, Light, Ultraviolet
    Radiation, Sound, Electromagnetic
    Radiation)
Environmental (Within Food,
    General Living Conditions)
Exposure To Natural or Man-Made
    Toxins and/or Chemicals

NUTRITIONAL
Environmental (Poor Diet,
    Food Lacks Nutrients, Drought,
    Famine, Financial)
Psychogenic (Self-Imposed:
    Starvation, Bulimia, Anorexia,
    Purging)

INFECTIOUS
Bacterial, Viral, Fungal or
    Parasitic Diseases

NON-INFECTIOUS
Non-Infectious Bacteria,
    Viral Illnesses

Parasitic Disease

STRESS
Allergies
Autoimmune Diseases
Emotional Injury
Hypertension

APPENDIX D - 2
TYPES OF ILLNESSES*
BIRTH RELATED ILLNESSES AND INJURIES

INJURIES
Home
Environmental
Self-Induced
Work Related
Physical Injury
Psychiatric Injury
   Stress-Related Illnesses
   & Disorders   (SRDs)
Word & Thought Related Disorders
Traumatic & Post Traumatic
   Syndromes

MENTAL & EMOTIONAL ILLNESSES
Birth Matrix Disorders
Birth Trauma
Degenerative Diseases
Emotional
   Anxiety
   Panic
   Depression
   Confusion
Genetic
Infectious Disease
Nutritional
Primary Psychosis
Relationships
Stuttering
Toxic
Trauma

SPIRITUAL
Sin Related
Spirit Possession
Word & Thought Related Disorders

MISCELLANEOUS
All Illnesses Which May or May Not Fit
Into Above Categories

STRUCTURAL DISEASE & ILLNESS
Development
Heart Attack
Inadequate Cellular, Tissue
   or Organ
Stroke
Unable to Function to Tolerances
Unable to Function Beyond
   Tolerance Levels

ENVIRONMENTAL
Lifestyle
   Poverty
   Risk Taking
   Sexually Promiscuity
Natural Disasters
Toxic
Weather

DEGENERATIVE DISEASES
Aging & Decay
Arthritis
Autoimmune Diseases
Environmental Forces
Improper Regeneration
Irreparable Trauma
Nutritional
Repeated Trauma
Tissue Breakdown or Injury
– Improper Repair or Healing

CANCER
Environmental
Genetic
Toxic Chemical (including smoking)
Radiation
Inflammatory
Foreign Body

www.ingramcontent.com/pod-product-compliance
Lightning Source LLC
Chambersburg PA
CBHW062159270326
41930CB00009B/1591